PSYCHIATRIC NURSING

PSYCHIATRIC NURSING

Mary Topalis, R.N., Ed.D.

Professor and Chairman,
Department of Nursing, San Francisco State University,
San Francisco, California

and

Donna Conant Aguilera, R.N., Ph.D., F.A.A.N.

Associate Professor of Nursing, California State University,
Los Angeles, California

SEVENTH EDITION

The C. V. Mosby Company

Saint Louis   1978

SEVENTH EDITION

Copyright © 1978 by The C. V. Mosby Company

Previous editions copyrighted 1953, 1957, 1961, 1965, 1970, 1974

Printed in the United States of America

Distributed in Great Britain by Henry Kimpton, London

The C. V. Mosby Company
11830 Westline Industrial Drive, St. Louis, Missouri 63141

Library of Congress Cataloging in Publication Data

Topalis, Mary, 1922-
    Psychiatric nursing.

    First-6th ed. by R. Matheney and M. Topalis.
    Includes bibliographies and index.
    1. Psychiatric nursing. I. Aguilera, Donna Conant,
joint author. II. Matheney, Ruth Virginia, 1911-
Psychiatric nursing. III. Title. [DNLM: 1. Psychi-
atric nursing. WY160 T673p]
RC440.M3 1978   610.73'68   77-13051
ISBN 0-8016-3148-3

GW/VH/VH 9 8 7 6 5 4 3 2 1

Foreword

No field of health care can claim greater diversity of determined approach than that of the behavioralists. Within the science and art of psychiatric and mental health nursing are the staunch freudians, neofreudians, biophysicists, and socioculturists, to cite but a few of the representative camps and their experts. Each is committed to its established formula for maximization of mental health, and each enthusiastically expounds only its found or chosen way of providing care. In the center of such a diversity in approaches stands the student in nursing required to know the basics of providing sound care to persons experiencing emotional distress. The confusion of all the options is often overwhelming and adds only greater stress for the learner. Qualified faculty reach out for meaningful resources to provide a sound framework and just, unbiased interpretation of the various theories and approaches to mental health; until now that search has largely ended in disappointment.

This work of Topalis and Aguilera creates order out of the confusion in the behavioral sciences today. As unequaled experts in psychiatric and mental health nursing, they deftly and in a quiet, orderly fashion lead the learner through the maze of the various patterns of behavior and therapeutic approaches based on various theories of psychopathology. The richness of the case studies presented allows the student to mentally experience clinical situations before entering the health care setting in a provider role. By the very process of visualizing such situations in a relaxed state, the student will find the actual clinical experience familiar even on point of initial entry.

The simplicity of the writing belies the complexity of the behavioral theories but well bespeaks the expert authority of Topalis and Aguilera in the field. Their work coaxes the reader to experience, as have they, the stimulating challenges and rich unequaled satisfaction of working with another human

v

toward enhanced mental health. The authors quietly transmit their absolute concern and unlimited respect for the clients in this area of nursing; such regard for persons is contagious to the reader and sets a solid foundation for delivery of holistic nursing care.

Psychiatric and mental health nursing is the most prominent area of nursing care that has as its only tool the nurse provider. Topalis and Aguilera in this work groom the learner to exploration and definition of one's own personality in extending itself to another human. In so doing, they have not only created order out of confusion but have reaffirmed nursing's role as a human response to another's needs.

Mary E. Reres

Dean, School of Nursing,
University of California at Los Angeles

Preface

Much has happened in mental health nursing since the publication of the previous edition of *Psychiatric Nursing;* therefore, much has been changed in this seventh edition. The development of the book takes into account the Standards of Psychiatric–Mental Health Nursing Practice. (See Appendix B.) It is intended that faculty and students incorporate these standards in their teaching-learning processes.

The format has been changed to make a more succinct and useful text for students and their clinical instructors. Case studies have been added to illustrate some concepts whenever they were applicable. Tables of major and minor psychotropic drugs have been included to provide students with rapid access to their recommended dosage, effect, and lethality.

Much of what appears in psychiatric nursing textbooks is applicable to all nursing situations. As we provide health services to the public, more attention is being paid to the effort to treat human beings as such—persons who respond holistically, with body and mind operating as a unit. Although progress has been made, actual practice in the field continues to range from the old custodial-control concept to the behavioral approach.

Chapter 1 presents the nurse's role in the mental health program. It establishes the general tone of the text and provides a comprehensive and updated overview of psychiatric/mental health nursing, both inpatient and outpatient. The balance of Unit one is devoted to the concepts of personality and behavior, to the *normal* evaluation of personality development, and to the *abnormalcy* of psychopathology.

Unit two deals exclusively with the principles of mental health nursing. It includes chapters on communication techniques, interpersonal techniques, and an expanded chapter on crisis intervention and community psychiatry, with examples of a case study and a paradigm of intervention.

Unit three discusses in depth a broad range of patients with dysfunctional behavior patterns. Totally new chapters cover patients with antisocial patterns and psychotherapeutic techniques. Ego functions, mental status, and current therapies are also presented in a new chapter. Numerous new case examples have been employed to help familiarize the student with nursing care.

Unit four presents organic behavior disorders. Topics included are the characteristics of aging and acute and chronic organic behavior. This material is exceedingly relevant to many current social problems.

Unit five encompasses the nursing interventions necessary for patients who depend on emotional crutches, such as alcohol and other abused substances.

Unit six concentrates on children, their behaviors, and their problems. Discussed are the developmental problems of children—both functionally based behavior problems and organic behavior disorders.

Many people have contributed to this seventh edition of *Psychiatric Nursing*. Students and instructors who have used earlier editions of the book have made scores of thoughtful and thought-provoking comments orally and in writing. Portions of the sixth edition that were pertinent and relevant were retained, and new material was added with special regard to these much appreciated suggestions.

We wish to acknowledge a very special debt to our many students—past, present, and future—and to the patients we have worked with and to those we will work with in the future. To our families, friends, and colleagues we express our gratitude for their patience and understanding while this edition was being written.

Mary Topalis
Donna Conant Aguilera

Contents

APPENDIXES

CONCEPTS OF PERSONALITY AND BEHAVIOR

CHAPTER 1

The nurse in the mental health program

It is infrequent that one finds an explanation of when and why the study of man was separated into physical-biochemical and psychosocial components that make up this complex, integrated phenomenon called man. The rationale presented is usually attributed to the need for facilitating the in-depth study of the intricate components that make up the total individual. It is important for nurses never to lose sight of the fact that they, more than any other persons concerned with care of people, must continuously integrate the compartmentalized knowledge components into the total care of the person in health and in illness.

In few clinical fields in nursing are the opportunities and challenges more interesting or greater than in the field of psychiatric and mental health nursing, and in few fields of nursing is the nurse in a comforting role more needed. Although the number of patients in psychiatric institutions is decreasing, the number in need of improved nursing care is still tremendous, and the opportunities to utilize creativity in devising and implementing new patterns of nursing care are numerous. Greater public acceptance of the real meaning of mental illness and deviate behavior, greater federal interest and financial assistance, increased knowledge about human behavior, an ever-widening scope of therapeutic approaches, and a greater emphasis on interpersonal skills in nursing generally are all having a strong impact on psychiatric nursing practice. As a result, the opportunities to actually help patients have increased markedly, and the satisfactions to be derived from psychiatric nursing have increased proportionately. Mental health and mental illness constitute a major social health problem and therefore present a major challenge to the health professions, including nursing.

A SOCIAL PROBLEM

Of all the health problems confronting the public, few have such staggering proportions as the problems of mental illness and mental health. Almost half of the hospital beds in the United States on any given day are occupied by psychiatric patients. Some physicians believe that at least half of all patients who go to private medical practitioners suffer more from psychologic and emotional problems than from physical ailments. In addition, there is a rapidly growing recognition of the importance of psychosocial factors in the development and expression of all health problems.

Many authorities believe that the extent of actual mental illness goes well beyond these overwhelming figures. Admission rates to psychiatric hospitals are influenced by many factors, including the presence of psychiatric facilities, the ability of family and friends to recognize the significance of unusual behavior, social attitudes toward psychiatric disorders, and economic status. With such factors influencing admission rates, many believe that the number of patients hospitalized or actually under private psychiatric care is only a surface indication of the extent of the problem.

While no exact figures are accepted by all, practically everyone in the health field agrees that mental illness and mental health constitute a major health problem—possibly the number one health problem. There is also general agreement that we do not yet understand fully or have a solid scientific identification of the cause-effect relationships that result in psychiatric and psychosomatic disorders. We do have a collection of theories, and the various theories do have some points in common. Nonetheless, we cannot yet identify specific causes and cures in the various psychiatric syndromes. In fact, we sometimes cannot identify with exactness what the specific psychiatric syndrome may be.

A number of related social problems also have implications for the mental health of the public. These problems, among others, include emotionally disturbed and psychotic children, mental retardation, juvenile delinquency, alcoholism, drug abuse, and the emotional problems of the aged. There can be no question that many children have relatively serious emotional problems and that the trained personnel and the facilities for identifying and treating such children are inadequate. The number of children and adolescents known to police and courts for law violation is increasing at a greater rate than their proportionate population increase, and the proportionate rise in juvenile delinquency continues each year. While the incidence of alcoholism, like mental illness, is difficult to pinpoint, estimates run as high as 6 to 9 million in the United States. In addition to the problems of organic brain disease, the elderly are subject to many difficult emotional stresses as a result of their aging process and reduced productivity and usefulness. The problems of the aged increase in importance as the percentage of the population over 65 continues to grow rapidly.

Mental health as a social problem must therefore rank as one of the major challenges to the health professions, including nursing.

PROBLEMS IN DEFINITION

In 1946 the sages of the World Health Organization struggled in their attempt to put forth an understanding of health in its Constitution. It reads as follows:

> Health is a state of complete physical, mental and social well-being and not merely the absence of disease or infirmity. (p. 1)

In 1947 the International Preparatory Commission tried its hand in defining mental health:

1. Mental health is a condition which permits the optimal development, physical, intellectual and emotional, of the individual, so far as this is compatible with that of other individuals.
2. A good society is one that allows this development to its members while at the same time ensuring its own development and being tolerant toward other societies.

Both of these definitions are idealistic in the face of world realities. The terms are value-loaded, subject to interpretations derived from the different norms viewed as appropriate by individuals and to particular societies. However, the idealism reflected in both of these definitions will hopefully serve as a positive stimulus toward the consideration of a people's goal in health.

Defining clearly what constitutes *mental illness* and *mental health* is not easy. Defining health and disease is difficult, since the concepts of both constantly undergo change and development. It is usually much simpler to identify the extremely healthy and the extremely sick than to distinguish between the borderlines of either physical or mental health. Of one thing we can be certain—the absence of disease is no longer an acceptable definition of health in either the physical or the emotional sense.

Mental health is even harder to define than mental illness, and the many experts who have attempted to clarify the concept do not always agree. In general, they tend to emphasize one aspect or another of what they consider to be mental health. After an extensive survey of the literature, Marie Jahoda (1958) indicated six general approaches to develop criteria for the existence or absence of mental health. These include attitudes toward self, personal growth and self-realization, internal psychologic oneness or unity, independence from social influences, adequate contact with reality, and environmental mastery. While the emphasis of various experts may differ somewhat, there seems to be general agreement that a mentally healthy person has a realistic knowledge of himself, accepts himself with his strengths and weaknesses, can be genuinely concerned for others, is more directed by inner than by outer values, can take care of himself without hurting others in the process, and can tolerate stress and frustration without personality disorganization. That a single, unifying concept of health and illness does not exist in the field of mental health is not surprising—it does not exist in the field of physical health either.

The definition of mental illness is a relative one and is usually based on what constitutes socially accepted behavior norms. Behavior that is normal in one culture is not infrequently considered abnormal in another culture.

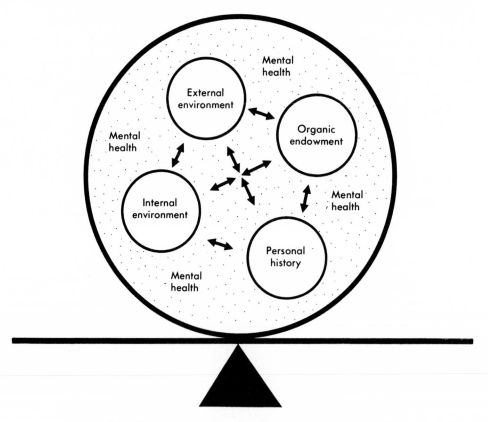

Mental health is the balance and interaction of many factors.

In mental illness, again, it is the extreme that is easiest to identify; the closer the individual is to the borderline between mental health and mental disease, the more difficult the determination of the state of health becomes. If one thinks of health as a continuum, with the extremes of health and sickness at either end, the closer one comes to the center of the line, the harder it becomes to determine whether a person is sick or healthy. It is certain that degrees of health and illness exist, but their clear-cut definitions remain elusive. That most well persons have a sick potential and that most sick persons have a well potential is also implicit in practically all current thinking about mental health.

Despite the fact that definitions of mental illness and mental health remain somewhat elusive, existing definitions need testing in practice and continued utilization until better definitions are developed. In spite of the semantic difficulty, the medical and nursing care of those patients labeled mentally ill by the social criterion of acceptable behavior norms constitutes an immediate problem of enormous magnitude.

CARE OF THE MENTALLY ILL

The old pattern. There can be no objection to the statement that the care of patients with psychiatric problems has lagged well behind the care of patients with other types of health problems and also well behind the currently available knowledge of human behavior. In general, this is usually attributed to public attitudes toward mental illness; the care provided is considered a reflection of public social concern. The historic development of the pattern for providing care for the social deviate on a psychologic basis unfortunately took such care out of the mainstream of community life and the medical and nursing professions. The result has made utilizing current knowledge more difficult.

Before the development of psychiatric hospitals, the major resource facility in psychiatric therapy, patients were often looked on as persons under the influence of evil spirits, and the basis of therapy was either driving the devil from the patients or driving the patient from the community. Therapy was largely punitive, a concept not yet entirely dead, although its demise should have occurred long ago. The next step was the creation of institutions for socially undesirable persons or misfits, where paupers, criminals, and the mentally ill were housed together. Society's lack of interest in anything other than the incarceration of undesirable persons and the protection of society from them supported a widespread pattern of abuse. The beginning recognition of the fact that some of the segregated persons were actually mentally ill, coupled with the work of pioneering reformers such as

Dorothea Lynde Dix, led to the acceptance of the principle of state responsibility and provision for the mentally ill in separate institutions. The shift in therapy was from a punitive approach to "moral treatment" based on showing kindness and consideration for the patient as a human being and providing the patient with an opportunity to behave like a human being. "Moral treatment" of the mentally ill actually developed first in Europe, when Dr. Philippe Pinel in France and William Tuke in England pioneered nonrestraint and humane treatment of patients.

Unfortunately, as a reflection of public opinion, state hospitals, which became the primary psychiatric treatment facilities in the United States, were built as large institutions away from the community and from medical and teaching facilities. Fresh air, quiet, and peace were provided for patients out in the country, but such patients were also placed out of sight and out of mind. The institutions focused on custodial care and patient control, and their very size forced impersonal attitudes. The state hospital's isolated setting and size hindered the recruitment of qualified personnel, made keeping abreast of medical developments difficult, and contributed to patient chronicity much more than to patient recovery. The care of patients deteriorated, and the "shame of the states" has been the subject of many studies and books.

There can be no doubt that in recent years many improvements have been seen in attitudes toward mentally ill patients, in the provision for social and recreational activities, in the patient's increased responsibility for himself, and in the therapeutic use of the psychiatric hospital environment. However, the well of misery has only been tapped. For each small step taken, there are many giant steps still to be taken. The largest percentage of all psychiatric patients is still in state hospitals where the physical facilities, traditions, location, organization, financing, and staffing patterns make the use of modern therapeutic techniques extremely difficult. In addition to state hospitals, mental patients are found in three other types of facilities— Veterans' Administration hospitals, small private hospitals, and psychiatric units in general hospitals.

The new pattern. Changes that promise real improvement for the care of the mentally ill are rapidly taking place. Current thinking and planning for mental health and for the care of the mentally ill are much more comprehensive and diversified in scope than in the past. The beginnings have already been indicated in the development of community, state, and regional planning bodies and in the development of new types of facilities for prevention, diagnosis, and treatment. Although much is yet to be done, the new era has begun.

Perhaps the most significant change that has taken place has been in the area of thinking which now is characterized by a much broader approach to mental health and mental illness and is focused on prevention, early diagnosis, treatment, and return to the community. Such thinking (and planning) envisions a wide range of services brought to the patient or potential patient when they are needed and when it is possible for him to utilize such facilities effectively.

Changes have also been made to improve the therapeutic posture of psychiatric hospitals already in existence. Among the most impressive of these changes are the institution of the open-door policy, patient government, the use of a therapeutic milieu, and decentralization of large institutions. The open-door policy consists of open units with unlocked doors where patients accordingly assume more responsibility for their own behavior. There can be little question that the locked doors of psychiatric hospitals contributed more to the security of society than to the therapy of patients. Nonetheless, it has taken courage to open doors that have been locked for so long, despite the fact that history makes clear the value of the open-door or nonrestraint policy. While the use of patient government is not yet widespread, it has been instituted in a variety of psychiatric hospitals or units and has proved itself to be a valuable therapeutic adjunct. In a program of patient government, patients help formulate the rules and regulations under which they live, air and settle grievances, participate in the decisions as to the patients' status, help each other, and sometimes participate in therapeutic decisions. The therapeutic milieu approach includes a variety of organized efforts designed to induce patient participation in activity programs that promote improved social behavior. These can range from habit training programs aimed at bowel training, eating habits, and physical hygiene to complicated activity programs supported by individual and group therapy.

Social movements outside the psychiatric hospital have made an impact toward an increased recognition and understanding of the rights of patients and their privilege to participate in the determination of their life-style. This opportunity for the patient to reconsider and to reassume, through participation, the responsibilities of daily living enhances his chances and courage to resume self responsibility. It can be the reassurance a person needs to demonstrate his capability to return to the demands of society.

Real progress has also been made by the current resistance to increasing or expanding the large state hospitals that now exist. Planning leans toward smaller units, closer to the patients and to medical centers. In addition, there has been a widespread movement toward decentralization of decision-making in large hospitals. Large hospitals are divided into relatively autonomous units, often serving specific geographic areas.

Another worthwhile development is the slow but steady increase in psychiatric units in general hospitals. Such units in an active, treatment-centered institution provide excellent facilities for short-term care of patients with psychiatric disorders and should contribute much to preventing the development of chronic problems.

Foster family care for psychiatric patients as a substitute for hospitalization or as a transitional stage in the return to the community is not a new idea, but it has received impetus with the recognition of the need for a broad scope of services to provide patients with necessary treatment facilities. The famous community of Gheel, Belgium, where patients were placed with families in the community rather than in a hospital, has functioned successfully in this manner for many years.

Halfway houses, although not yet widespread, have been developed to help patients during the transitional period from hospital to community. These houses vary in the services offered, ranging from a boardinghouse-type setting to a house with intensive individual or group therapy.

Daycare and nightcare centers have also been established, although these are not yet widespread. Daycare centers provide acitivity and therapeutic services for patients and permit them to stay with families in the community at night. Nightcare centers provide a therapeutic program for patients who can continue employment. Both have the advantage of keeping the patient in contact with his community while receiving therapeutic help.

The establishment of community mental health clinics was begun some time ago and has gained rapid momentum. Their major problem has been overcrowding and long waiting lists. These clinics provide diagnosis and treatment and sometimes assist with the return of patients to the community. The ultimate value of mental hygiene clinics is unquestioned, but their current value is somewhat limited by the extensive demands made on them.

Aftercare clinics, designed to assist in patient return to the community, are also being established. Here again, the clinics are not yet widespread, but a beginning has been made.

In some communities, emergency services on an outpatient basis (sometimes called walk-in clinics) are being developed and are open 24 hours a day. This type of emergency service has not been available on an outpatient basis before, and it holds a real promise.

The telephone has become a therapeutic tool for suicide prevention; for giving psychologic support for drug abusers, alcoholics, and child-abusing parents; for helping adolescents with venereal disease and crises situations; and for assisting elderly persons experiencing mental, social, and/or economic problems. The type and amount of telephone services vary in each community and are directly related to the interest and needs of the particular community. The resources available and the persons prepared with the knowledge and skills needed are also significant in the quality of these telephone services. Student nurses with psychiatric nursing knowledge and experience are often called on to participate in such activities. However, unskilled personnel, prompted by enthusiasm and good intentions, can cause serious harm to desperate individuals.

Nursing homes, though they have enough problems of their own at the present, are also a potential source of help with the less seriously disturbed psychiatric patient and with the elderly person with emotional problems. Many elderly persons housed in psychiatric hospitals really belong in nursing homes. Convalescent nursing homes could also help with patient transition from the psychiatric hospital to the community.

Sheltered workshops offer the possibility of a real contribution to the psychiatric therapy battery. Although the acceptance of psychiatric patients, recovered or not, in sheltered workshops (where the handicapped are gainfully employed) is not widespread, some beginnings in this direction have been made, and it is anticipated that the movement will grow.

Another slowly developing resource is expatient clubs ranging from social groups through problem discussion to actual continuing therapy groups. Such patient clubs have been effective in areas of other health problems, and with professional direction they would be most valuable for former psychiatric patients.

Stress is now being placed on prevention, both primary and secondary. Primary prevention is somewhat vague since it is devoted to improving mental health, and mental health, or what produces it, is not absolutely clear. Nonetheless, the emphasis on the potential mental health contribution of schools, churches, health departments, welfare departments, courts, and public recreation programs may increase their effectiveness. Alertness to the problem certainly should improve their contribution to secondary prevention, the early recognition and treatment of persons with emotional problems.

With the increase in the scope and variety of services available for persons with emotional problems, the health professions and the community must necessarily come to grips with the difficulty found in all health services—the need to coordinate efforts on a community level to provide continuity of care for individual patients.

GOVERNMENTAL AGENCIES AND LEGISLATION

One of the most encouraging developments has been the interest of and the actions taken by the federal government. A national problem with the scope of the mental health problem needs a national approach. The practice of having the states primarily responsible for the care of the mentally ill ignores hard realities such as the differences in state financial incomes and the resulting variations in the ability to provide care for such patients. Mental health is a national resource and a matter of national concern.

The Mental Health Study Act of 1955 led to the appointment of the Joint Commission on Mental Illness and Mental Health, which published its famous report *Action for Mental Health* in 1961. The report recognized the continuing underlying problem of public rejection of the mentally ill and identified the key resources needed to provide both adequate treatment and prevention—manpower and money. Funds made available for planning on community and regional bases, for the preparation of personnel, for research, and for construction should make substantial improvements in the mental health services available to Americans.

The Community Mental Health Centers Act was passed by Congress in 1963. It provided funds for the development of community comprehensive mental health care centers where varieties of services would be available to individuals and families requiring mental health and psychiatric care. It was intended to bring within the reach of the people of the community those services usually provided by the large state mental hospitals. Federal funds were awarded to those facilities that agreed to offer at least the first five of ten important services.

1. Inpatient care unit for individuals requiring observation, treatment, and care as residents of the facility for a specified, limited period of time.
2. Outpatient care unit for individuals of all age groups and their families requiring ambulatory–clinic type services.
3. Daycare and nightcare services for individuals who could continue their activities in the community but who could benefit by a planned, consistent program of therapy.
4. Emergency care services for individuals requiring immediate attention because of crises or circumstances precipitating a situation necessitating urgent assistance.
5. Educational and consultation services to be provided as identified by community agencies and related groups.
6. Diagnostic services to assess the individual's status and to provide the basis to a therapeutic care plan.
7. Rehabilitative services for individuals needing assistance with social adjustments, job training and placement, and other related problems.
8. Precare and aftercare services to assist individuals and families with problems associated with planning for admission to a hospital and/or for after discharge in order to help with these adjustments.

9. Training of mental health personnel to facilitate the services offered by the units of the community mental health centers.

10. Research and evaluation, an integral part of the ongoing functions of the centers.

This federally funded program was directed to provide essential services to the people of a community and thus prevent the usual separation and isolation of the state mental hospital system. The therapeutic milieu included concern for the individual and his family and provided care modalities appropriate and necessary for continuity in treatment and care.

Community mental health centers are the most promising development of all. Such centers, found at various locations within the United States, are quite different from other existing facilities for mental health. Instead of merely being available when the community or its members need it, the center reaches out into the community to take primary and secondary prevention measures, in addition to providing treatment. The primary measures, which deal with factors concerned with mental health, make such matters as poverty, conditions of family life, and many other social conditions of concern to the center. The secondary prevention measures, dealing with the early diagnosis and treatment of behavior disorders, are usually accomplished while the patient remains within the community. Roles of the different members of the community mental health centers are not yet clearly defined. Such centers use indigenous workers who know and are accepted by the community. Since both the physical and mental aspects of health are inextricably interwoven, such an approach seems to promise much for the future.

PSYCHIATRIC NURSING EDUCATION

The nurse's role in the care of the mentally ill has been a kaleidoscopic one. As nursing changed from era to era, social and economic forces were important determinants in the patterns of psychiatric nursing care. The degree of social conscience of society, the political interest in welfare, the concern and emphasis on educationally prepared personnel, the number and variety of needed personnel, and the resources for a therapeutic environment are all factors that influence the quality of nursing provided for the mentally ill.

As late as the 1950s, psychiatric nursing education was just being incorporated into basic nursing programs in some states. It was not until after World War II that psychiatric–mental health nursing was added to most nursing curriculums. The educational experience took place during a specific period of time, usually 3 months, in an isolated setting away from the home, hospital, or school, and was added onto the curriculum somewhere near graduation. This emphasis on psychiatric nursing as an appendage, rather than a component of nursing, continues in a few nursing programs to this day! The responsibility for this falls squarely on the shoulders of teaching faculty in all areas of nursing.

From the start, the focus of this training was to understand people, but the control and management of disruptive behavior patterns retained their prominence. It now seems ludicrous that the study of understanding people was left until so late in nursing education and dealt mainly with the chronic institutionalized mental hospital patient. In some mysterious way nursing students were expected to integrate and transfer knowledge about understanding people to all areas of clinical practice.

In recent years more emphasis has been placed on students' developing the ability to provide nursing care for psychiatric patients in a wide variety of mental health treatment and prevention centers. Their experience takes them from the traditional state hospital setting, to psychiatric units in general hospitals, to satellite clinics, to rehabilitation centers, and into the community itself. Increasing emphasis has also been placed on understanding general hospital patients' emotional response to their illness and to the effects of hospitalization. Concepts of mental health nursing are being integrated throughout many associate degree and baccalaureate degree nursing curricula. The process of death and dying has become in itself a field of specialization. In many hospital settings there is a psychiatric consultation liaison team with a nursing member whose role is to assist other nurses with understanding patient behavior when that behavior interferes with the treatment plan. The old barriers separating the treatment of mind and body are slowly beginning to fade as we acknowledge their effect on each other and as we see the person who is our patient as a more integrated whole.

While this change in emphasis is taking place, innovations in health services, educational patterns, and the broad field of nursing itself have caused considerable confusion. Exactly what constitutes psychiatric nursing is not clear as it used to be, just as what constitutes nursing itself is not as clear as it was once assumed to be.

PSYCHIATRIC SETTINGS

Not too long ago, nurses and physicians, like the general public, tended to avoid psychiatric patients, mostly because of fear, misunderstanding, and limited exposure. Today, societal attitudes, related legislation, and educational focus have influenced changes among the public and professions with respect to psychiatric patients and their treatment. Psychiatrists and psychiatric nurses find themselves granted increasing respect and acceptance, particularly by their colleagues. Their services are in increasing demand by the public and by hospital staff members who are attempting to understand their patients' emotional reactions to illness. In some settings, the psychiatric clinical specialist serves as a consultant to nonpsychiatric units of the general hospital where some patients' behavior or emotional responses to their illness may require psychiatric nursing expertise. However, the single most serious problem in the provision of health care for psychiatric patients, and still the most pressing problem in mental health, is the inadequate supply of qualified personnel— physicians, nurses, psychologists, social workers, and the many others who provide care, treatment, rehabilitation, and hopefully prevention of illness.

The psychiatric setting for services and treatment has shown considerable change during the past decade. In 1973 the Department of Health, Education, and Welfare reported that 41.9% of psychiatric cases were served by inpatient agencies, including state and county mental hospitals, general hospital psychiatric services, Veterans Administration hospitals, community mental health centers, and other inpatient facilities. Outpatient services in communi-

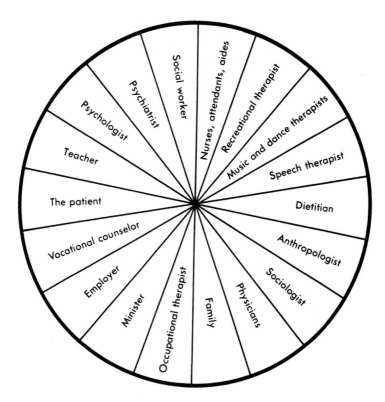

The major health team components.

ty mental health centers and other agencies provided 55.3% of the services and 2.8% in daycare type of services.

In the publication "Baselines for Setting Health Goals and Standards" (1976), several factors are indicated as probable influences on the future.

> The proportion of people age 45 or over will increase slightly from about 31% in 1974 to 34% in 2000. The median age will rise gradually from 28.6 years to 34.8. Adults will outnumber children by 2.7 to 1 in 2000, compared to 2.2 in 1970. The "dependency ratio" (population 0-17 and 65 & over per 100 persons age 18-64) will increase from 17.8 in 1974 to 19.0 in 2000. Also, as the population over age 65 increases, the gap in numbers between the sexes will increase; by 2000, there will be 6.5 million more women than men among the elderly, as contrasted with an estimated difference of 3.9 million in 1974. (p. 101)

These changes in the population picture, economic pressures, job opportunities, housing and living conditions, and other related factors are expected to influence people's life-styles. The trend is for more women to enter and remain in the labor force, which could result in an increase in the need for home health services, particularly with respect to the care of invalids who will be part of the household. The report goes on to caution:

> A sense of "bigness" and depersonalization will pervade the society and there may be pronounced separations between unequal population groups, e.g., healthy young people and the elderly incapacitated. There is also likely to be an increase in self-damaging behavior, and neglect of helpless individuals. Therapy groups may gain in popularity as people attempt to restore consciousness of individual worth and sensitivity to others. Interests in decentralizing authority within bureaucrasies may grow in order to make institutions more responsive to both their staffs and users. (p. 104)

Numerous stresses emanating from the future trends cited and societal changes are expected to contribute to emotional disorders, particularly among youth and the elderly. It is predicted that the changes in the population composition could increase "the incidence and prevalence of mental illness, especially schizophrenia." There will be a greater demand for geriatric services as larger numbers of people live beyond the age of 70.

By 1990, the supply of registered nurses is expected to more than double (1,466,000) from the number reported in 1970 (723,000). The expanded role of the nurses is predicted to include more concern for the care of the mentally and/or chronically ill, delivering primary care and home care, and counseling on prevention.

Home health care services are expected to replace institutional care for a fairly large number of clients. The opportunity for nurses to use their extensive knowledge and skills in the home and community setting will require innovative and creative approaches with less constraints like those currently imposed by community health nursing services. It may be that nurses with different specialties will form teams and function cooperatively to meet the total needs of individuals and families with physical and emotional problems. Hopefully, such nursing services will be localized to serve reasonable numbers of people within a defined area and thus provide the means of effective care. The effectiveness and quality of services rendered are strongly influenced by the ratio of persons served by the professional nurse or team.

PSYCHIATRIC NURSING: WHAT IS IT?

Psychiatric nursing can be seen as a dynamic interplay between nurses and patients that encompasses knowledge and skillful application of the concept of behavior, personality, the mind, psychopathology, and, most importantly, the process of interpersonal relationships. This implies that nurses must have an awareness of self, their behavior, their needs, and their ways of relating and handling stress if they are to see clearly where their problems and responses end and where the patients' begin. This is of prime importance because the identification and evaluation of patients' behavior are paramount in establishing an effective nursing care plan approach. The nurse-patient relationship is now being recognized as perhaps one of the nurse's most important therapeutic tools. Intervention—disruption of pathologic or nonfunctional behavior—is intended for reeducation and remotivation purposes. We no longer interfere just for the purpose of interfering. There must be sound judgment underlying all our actions. The days of punishment for behavior that is not within our own value system must be over. Punitive reactions have never been a way for meaningful learning and long-lasting change. Psychiatric nurses must use themselves and their total personalities as the main implement for effective care. Physical manipulative skills are limited here, since nurses meet patients on a communication level. Social and recreational activities serve as a bridge to open communication, yet in the final analysis, when all the props are gone, communication is still person to person. The intensity of this interpersonal relationship may be difficult and threatening to some, but to others it is the most challenging and rewarding field in nursing. The therapeutic nursing relationship is the basis upon which nurses can truly effect a helping relationship.

Psychiatric nursing is comprehensive nursing care. This suggests the acknowledgment of a patient as a total person who possesses needs covering all aspects of life—including biopsychosocial, environmental, religious, occupational, and recreational. Such an approach alleviates the medical profession's habit of seeing patients primarily as disease entities or, in this case, as having defects in personality adjustments to life. The interpersonal nursing relationship temporarily places us in the patients' social sphere. It is here that we can effect a change in a person's identified psychiatric problem by relating to his disturbed patterns of need gratification in a healthier fashion. Through this process patients can relearn more successful means by which to identify their inner needs and can find new, creative, and nondestructive outlets for their expression. To illustrate this point an effective nursing approach would be to assist patients in dealing with reality at the moment when their defensive symptoms are in effect attempting to protect them. A patient who starts to hallucinate does so for a specific reason. Clarification at that moment helps that person identify the underlying stress, thus giving the opportunity for reversal and nonreinforcement. In essence nurses then become sounding boards, reinforcing reality and offering a basis on which more successful patterns can be learned. Defensive symptoms are then no longer necessary. It is hoped that this process, once begun, will be transferred to the outside world and used in the patient's daily life.

This is a far cry from the psychiatric nurses of the not too distant past whose job it was to "take care" of the hospitalized mental patient. Their functions were mainly organized around custodial care and management of the patient and the ward. Suppressive treatment, including sedation, restraint, and punishment, was the only tool available for effective patient control. Psychiatric nurses were *not* to develop therapeutic relationships with their patients because this treatment was reserved mainly for the physician. It was strongly believed that any relationship outside of the medical one would interfere with the treatment process. Staff members such as social workers, psychologists, and occupational and recreational therapists remained isolated and mainly functioned independently and on a referral basis. Nurses and nursing care remained essentially a supportive function, retaining a handmaiden role, thus increasing the dichotomy between the professions. This is called the medical model approach to psychiatry. It exists today, along with other new, challenging theoretical frameworks. However, its influence is still strong since the majority of treatment settings operate under this method. Note is starting to be taken of the extent of the commitment to this idea in some people today.

When psychiatry was a new science, it was based on the descriptive approach, the identification of patient symptom syndromes. Treatment was medically based, because psychiatrists with their original formal education in medicine translated that conceptual framework to psychiatry. Thus we have diagnosis, symptoms, treatment, management, and other medical words. Treatment followed the medical influence with the use of medication, shock treatment, and hospitalization. The patients whose symptoms did not "disappear" were kept institutionalized. Psychiatry failed to recognize, however, that the process of long-term institutionalization itself led to more pathologic symptoms. Patients remained hospitalized, developed more symptoms, and still remained hospitalized, hence the beginning of the vicious cycle of chronicity that we still see in evidence today in our large overcrowded mental hospital systems.

As the emphasis in psychiatry shifted from a descriptive approach to a behavioral approach, understanding the meaning of symptoms became the focal point. Gradually ideas about the causes of mental illness became broadened to include the effects of interpersonal relations as not only the result of mental illness but also as possibly the cause. Logically a change in nursing philosophy and function has followed. Today we are still in transition as nursing takes steps toward becoming its own science based on its own growing body of knowledge, not just on the utilization of knowledge from allied fields.

Greater attention is now being focused on the scientific utilization of interpersonal relationships and on the use of the nurse as a person in a therapeutic sense. As the social aspects of psychiatric disorders are receiving increased emphasis, skills in using group relationships and manipulating the environment, including its social organization, for therapeutic purposes are being added. These changes are taking place at very uneven rates, and actual psychiatric nursing practice at present runs the full gamut from the old custodial-control approach to settings where nurses participate actively in individual and group patient therapy. This state of affairs has led to the objection that nurses do not necessarily function as psychiatric nurses even though they work in a psychiatric setting. Such an objection is legitimate.

Changing patterns of major health problems have influenced the concept of what constitutes psychiatric nursing today. For many years the psychologic aspects of nursing were considered the exclusive property of psychiatric nursing. The dichotomy between mind and body reigned supreme as both fields of specialization failed to recognize just how dependent each one was on the other. How could the effects of the mind and body have been separated for so long and, in certain instances, have been the media for hostilities to develop? It is now widely accepted that the physiologic disease process influences the person's psychologic state. Cancer, heart disease, diabetes, or any pathophysiologic stress on one's body has some degree of emotional stress as an inherent component. Meeting the ill person's inevitable psychologic needs has made skillful interpersonal relations necessary on general medical-surgical units, as well as in the emergency room, labor and delivery rooms, pediatrics, rehabilitation, geriatrics, outpatient clinics, public health, and in essence any area where nurses come into contact with patients. We are gaining increasing knowledge about the effects of hospitalization not only on our identified patients but also on their families, friends, and the social system itself.

Disease and injury are crisis situations emotionally as well as physically. Often during such crises, disorganization of the personality is seen in either the patient or the patient's family. During this period of stress many people are unable, unaware, or perhaps unwilling to express their reactions directly. It takes sensitive and aware nurses to see beyond some of the indirect expressions of people in this state. It also takes a willingness to deal with these reactions rather than giving in to the fear of getting too involved. In situations where these expressions are of an angry, withdrawn, or demanding nature, the patient too quickly is categorized and stereotyped as an "uncooperative" patient. In other words, the patient is not following the acceptable role model of a "good" patient. Once this happens, the interpersonal forces are set into motion for continual estrangement of the patient and the nurse—both becoming mutually withdrawn or aggressive toward the other. Accurate evaluation of the situation becomes difficult because it appears to be a personality conflict. In most cases, however, the patient is usually the one who is seen as having the problem. Throughout the entire process the patient, whose behavior is a response to the original reaction, is further away from expression than he was before the situation occurred. Hence, the patient's needs are not only unmet but also often thwarted. On the other hand, nurses have to deal with their emotions, which are ambivalent, that is, angry and caring at the same time. The reaction pattern described above is basically opposed to nursing values and ethics and does take its toll in frustration and perhaps guilt for the nurse. Unfortunately such situations as the one described happen more frequently than nurses are willing to admit. Skillful interpersonal relations based on an awareness of the patient's emotional response to illness and an understanding of one's own response patterns bring general nursing closer to the goals of psychiatric nursing.

Meeting the patient's needs has always been a catchall phrase for nursing intervention. Too often only lip service and the written statement in the Kardex have been paid to this ideal. Process-oriented recording is being instituted in many health agencies as a means of providing a basic structure for appropriate action. The work realities of understaffing and overcrowding have made the time and effort needed seem inadequate and frivolous. In the previously described situation, meeting the emotional needs of the patient would have taken more time and effort initially. But in the long run, less time and effort would have been spent than was required for the problem patient, not to mention the cost in unnecessary stress placed both on the patient and the nurse. We must consider the "problem" of the problem patient. Is it his problem alone,

ours, or an intricate combination of both? If the answer is the intricate combination of both, then we must be responsible for our part in that process. An
error in judgment or response is not a crime, but the refusal to acknowledge it
is. Errors in judgment can be rectified, and new patterns of response can be
learned. But nothing can be done until we admit our part.

Recognizing the emotional component of the pathologic disease process is
only one half of the body's influence; we must also consider the reverse, the
influence of the mind on the body. The word "psychosomatic" is very old in
medicine. It has been subject to flippant attitudes, confusion, and misuse. We
refer to psychophysiological patterns here as a group of somatic disorders of an
unknown specific etiology in which psychologic factors play an important role.
Used in another sense the term "psychosomatic" is unfortunate, for it implies
a dualism that does not exist. No somatic disease is entirely free from psychic
influence. While it is generally recognized that many symptoms and diseases
occur in the setting of difficult life situations, no acceptable answer has been
found as to why some people get one disease and some get another. Various
hypotheses suggest the possibility of personality pattern types common to all
patients with the same disease; others try to demonstrate a single personality
trait; some maintain that a specific conflict is unique to a particular disease;
and still others emphasize the influence of past developmental patterns. However, none of these has been totally satisfactory as an explanation because not
all patients fit specific patterns of response. Many patients show more than
one illness; others show specific conflicts without developing the disease.
There is often little similarity between life situations that provoke similar
illnesses.

These disorders are often chronic and relapsing diseases, such as bronchial
asthma, essential hypertension, peptic ulcer, ulcerative colitis, migraine headaches, and neurodermatitis. The degree of personality disturbance is often
correlated with the severity of the actual observable tissue pathology. These
disorders share the following four criteria. First, the organs involved are in-
nervated by the autonomic nervous system; hence, they are not under conscious voluntary control. Second, the disease process does not relieve the basic
psychologic problem, which is anxiety. Third, the symptoms are physiologic
rather than symbolic in nature. Fourth, tissue structural changes that may
threaten life are frequently produced (Nodine and Moyer, 1962).

Various theoretical approaches will help in understanding the influence of
the mind on the body. Selye (1956) has introduced the idea of the general alarm
system. His theory deals with a sequence of events that affect the organism,
the main key being stress. Over a period of time the person responds first with
an alarm reaction, second with a stage of resistance, and third with a stage of

exhaustion. Thus the disease process is seen as the person's failure to adapt to stress. The psychoanalytic approach to the psychosomatic process is widely accepted. It postulates that basic human conflicts occur between passive receptive wishes and active aggressive ones. As an example, a girl goes shopping with her father for a car, which is to be a gift. It then occurs to the girl that the father purchased a better car for her sister. The wish to receive becomes incompatible with the existing angry feelings. Therefore each side of the psychologic conflict has its own physiologic component. The receptive, regressive wishes are expressed in parasympathetic nervous system tone and are linked to peptic ulcer, diarrhea, ulcerative colitis, and asthma. Sympathetic nervous system stimulation occurs whenever the expression of competitive, aggressive, and hostile attitudes are inhibited. Symptoms result from sustained sympathetic excitation, and no discharge of the flight-or-fight mechanism is achieved. This response is linked to essential hypertension, migraine headaches, hyperthyroidism, and diabetes. Organ dysfunction then is seen in this theoretical approach as the antagonism between the two systems upsetting the physiologic balance. It is important, however, to acknowledge that no one mechanism or agent is responsible for the psychophysiologic disorders. Understanding the patient's entire way of life is generally more rewarding and beneficial than searching for a magic key.

Conversion reactions comprise a major category of mind-body influence. However, they are quite different from the psychosomatic disturbance because conversion reactions do not have any tissue alteration, change, or pathology. There is no organic defect. They represent a psychologic means of dealing with stress by symbolic expression through body activities and sensations. This reaction occurs when the wish, idea, or fantasy cannot be expressed or acknowledged. Therefore this idea or wish attains expression in the form of symbolic body language. It is a means of compensation at the expense of some abnormal utilization of the body part. The symptoms affect a great variety of body parts and systems. Some include motor paralysis, which results in seizures, tics, tremors, ptosis, and abnormal postures, and sensory disturbance of pain, anesthesia, blindness, and deafness. Symptoms may involve the major body systems, including the gastrointestinal, respiratory, cardiovascular, genitourinary, and dermal systems. It can also affect the person's level of consciousness.

Hypochondriacal symptoms present still a different picture, for they refer to a habitual overconcern with health. Hypochondriacs are apt to exaggerate and misinterpret harmless and meaningless signs and symptoms. Characteristically they have an insistent, demanding, nagging, torturing, and even persecuting quality and are a great source of discomfort to other persons. Severity of the condition can be gauged by the person's inability to convince himself of the falseness of the symptoms. Hypochondriacal behavior often provokes anger, and at times it can be noted that retaliation occurs. These patients are often rejected, punished, or ridiculed. They move from physician to physician, clinic to clinic, and are those patients to whom staff members are reluctant to give care. Attitudes of disinterest and disgust accomplish the worst result—alienation; hence the vicious cycle continues.

A recent trend—the development of mental health community centers where teams of well-prepared health personnel and their assistants attempt to bring their services to people in the community—is contributing to a broader definition of the psychiatric and mental health nurse.

Community mental health was a revolutionary idea when it was introduced in the early 1960s. Its overall goal was helping people in their own community or neighborhood to reach and maintain more satisfactory levels of functioning. In community mental health today, psychiatric nurses with a generalist background are prepared to attempt to meet the needs of the "total patient." Their flexibility enhances the developmental nature of this growing specialty. Community mental health nurses are action oriented. As in all community health, the focus is on primary prevention. The nurse does not wait for the patient to become "ill" first; rather, the emphasis is on prevention. Problems are dealt with in the setting where they began; an attempt is made not to remove the person from the community. The nursing role may include any conceivable function as the specific needs of the community and the patient are matched to the ability of the team members. There is more role diffusion here as each member of the interdisciplinary team works in a complementary relationship. The nurse who is a clinical specialist in psychiatric nursing serves as an individual and group therapist and a consultation and liaison person to community agencies and hospital units, makes home visits, and serves as a resource person, educator, administrator, and researcher. Nurses in particular define and develop their role. They must communicate clearly with the other health team members to maintain their significant professional contribution. Communities have growing needs, and citizen awareness has increased the demand for service. For greater outreach nurses will have to further expand and develop their role, especially in the areas of mental health consultation and community organization. There must be an awareness of the political and economic trends, as these alter considerably the availability of services and therefore affect health trends.

Psychiatric nursing today faces the challenge of what constitutes its practice. We face a problem common to all nursing—that of the differentiation of competency levels related to the variety of educational levels.

Services contributing to community mental health other than psychiatric

Goal	Mental health for individuals, families, and community
Need	Coordination of broad range of services on community level
Emphasis	Prevention, early diagnosis, treatment, return to community

Services Churches
Schools
Courts
Welfare departments
Public health departments
Expatient clubs
Aftercare clinics
Industrial health services
Other inpatient and outpatient services
Community mental health associations
Community interest groups
Public relations programs
Sheltered workshops
Daycare centers for adults, children
Nightcare centers
Halfway houses
Group sessions for patients, families
Home care programs
Nursing homes for elderly, convalescent
Foster family care for adults, children
Well-baby clinics
Mental retardation services

We have graduates of basic nursing with associate degrees, baccalaureate degrees, master's degrees, and diplomas from schools of nursing. We have graduates with master's degrees prepared for teaching, administration, consultation, and more recently expert clinical psychiatric nursing. We also have a small number of nurses prepared for psychiatric nursing at the doctorate level. Recent trends, however, suggest a reversal away from specialization to more generalist graduate nursing education. Many times outnumbering all of these combined is the group of psychiatric aides and attendants who comprise the largest core of personnel involved in the care of psychiatric patients. The levels of roles, functions, and responsibilities of all these groups have been defined and accepted no more clearly in psychiatric nursing than in any other clincial field of nursing. Thinking ranges from the belief that all these varied groups have a place in the provision of psychiatric nursing to the belief that only a nurse with a minimum of a master's preparation for the field is competent to give psychiatric nursing care.

The response of higher education to the shortages that exist in the health services, including the shortage of nurses, appears to be going in the direction of an already well-established trend. That trend is the development of an ever-expanding number of occupational groups to meet health care needs. At the technical level, for example, community colleges are undertaking the preparation of mental health technicians. The current projects are going in two directions—the preparation of generalists who can function in many settings and the preparation of technical specialists who are more deeply prepared in narrower categories, such as vocational rehabilitation or the care of the mentally retarded. At higher levels, community health leaders, biomedical technicians, and other occupational specialties are being developed.

NURSING AND MENTAL HEALTH

Mental health focuses on primary, secondary, and tertiary prevention of mental illness. Primary prevention involves the promotion of positive mental health, secondary prevention involves early diagnosis and treatment of mental illness, and tertiary prevention involves rehabilitative aspects of mental health. One thing is certain: mental health care is not and cannot be the exclusive province of psychiatric nurses. There are several practical reasons for this. From a realistic point of view, simply not enough psychiatric nurses are available to undertake the task. Another reason is that many nurses in other clinical fields and in varying specialties are already in key settings for the detection of significant signs and symptoms that could lead to early diagnosis and treatment. Additional methods must be found to extend further educational preparation to those in the key settings. One must move delicately here so that one's preparation and position are not offended. Yet realistically, continual educational enlightenment—both formal and informal—is the responsibility of nurses. In some cases a shift in attitude is the first step.

Public health nursing is an excellent example of the smooth incorporation of psychiatric principles into daily practice. The concept of community mental health has its roots in the field of public health. In the territory of the person's own home, nurses can see the dramatic interplay between the forces of the mind and the body and their effects on each other. The home and the family are the arena in which illness is usually first established, and there patterns of response to it are learned. The early recognition and referral of patients with

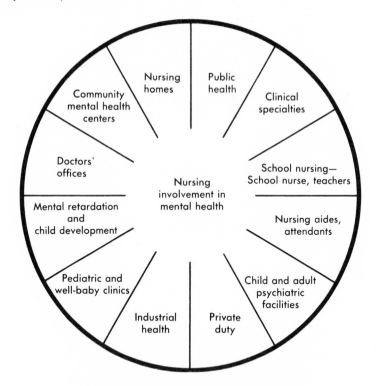

Involvement of nurses in mental health.

emotional problems have in countless instances prevented the debilitating effects of mental illness. By the nature of their position and entrance into the home, public health nurses are often trusted with confidences that unfamiliar hospital personnel work hard to learn. They are in a position to offer support, guidance, and referral. They are often available in family crisis situations and assist in working with the problem child, the acting-out teenager, marital and sexual problems, geriatric family problems, returning hospital patients, and countless other situations.

In well-baby and pediatric clinics, as well as in the general physician's office, nurses are in a strategic position to make observations and evaluations of erupting problems. Patients are well known for giving key information to nurses both immediately before and after their medical interview and examination. Many are afraid or embarrassed to ask questions of or relate information to the physician; many just freeze or forget. School nurses and camp nurses are invaluable with their contacts with children and parents. Again in nonformal, nonmedical situations nurses can often observe budding problems before they give rise to an aggravated syndrome of responses.

Other nurses in a key position to make a mental health contribution are industrial nurses. Stress associated with poor working conditions often shows itself in vague physical symptoms. Aware nurses with a good "ear" can do more than any two aspirin. Those nurses who function in the clinical specialties of medicine, surgery, obstetrics, and pediatrics have valuable opportunities to observe, identify, and refer for help persons with emotional conflicts and symptoms. Clinical specialty nurses also can make a significant contribution to mental health through making the sick role more palatable and through helping patients with emotional support through the crises of hospitalization. Private-duty nurses have the same opportunities. This is not to say that all nurses are prepared to assume the responsibilities of mental health nursing; it is only to say that in the future they must be. Mental health nursing is the responsibility of every nurse, not of psychiatric nurses alone.

There is a trend in medicine today that may achieve our unmet mental health goals—it is the concept of accountability. In essence the health professions are now held accountable for the success or failure of their methods of performance. This refers to nursing in general, as well as to psychiatric specialization. We are held accountable by the public whether we choose to assume the responsibility or not. In other words, we can no longer close our eyes to the existing problems and pretend that they are not there or that somehow someone else will make them go away magically. The time has long passed for such an attitude to continue; the system has to be changed.

REFERENCES

Baker, F.: From community mental health to human service ideology, Am. J. Pub. Health **64:** 576-581, 1974.

Baker, J., and others: An alternative to process recording, Nurs. Outlook **24:**115-118, 1976.

Baselines for setting health goals and standards, U.S. Department of Health, Education, and Welfare, Public Health Service, Health Resources Administration, DHEW Publication No. (H.R.A.) 76-640.

Bayer, M.: Easing mental patients' return to their communities, Am. J. Nurs. **76:**406-408, 1976.

Berry, C., and others: Community care for the mentally ill, Nurs. Times **72:**804-805, 1976.

Brown, F. G.: Social linkability, Am. J. Nurs. **71:**516-520, 1971.

De Young, C. D., and Tower, M.: The nurses' role in community mental health centers: out of uniform and into trouble, St. Louis, 1971, The C. V. Mosby Co.

Elwell, R.: Community mental health centers, Am. J. Nurs. **70:**1014-1018, 1970.

Engel, G.: Psychological development in health and disease, Philadelphia, 1962, W. B. Saunders Co., pp. 368-375.

Fagin, C.: Accountability, Nurs. Outlook **19:**249-251, 1971.

Jahoda, M.: Current concepts of positive mental health, New York, 1958, Basic Books, Inc.

Janzen, S. A.: Psychiatric day care in a rural area, Am. J. Nurs. **74:**1632-1635, 1974.

Joint Commission of Mental Health of Children: Crisis in child mental health: challenge for the 1970's, New York, 1971, Harper and Row, Publishers, pp. 477-481.

Klonoff, H., and others: A problem-oriented system approach to analysis of treatment outcomes, Am. J. Psychiatry **132**:836-841, 1975.

Nodine, J. H., and Moyer, J. H.: Psychosomatic medicine, Philadelphia, 1962, Lea & Febiger, p. 10.

Numeier, D. F., and others: Nurses can be effective behavior modifiers, J. Psychiatr. Nurs. **14:** 18-23, 1976.

Osted, A., editor: Are you competent to do what you are allowed to do? Can. J. Psychiatr. Nurs. **17:**6, 1976.

Randolph, G. I.: Experiences in private practice, J. Psychiatr. Nurs. **13:**16-19, 1975.

Regester, D.: Community mental health for whose community? Am. J. Pub. Health **64:**886-893, 1974.

Santopietro, M. C., and others: Teaching primary prevention in mental health, Nurs. Outlook **23:**774-777, 1975.

Selye, H.: The stress of life, New York, 1956, McGraw-Hill Book Co.

Selye, H.: The evolution of the stress concept, Am. Sci. **61:**692-699, 1973.

Smith, D. C., and others: The national health planning act: significance for mental health agencies, Hosp. Community Psychiatry **27:**393-397, 1976.

Statistical note 92, Department of Health, Education, and Welfare, DHEW Publications No. (HSM), 74-655, 1973, p. 1.

Vaughn, W. T., and others: Family mental health maintenance: a new approach to primary prevention, Hosp. Community Psychiatry **26:**503-508, 1975.

ADDITIONAL READINGS

Bayer, M.: Psychiatric patients are people too! Nurs. Care **9:**22-24, 1976.

Brown, B. S.: The federal mental health program: past, present, and future, Hosp. Community Psychiatry **27:**512-514, 1976.

Carter, A. B.: Rural emergency psychiatric services, Am. J. Nurs. **73:**868-869, 1973.

Christie, L. S.: Conflicting needs and concepts in psychiatric hospitals, Nurs. Times **71:**2036-2037, 1975.

Krall, M. L.: Guidelines for writing mental health treatment plans, Am. J. Nurs. **76:**236-237, 1976.

Lamb, K. T.: Freedom for our sisters, freedom for ourselves: nursing confronts social change, Nurs. Forum **12:**328-353, 1973.

New ways to heal disturbed minds: where will it all lead? U.S. News and World Report **80:**33-36, 1976.

Zahourek, R.: Nurses in a community mental health center: functions, competencies, and satisfactions, Nurs. Outlook **19:**592-595, 1971.

CHAPTER 2

The evolution of personality

In recent years, we have witnessed many events that demanded the attention not only of government but of particular groups and individual citizens as well. Sociocultural issues have been most prominent in governmental and community actions. American Indians, blacks, Chicanos, Puerto Ricans, and many others have made their needs known as individuals, as families, as cultural groups, and as socioeconomic classes. Nursing and nurses in particular have recognized that a holistic concept must be employed to assist people in the maintenance of health, in the prevention of illness, and in the curative, therapeutic aspects of health care.

The behavior of any given individual is an extremely complex phenomenon. Human behavior is learned; it is not innate; and it carries with it its own specific meanings. We also learn fears, guilt, and social motivations, and some suggest that we even learn symptoms. Learning is reinforced both internally by ourselves and externally by significant others. Reinforced learning leads us to behavior patterns established early in our development. Thus the behavior patterns of individuals have a dynamic development with roots into the past and influence on the future. Personality, of which overt behavior is one aspect, goes through successive stages of development on the road to maturity. Some understanding of this development process is necessary to understand behavior.

BASIC CONCEPTS

Regardless of the basic theory to which there is allegiance—and there are differing theories—certain concepts regarding personality development are shared by almost everyone. Those concepts will be presented first.

29

Definition. We are speaking of personality in a technical sense and therefore must dissociate it from its common meaning. Personality is the characteristic and somewhat predictable behavior response patterns that each person evolves as his life-style. It is all a person is, feels, and does, both consciously and unconsciously. Personality is a compromise between inner drives and needs and internal and external controls. The internal controls are characterized as the conscience or superego, and external controls as the demand of reality. Personality then serves to maintain a stable relationship between the person and his environment.

Personality development unfolds in phases and not always at a steady pace. Its greatest influence is during the formative years. The child goes through periods of relative quiescence and then erupts in marked change. As the child moves into new phases of life, he finds new potentialities, new areas to explore, new challenges to master, and new skills to acquire. Physical or biologic maturation plays an important role in this development process since acquisition of certain abilities depends on physical development. Personality is not a system of traits existing solely within the capsule of a person. It is the inward organization of an individual in interaction with the outward organization of his environment, the most important parts of which are the significant persons in it. Personality is something always in the process of becoming something else, yet retaining a continuity that makes it ordinarily identifiable from situation to situation, from year to year, and from birth to death. Behavior, in both its outward and inward manifestations, is a function or expression of personality.

Motivations of behavior. What are the potentialities of any given individual as a person, and what determines which potentialities shall be developed and which shall remain latent? How much *do* we know? First, we must accept that what we know is not all and that there is more to learn than has yet been learned. The theories we now hold concerning behavior are the most adequate explanations we have been able to devise up to the present.

Although an infant emerges into the world without being asked, he is committed to the world and the life that he has ahead of him. At birth the child possesses a genetically determined biologic endowment, which is uniquely individual and yet common to all mankind. Already having been influenced by the intrauterine environment, the child will be further affected by culture and environment in the developmental process. Each individual then is unique, even though most people live through similar life experiences.

Because of this highly complex human nature, diagnostic procedures and categories are inexact. Present personality testing gives only a description of dynamic forces based on the examiner's interpretation of responses. Unlike general medicine, psychiatry has no precise tools to measure or diagnose personality. Psychiatrists are not dealing with an organ or system but with a human being in unique totality. The element of the unknown, the unexpected, and the unpredictable is always with those working in the psychiatric field.

One of the things we do know is that the entity we call a human being is endowed with biologic energy that apparently must be discharged with some degree of comfort to the organism. The human organism strives to maintain a state of equilibrium. Discomfort felt as frustration, urgency, tension, or want is met with biologic activity to relieve discomfort and its symptoms, leading to a state of gratification and restfulness. Thus, for example, hunger is relieved by behavior that leads to ingestion of food. Besides behavior's being influenced by physiologic drives to sustain life, psychologic drives also influence behavior by affecting one's conception of oneself and how one stands in society. The meeting of psychologic drives is more complex and less obvious than meeting most physiologic needs. The behavioral patterns with which we learn to meet these needs are significant aspects of our personality and influence our state of mental health. Again behavior is reinforced. Even behavior that is maladaptive, not leading toward gratification, may become fixed, eventually leading the person to show obvious pathologic symptoms. Human beings, however, strive for fulfillment, satisfaction, and security. Awareness of maladaptive patterns with proper emotional reduction and reinforcement can and does effect a change in behavior. This tendency toward self-realization—that is, the use of personal talents and skills with satisfaction and the ability to reach out freely and find fulfillment with others on a realistic basis—seems to be an important force in all of us.

Along with the need to expend energy, we recognize the need for adequate stimulus from the environment to maintain any individual's ability to function. There must be input as well as output. A person needs the physical and social stimulus of the surroundings to maintain himself. Herein may lie one of the major inadequacies of the custodial-oriented psychiatric hospital. Long-term isolation and control of a person with maladaptive or pathologic patterns of behavior does nothing but reinforce those patterns. According to the self-fulfilling prophecy, a person will behave as expected. Once that behavior is learned and reinforced, it will remain until new patterns of behavior are learned.

Anxiety. Anxiety, with its influence on growth and the achievement of maturity, is a central problem in personality development. It is a strong motivational force in normal behavior and the crucial problem in emotional and behavioral disorders, for these are both an expression of and a defense against intolerable anxiety.

Patterns of maladaptive behavioral responses are often linked with attempts to deal with this state of dreaded apprehension. Anxiety may be experienced as conscious, preconscious, or unconscious. Hence many people are not aware that anxiety is influencing their behavior. When consciously experienced, anxiety is felt as an extremely uncomfortable state with both physiologic and somatic responses. The physical symptoms of anxiety may include disturbances in motor and visceral responses characterized by palpitations, tachycardia, change in blood pressure, hyperventilation, dryness of mouth, anorexia, vomiting, gastric hyperactivity, "butterflies," constipation, diarrhea, diaphoresis, and urinary frequency. Some persons become overactive and agitated or show motor tension and tremor, while others are unresponsive, immobile, or frozen. The emotional response may include a peculiar, feeling state of consciousness. It can be characterized by mentally painful awareness of the feeling of powerlessness, by a feeling of persistent or inevitable danger, by physically exhausting alertness, by apprehensive self-absorption that often interferes with problem-solving, and by a feeling of doubt. Anxiety can also be characteristic of neurosis. This is called signal anxiety; it is a learned pattern of response in anticipation of a traumatic event. Thus the person reacts with anxiety before the situation actually takes place. Fear is different from anxiety in that fear is a response to a real or threatened danger, while anxiety is more typically a reaction to unreal or imagined danger.

No one is permanently free from anxiety. A mild degree can be constructive when it provides a stimulus to action that deals directly with anxiety or removes the cause of it. It can, for example, motivate a student to do the necessary studying to pass an examination or, an even more healthy reaction, motivate him to learn something he recognizes a need to know. On the other hand, anxiety can be destructive when it either leaves the concerned individual helpless to act or overwhelms the personality. Anxiety can be aroused by external or internal danger. The power to arouse anxiety from within lies in unacceptable thoughts, feelings, wishes, or drives that entail the loss of love or approval and the expectation of punishment. The anxiety connected with rejection and disapproval is used by adults in teaching children behavior patterns. The dangers and the potentials for the healthy development of children are implicit in this process. How parents or parent-surrogates use anxiety, how they balance it with love and affection, and to what extent they themselves are the carriers of intense anxiety are profoundly important for the child's developing personality. Severe and consistent disapproval by significant people is quite enough to account for lifelong severe anxiety.

Some of the source of anxiety in patients may well be related to the times in which we live. This era is often called the age of anxiety. It is a complicated world with the threat of atomic warfare close and immediate. We are in a period of rapid social change in which old, accepted values and standards of behavior have not been replaced with others of equal authority, and the result is uncertainty.

Sexual mores, values, and trends are in rapid transition in this age of the sexual revolution. The communications media, including television and movies, portray sex in an open fashion. There is a pressure to seek membership in and to conform to a variety of self-styled groups. Anxiety associated with nonacceptance, rejection, and isolation is more intolerable than the anxiety related to the actions themselves. Thus a better insight can be gained into the motivations of certain deviate patterns of behavior. Unfortunately, the person does not "win" either way. Both roads often lead to internal stress since lifelong attitudes reinforced by society, culture, religion, and significant others do not yield with ease.

Student unrest, as exemplified in the peace movement against the Vietnam conflict, reached its peak as the credibility gap between leaders and followers became more obvious. Values became confused and attitudes embittered, as students could no longer deal with the inconsistencies of killing, wanton destruction, poverty, and disease and still maintain a sense of social consciousness. The pieces of the puzzle no longer fit, so new pieces are being explored and crafted by the restless. An example of this can be found by this decade's growing awareness and concern about the ecology. Interest here is stronger and more organized than in previous history. With the formal end to the Vietnam conflict, energies are now being turned to our own environment. The restlessness in all probability has not gone; it is just wearing a different face, perhaps a face more able to respond and function in the midst of the age of anxiety.

More recently, however, the exposés of illegal governmental activities have dealt another blow to our society's already shaky value system. Whatever the outcome, one must deal with the knowledge of and the feeling of individual powerlessness. Inner security is violated when beliefs are shattered so mercilessly, as power, control, and deceit seem to be worth more than personal ideals. Some may deal with these situations by avoidance, denial, anger, bitterness, or resentment as means of handling anxiety. Our highly advanced technologic society has also created a similar sense of confused values as man becomes alienated from himself in endless nonrewarding, boring occupational tasks. Economics and the pull toward greater financial gain, although important, cannot fulfill the individual's total inner needs. There seems to be less use for the individual as such, with a resultant threat of a meaningless existence. Almost everyone experiences insecurity in the face of the complexities of today's world. However, anxiety so generated can be constructive as well as destructive. It can be used as an instrument for improvement and progress.

Raymond B. Cattell (1963) and other psychologists have been working with a new statistical technique, factor analysis, in the study of personality traits. As a result of their work, they conclude that anxiety does exist both as a temporary state of being and as a personality trait. Anxiety as a personality trait is marked by a high susceptibility to annoyance, ego-weakness, guilt-proneness, easy group inhibition, and rapid body tempo along with the physiologic manifestations. Two physiologic responses usually associated with anxiety as a temporary state of being, dry mouth and general muscle tension, were found to be missing. Instead, salivary output increases, and muscle tension is found primarily in the trapezius muscle. In other words, anxiety may exist as a temporary state for the individual or may be a chronic anxiety reaction, with slight physiologic differences between the two states. In response to anxiety, the individual may use effort stress to overcome its source, or he may use neurotic adjustment as a coping mechanism. In effort stress the individual grapples with difficulties and shows strong concentration and awareness of effort. In neurotic adjustment the individual may retreat and attempt to escape. The researchers suggest that this may be an age of effort stress rather than an age of neurotic adjustment. It is difficult to assess the significance of such findings at present, but the ideas do raise some interesting questions.

Combined research in this area supports the idea that an initial anxiety reaction may be either an inability to cope with the presenting difficulty (rising anxiety) or an organization of the individual's resources to cope effectively (stress response).

Organic endowment. The newborn infant is endowed with a certain physical makeup. He is an extremely complex organism maintained by the balance of tissues, organs, and systems, their interaction with each other, and their combined interaction with their environment. Life is, first of all, a biochemical fact. No infant could exist without the oxygen in the atmosphere that surrounds him any more than he could exist without lungs to absorb it, without blood to distribute it, or without tissues to utilize it. All this is organized into the unit that is the infant.

We usually call what is programmed in the chromosomes genetics or heredity. The sum of what is biologically given by genetics or through the intra-uterine environment is referred to as constitution. Maturation, then, is the unfolding of these biologically given factors at critical periods of development as if on a schedule. As the person matures, he interacts with the internal physical environment and the external psychosocial environment in a process called development. The role of environment and constitution must be seriously considered as each is important in understanding the precipitating and predisposing factors of mental illness.

The type of organized physical unit that the infant possesses will play a part in his personality development. Some biologic needs may be stronger than others and may cause him to select from his environment certain factors to which he will respond more readily. The predominance of one type of tissue over another—ectodermal over endodermal and mesodermal—may endow him with handicaps or attributes in his search for satisfaction. His very physical appearance may have much to do with his feeling of security since practically all cultures have strong attitudes about personal appearance against which a person will be measured and found acceptable or wanting.

Suffice it to say that the organic matrix from which personality develops will have a very definite influence on the direction of personality development.

Cultural influences. The society into which an individual is born will unquestionably be a profound factor in the kind of personality he will develop. Character and personality take shape in a social setting. One is born with a set of potentialities for personality development, but the environment will indicate those particular traits to be developed and those to be discouraged. In fact, probably the most characteristic trait of the human being is his plasticity.

Undoubtedly, the most important part of life as far as personality development is concerned is early childhood. It is within family life that the foundation for the adult personality is laid. Here basic drives or directing tendencies are modified by early interaction, and here the awareness of self is learned in relationships with others. Society determines the basic pattern of family life. The cultural pattern into which an individual is born provides and defines his behavior expectations and the roles that he must learn to fill. The system of values, the definition of behaviors that will win acceptance, and the types of life goals that will be important aspects of the dynamics of individual personality development are derived from the social culture.

Individuals and their families are the components of the community. Depending on the size of the community, the social culture or cultures manifested are an aggregate of the values of the individuals of the community. Multicultural communities are more characteristic of large cities than of small towns or villages. For many individuals the interrelationship among people of different cultural derivation brings enrichment, color, and creative interests and responses to the experiences of daily living, while for others these cultural differences stimulate insecurities, suspicions, irritations, and hostilities. The latter responses can become the focus of rationalizations for judging the superiority of one culture, race, or creed over another.

Attitudes toward race, creed, color, sex, and cultural background are an integral part of the setting within a community. Obviously, these influence those who live and develop within each community. The individual's attitude toward himself, as well as for those around him, are formed by each day's experiences in that community: in the playgrounds and the schools, in the offices, in the factories, and in the shops he frequents to maintain and supply his daily needs.

Social-class concepts have recently been applied to psychiatry in an effort to further understand the individual. Social class is defined by sociologists as a large segment of the population with certain common socioeconomic characteristics. These characteristics include the following objective criteria: occupation, education, residential area, type of housing, income, recreational patterns, and food habits. Studies about the relationship of social class to mental illness have suggested a significantly larger proportion of mental disorder in the lower socioeconomic classes of treated patients. Neurosis was found to be more common in the upper socioeconomic classes. To avoid misunderstanding, it is stressed that these studies are based on patients under actual treatment. However, information suggesting prevalent trends can be utilized constructively in focusing on prevention. It is suggested that the grim living conditions of the lower classes, the loneliness, and lack of therapeutic facilities contribute to these statistics. Criticism has been directed at the criteria used in evaluation of mental illness and at those who formulate the criteria. Cross-cultural psychiatry, the study of cultures influence on behavior patterns, is gaining stronger recognition as it strives for a more culturally sensitive evaluation of symptoms and diagnosis. Only the thorough study of determining factors will be able to suggest just what is the impact and influence of culture. To date, we know that severe behavior disorders occur in all known cultures and that social, economic, and ethnic factors alone cannot explain them fully.

Leininger is recognized as the first nurse-anthropologist. She studied an urban American community (1973) and demonstrated the effect of witchcraft beliefs on hospitalized patients with mental illnesses who belonged to a subculture group within that community. She found that patients who expressed these beliefs had been diagnosed as paranoid schizophrenics. Leininger states, "The traditional psychiatric therapists had focused upon the usual problems of nosology, failing to recognize the cultural beliefs underlying their patients' problems." After identifying these factors, she proceeded to deal with them by using family therapy as a means of returning the "bewitched" victims to their families and community.

Osborne (1973) describes the anthropologist's focus in a most significant way.

> For the anthropologist, people who manifest these strange behaviors are informants, not patients. The treatment of infirmity is not the important factor

for the anthropologist; his job is to understand the social culture, and psychological components of behavior, and the study of psychiatric illness provides a strategic point of entrée for the analysis of the structure of societies and for the development of their cultural theories.

As a practical point, nurses need to learn enough about the cultural backgrounds from which their patients come to use this knowledge in understanding behavior. Evaluation of identified behavior can only be accurate when all the factors influencing that behavior are taken into account. Then an appropriate care-plan approach can be instituted based on understanding of the total patient. Certain ethnic groups, as part of their cultural background, learn to freely verbalize their physical complaints and pains as an accepted pattern of behavior. In contrast, others tend to withhold their expression of pain, thus affecting the type of care received. An experience in labor and delivery rooms can substantiate this fact, as women of different cultures, backgrounds, and ethnic groups express their pain differently. Nurses who sit in judgment of behavior that is different from theirs or not acceptable by their value system unfortunately "miss the boat" for the patient, as well as for themselves. Another interesting example about how life situations affect the total functioning of the person comes from the Hopi Indians. Their belief is that thinking and concentration can cause something to happen. Thus relatives and friends have affectionate thoughts about an ill person, wishing for his recovery. Should the person remain ill or worsen, those around him become enraged and berate him for disregarding their wishes. Eventually they may even beat the person physically to make him change his attitude. Although such ideas and behavior seem ridiculous and cruel to us, they contain a certain wisdom that has escaped medical science. Psychologic theory suggests that the depression, giving up, and the states of helplessness and hopelessness associated with illness contribute to the onset and worsening of disease. These background influences need understanding since they are almost certain to conflict with the social values of the nurse.

Dr. George Carstairs (1973) points out that in many countries in the world "age old concepts based on religious faith or superstitious fears, which have, from time immemorial, offered their traditional versions of mental illness and its treatment." Many observers have reported that mental disorders take on the forms related to the cultural contexts of the people. These have been described for China (Dr. P. M. Yap), the Hindu society (Dr. Surya), and Japan (Dr. Takeo Doi). In the Sudan, Drs. Mahi and Bansher were able to establish a cooperative plan with the "Mollahs" or learned men of the local community to refer cases of schizophrenia to the local psychiatric clinic. In this society, the Mollahs are consulted by individuals and families with respect to illnesses and many varied problems. In West Africa, Dr. T. A. Lambo was one of the first to establish "a cooperative relationship with the local witch doctors who specialized in helping the mentally afflicted." Dr. Lambo states, "Health as a medical interest cannot be separated from human well-being in the social, economic and political sense. All these segments of human activity have, in fact, the same objectives, that of total human well-being, although by tradition and by definition they are influenced by considerations that seem at first sight, and often are in practice, divergent in their immediate aims."

Actually, health behavior and attitudes in general differ in varying socioeconomic levels. The lower the social class, the less likely is the individual to seek medical help early and to utilize available health services. Also, the lower the social class, the less likely the individual is to recognize and to understand the significance of the more serious symptoms of illness.

A social study done by Hollingshead and Redlich (1958) in New Haven, Connecticut, indicates that social class itself is reflected by differences in types of diagnoses made and types of treatment given psychiatric patients. No cause-effect relationship was definitely established. One of the most disturbing facts uncovered was that patients from the upper socioeconomic classes in the community received considerably more in the way of psychotherapy, whereas patients from the lower socioeconomic classes tended to receive more organic therapy, especially electroconvulsive therapy. That value differences between high-status physicians and low-status patients were obstacles in therapy was pointed out. The need for understanding the impact of cultural patterns on behavior becomes obvious if personality development and patient behavior are to be understood.

Several sociologists have raised some cogent arguments against the medical model for psychiatric illness as opposed to reactive disturbances to or within the social setting. In the sociologic model of mental illness, it is implied that abnormal behavior is reactive to a situation and, therefore, limited. It is believed that it is reversible, that it is mostly a process of learning and adaptation. On the other hand, the medical model is described as a "within-self" model and describes the patient as sick, as determined by the medical profession. The sociologist sees the person as a client.

One of the early sociologists concerned with the field of psychiatry was Lemert (1946). He proposed that the psychiatrist's role was mainly one of "social control on a socially deviant person." He indicated that the pattern of behavior becomes fixed when the person is labeled or set in a situation, such as hospitalization. The traditional state hospital setting, which imposes adaptation to the routine, results in the reinforcement of the abnormal behavior. The longer the period of hospitalization, the greater the learning of this life-style.

The result may be that the patient finds some comfort resulting from the situation to which he is confined and begins to accept it as a pattern of survival.

Scheff (1967) studied the legal aspects of hospitalization and commitment of the mentally ill. He indicated that the courts were not discriminating with respect to judging disturbed behavior and as a consequence hospitalization and commitment were fairly automatic pronouncements. He also argues that there are data supporting the fact that some behavioral disorders do not necessarily worsen and that certain episodes are self-terminating.

Emotions. An emotion is a feeling, a mood, or an affect. It is a diffuse combination of physiologic states and mental sets that pervade thinking and influence relationships and one's sense of well-being. The list of human emotions is endless. Many are perceived as conscious feelings, including fear, anger, aggression, hurt, rage, sexual feelings, envy, anxiety, guilt, pride, dejection, and loneliness.

Frequently identification of emotions is difficult because they are often blurred and fused. It is common that individuals are not taught to discriminate their feelings, since many are associated with negative value judgments. Intricate patterns of emotion denial or emotion suppression are established. When anger, jealousy, and rage are labeled bad, then to experience them is also to be bad. Ambivalence, two opposing emotions existing at the same time, also makes differentiation difficult; feeling the powerful emotions of love and hate simultaneously is an excellent example of this concept.

As observers of human behavior, nurses are in a good position to assist patients in the identification of their emotions, as well as in their healthy expression. Emotions can be observed from the person's behavior, from motor activity, from the person's subjective reports, and from our own empathy. Frequently, and often in mental illness, the person's actual verbal message is contradictory to the affective message we receive. As good detectives, we must learn to pause frequently to sort out and respond to the affective messages sent. Thus decoding the intricate patterns of defenses and behaviors can be instituted, and healthier, more adaptive patterns can be learned.

Defense mechanisms. Mechanisms of defense are psychologic processes that defend the person against anxiety and provide temporary security. When there is a threat to satisfaction or security, a warning signal throws a switch, and unconsciously one or more mechanisms of defense are brought into action. Some serve to alter the perception of danger or to block out some temptation. Others block out memories of disturbing experiences, and still others transform wishes into a form more acceptable to the person's conscience.

The mechanisms of defense begin during childhood developmental phases. They become complex parts of our character structure. Defenses are *not* in themselves pathologic. They go through changes in development and can become adaptive for the person. These mechanisms may help to provide stability, but they can also create problems and disturbed behavior when they become rigid, or fixed. They profoundly influence thought, behavior, and personality development. An understanding of defense mechanisms is paramount in understanding human behavior and psychopathology.

Denial, plain ordinary rejection, is a method of resolving conflict that all persons use to some extent. We simply do not acknowledge the existence of something disturbing. A person may insist that he is not hurt or angry. A man is not a coward to himself, no matter how cowardly his behavior. He may go further and reinforce the denial, but it is often the only step taken. A thing is just not so if it produces pain or conflict for it to be that way. In fact, the denial of illness is a fairly common behavior pattern on medical and surgical patient care units. The rejection of physical illness can have serious consequences for a patient with a major health problem.

Repression is a more complicated mechanism in which unpleasant or unacceptable experiences, emotions, or motivations are actively forced into the unconscious and kept there. It includes the barring from consciousness all memories, perceptions, and emotions that arouse forbidden impulses. The emotional context of repressed material may be a powerful source of motivation for behavior, but the individual is never aware of the true source or association of the emotion. A child frustrated and downtrodden by a severe parent may spend his life as a rebel against authority, always thinking he is activated by altruistic motives yet always acting out his conflict with his parent. He is sure that he loves and has always loved that particular parent. Repression operates wholly on an unconscious level.

Conversion is exactly what it says: strong emotional conflicts are expressed as or converted into physical symptoms. The boy who hates his father and is torn between the desire to strike him and fear of the consequences if he does so develops a paralyzed arm. The conflict is resolved. He cannot strike his father even if he wishes to, and the situation carries no threat of retaliation. In addition, the boy secures sympathy and attention for his symptom. The mechansim of conversion also operates wholly on an unconscious level. Interestingly, the utilization of the mechanism of conversion is strongly influenced by cultural factors. A better educated public now uses the mechanism more subtly than was true in the past.

Regression is a retreat from the present pattern to past levels of behavior. It occurs when discomfort becomes intense. The individual returns to patterns of behavior that were successful in earlier stages of development. All people use this mechanism sometimes, usually under temporary stress when they resort to childish methods to obtain their goals. Tears and temper tantrums in adults are sometimes very effective, even though they may not be adult forms of behavior. Actually, some degree of regression frequently accompanies physical illness, and regressed behavior of varying degrees of intensity is found in most patients in general hospitals. It is almost a necessary component of placing oneself in medical hands.

On admission, the medical regimen of most hospitals requires the patient to adapt to the routine care by submissively regressing to a dependency relationship with physicians and nurses. Sick persons are often misjudged for their expression of childish, petulant, and demanding behavior. The difficult patient is often found to be the one who resists the demand to regress to dependency. We have not given adequate attention to this factor as an impediment to the principle of self-care and to the dignity of self-esteem. Regression is a mechanism exhibited to an extreme degree by mentally ill patients who may retreat all the way to the infantile level. Its ultimate illustration is the severely ill patient who curls into fetal position and remains there obstinately.

Sublimation is a rather constructive method of resolving conflict if it is successful. The mechanism consists of using the energy involved in a primitive impulse not acceptable in its frank and direct expression in an activity that is socially constructive. A man who has strong sexual drives and who utilizes that energy in writing poetry or painting nude women, doing it well and thereby contributing to the arts, is an excellent example.

Reaction formation or overcompensation is an interesting mechanism. It is a means of disguising from the self the possession of an unacceptable desire or drive by developing its exact opposite to an extreme degree. It often, however, reveals its nature to the alert observer by the many slips made and by the extreme degree of the trait, which seems uncalled for. The person who is excessively sweet and polite under any and all circumstances is often a very hostile person who finds it necessary to disguise his hostility from himself and others. He usually makes others uncomfortable in the process, which hints at the underlying hostility. An interesting illustration of reaction formation is to be found in letters to the editor from some public-spirited citizens who are opposed to the vivisection of animals in the study of disease. Such letters, with their description in cruel and bloody detail of what ought to happen to the persons involved, reveal their writers' basic hostility.

Rationalization is the joy and delight of the average human being. It is simply finding a logical reason for the things one wants to do and is self-deception at its subtle best. The woman who buys a dress she could well do without and cannot really afford, but who can explain its purchase satisfactorily to her husband and herself, is a good example. The self-deception is in regard to the real motivation for behavior.

Identification is a very important mechanism in the process of adjusting to culture. Closely related to it is the mechanism of *introjection*, and since the difference in the two seems to be mainly one of degree, their definitions may be considered together. The basic process in both mechanisms is the acceptance of persons, ideas, or ideals outside the self, feeling with them as though they were part of the self, and finally integrating them into the core of one's own personality. If there is a difference between identification and introjection, identification would include the first two elements in the definition, and the addition of the third would make the mechanism introjection. Accepting parents' standards and molding behavior to meet those standards on one's own initiative is both identification and introjection. The parents have been identified with, and their standards have been introjected.

Projection is a very popular method of resolving conflicts and one that dominates the behavior of certain personality types. It sees thinking, feeling, and motor activity as having their origin outside the self, when in reality their origin is in the personality of the perceiver. Its purpose is obviously self-protective since that which is unacceptable to the self can be projected on the environment, and self-esteem can thereby be maintained. For example, who is always wrong in a heated argument? The other fellow, of course. In the severely mentally ill patient, auditory hallucinations can and do occur; that is, the patient hears voices when there are no voices to hear. The only source for such voices is in the thoughts of the patient himself, which, being too unpleasant to tolerate as coming from the self, are perceived as coming from the environment. This wholly uncontrolled projection is a danger signal. Actually, strange as such behavior may seem, it is not different in nature or process from the common projection that operates when we place the blame for our difficulties on others. We project faults or failures that are our own. When grades are low, it is the teacher's fault; when the boss loses his temper at a mistake, it is because of his nasty disposition. Used too extensively, the mechanism of projection can grow to dominate behavior and lead to serious maladjustment.

Displacement is the transference of emotion from one object, situation, or idea to another. Being angry with one's wife and kicking the dog, missing a shot and breaking the golf club, and being angry at the charge nurse and snapping at a patient are all examples of displacement.

Transference is in a sense a form of displacement, except that its meaning is more restricted. It means the shifting of feelings of strong positive or negative emotional attachment from one object or person to another. If the feeling is love, we speak of a positive transference, and, if hate, of a negative transference. Transference forms the basis for most therapeutic relationships.

Symbolization, without which none of us could ever adapt to our culture, means that one idea or object stands for another. The distinction between a symbol and the thing symbolized and how they stand for and represent each other is one of the most confusing lessons a child must master. Many mentally ill patients appear to be in exactly this state of confusion. WORD is only four printed letters, but it means one of the tools of language. A single gesture can symbolize or hold the entire meaning of loved person. Symbols have both general and personal meaning. This must be remembered since symbolization is used extensively in organizing experience within the personality, and the method of using symbols is one key to the personality.

Humor, wit, and *comic devices* are also considered examples of normal defenses. They can reduce anxiety, relieve grim reality, and gratify forbidden impulses. Humor has also been used as an acceptable outlet for hostility and anger.

Fantasy formation has its roots in childhood development. Creative fantasy is considered an asset and usually prepares the child for future reality. Under certain conditions fantasy or daydreaming permit instinctual gratification without anxiety. Excessive daydreaming, however, may interfere with normal reality.

THEORIES OF PERSONALITY DEVELOPMENT

Varying schools of thought or disciplines exist in the field of psychiatry. Although the general trend has been eclectic in nature, many schools with varying interpretations of personality development do exist. Among the more important are the schools of psychoanalytic thought, all based on what have become the orthodox views of Sigmund Freud. Since psychoanalysis has been profoundly important historically, a brief outline of its major points and contributions will be included here. Sigmund Freud revolutionized the thinking of the profession about mental illness, personality development, and the treatment of personality deviations. Most psychiatric thinking today rests on the groundwork of his insights into human behavior. Over the years, other theories have resulted in significant consequences to psychiatric practices.

Freud is the founder of the psychoanalytic movement. Since Freud was a Viennese neurologist, he came into contact with neurotic patients. The acceptable treatment of this period (the late 1880s) proved unsuccessful, and he began to search for the causes of his patients' problems when his colleagues gave up. He became impressed with his early successful results as he explored areas of the mind that, in his day, were uncharted courses. He was responsible for the process of free association, the process of suspending censorship and saying anything that comes into one's mind. He developed dream theory through the discovery of the unconscious. The dynamic concepts of human drives were categorized as eros, the instinct of love and life that tended toward unity and thanatos, the forces of death and destruction. Libido was constructed as the psychic energy force of the sex instinct. Freud postulated that the organism tended toward tension reduction, resulting in the pleasure principle. The term "primary process" is characterized as that thinking, essentially magical and wishful, which short-cuts reality. It is oblivious to time and logic and is infantile in nature. Secondary process thinking corresponds more to the mature, reality-oriented, categorical thinking of adults. Freud did not admit to chance faction; thus he was led to the discovery of symptom formation to explain the cause of strange, bizarre, and self-defeating behaviors. He was subject to professional attack and personal ridicule as the repressive society of his time resented his suggestion of the innate sexual instincts of children. Freud saw himself as a discoverer and a scientist, not a genius. He had the courage and perseverance to convert the gift of his insight into a detailed and extensive body of knowledge. The following discussions are more detailed explorations of his most important contributions.

Structure of personality. The structure of personality, according to Freud, consists of three basic parts whose internal conflict and balance are the factors that produce what we call behavior. These three components of personality are the id, the ego, and the superego.

Concerned only with striving after pleasure and satisfaction, the id is the raw stuff of personality, the primitive, biologic drives and urges. It is also the reservoir of psychic energy, called the libido by analysts. The id is that part of the personality with which we are born, a personality ruled only by the pleasure principle.

Chronologically the ego is developed next and arises from the experiencing of frustration or thwarting of immediate satisfaction as the infant distinguishes himself from the surrounding world. It is the part of the self most closely in touch with reality and is roughly equivalent to what is meant by self, or I, or conscious awareness. The ego has the executive functions of integration, perception, thought, feeling, drive, and action. It protects the person from dangerous impulses by utilization of the defense mechanisms. The ego develops to mediate between the strivings of the id and the demands of the environment, so that satisfactions may be achieved in a manner coinciding with physical and social reality. As the ego develops, the reality principle supersedes or operates in concert with the pleasure principle in guiding behavior. The relative strength of each will be determined by the comparative strength of the id and the ego in the total personality.

The superego develops during early childhood at the resolution of the oedipal complex, later than the other two aspects of personality. It represents the individual's acceptance of responsibility for the regulation of his own conduct.

The superego is roughly equivalent to conscience, or the sense of right and wrong. Beginning primarily with the acceptance early in life of the standards of the persons who are most important to the child, it is first evident when the child feels within himself that his behavior is right or wrong.

The id then is primarily biologic in nature and biologically conditioned. It is the id that says "I want." The ego is derived from physical reality and says, "Better not because you will get hurt." The superego is social and cultural in origin and says, "You can't do that because it is wrong." There is constant conflict between the id and the superego and potential conflict between any two of them. From these conflicts comes the source of behavior, and the resolution of conflicts is in the direction of growth. Without conflict and frustration, there would be no growth.

Topography of the self. Conflicts do not always occur in the individual's awareness. One of Freud's greatest contributions to an understanding of human behavior was his popularization of the concept of the unconscious. Not all mental activity—in fact, only a small part of it—is conscious. The mind consists roughly of three overlapping divisions—the conscious, the subconscious, and the unconscious. These divisions are not actual physiologic separations but are conceptual regions of the mind. The conscious is that part of the mind immediately focused in awareness. The subconscious or preconscious is that part recalled and brought to awareness at will. It can be demonstrated by forgetting a person's name and later recalling it or in slips of the tongue. The unconscious is the reservoir of memories, experiences, and emotions that cannot be recalled. This part is by far the largest part of mental activity and is proportionately equivalent to the submerged part of an iceberg. Parts of the id, ego, and superego exist in all strata of the conscious and the unconscious, although the larger part of the id is in the unconscious.

Personality development. The freudian psychoanalytic school equates personality development with psychosexual development. Freud advanced the very unpopular theory that the sexual instinct does not spring into being suddenly and completely mature at adolescence. Rather, he held that its appearance at this period was the culmination of all the stages through which the individual had passed. Sex is interpreted more broadly than it tends to be in our culture, in which the meaning of the word is frequently restricted to genital activity. Freud saw the maturation of the sex instinct as the last step in the maturation of emotional development. Therefore personality development is explained through its core or center, psychosexual development.

The actual process of birth, the individual's first traumatic experience, does have psychologic significance, but its depth and extent are not clearly defined. The newborn child is a helpless person, largely id and primarily physiologic in expression. Feeding at the breast is his most important activity and source of greatest pleasure. Tension relief is achieved by sucking or swallowing, and there seems to be a sucking need that is independent of hunger satisfaction. For that reason, the earliest stage of development is called the oral sucking stage. The child is a passive dependent person, ruled completely by the pleasure principle. He derives satisfaction that is autoerotic in nature; he experiences pleasure without any knowledge of self and hence no self-love. The oral sucking stage is brought to an end by the frustration involved in weaning, which produces the first major trauma and the first major conflict.

By the process of weaning, the child is forced to develop a more differentiated personality to cope with his conflict. He begins to recognize reality and its demands and to develop ideas of himself as an individual. His ego begins to emerge, and he shows evidences of narcissism or self-love. He cuts teeth and now has the equipment to exhibit aggressiveness. The conflict over the frustration of weaning is resolved through the development of oral aggressive behavior. Pleasure is found in biting, as well as in sucking. At this time the infant shows ambivalence toward his mother—she is both a source of pleasure in feeding and physical comfort and a source of dissatisfaction because of the weaning process. Also at this time come further demands for conformity in the beginning of training in habits of personal cleanliness. The final weaning, the training in cleanliness, and the possible appearance of another child combine to produce the second major traumatic experience. The resolution of this conflict results in strengthening the ego and developing the reality principle as a factor in the motivation of behavior, although the pleasure principle continues its domination. This period of development, the oral aggressive stage, overlaps markedly the stage that succeeds it, the anal expulsive stage.

The child learns early to enjoy the release of tension that accompanies the evacuation of the bowels and the bladder. He also comes to learn that his parents place tremendous importance on urine and feces being deposited at specific places and times. He learns to recognize urine and feces as being something dirty on one hand and as something valuable to be retained on the other hand. Since the ego and the sense of reality become well developed during this period, the child achieves a sense of power through control of evacuation. Urine and feces not only are a means of securing rewards and affection but also are amenable to being used for aggressive purposes. The child reaches the stage at which he goes through a phase of reality-testing. He perceives the consequences of giving in to the pleasure principle under certain circumstances. If the course of his development has been relatively normal, from here on pleasurable acts generally will be carried out with a certain respect for reality and the probable consequences of the act. Two effects of the toilet-training period are, (1) development of the anal retentive period and (2) the vague beginnings of the superego or conscience. The child realizes the social value and power of retaining, controlling, and possessing feces. In addition, all excreta have an independent value for him. On the one hand, they are valuable as gifts to please the parents, but under certain conditions they are dirty and may be insults. Some of this childhood confusion may well continue throughout life. The final frustration of the anal period occurs about the end of the fourth year, when the child must finally give up the pleasures of the particular period. At the same time, reality has taught him that he is an individual, and, worse yet, it now dawns on him that he is not the most important individual in existence or even in his own family. In fact, he realizes dimly that his parents may even be more important to each other than he is to either of them. This is a blow. The realization of his relative unimportance is the conflict that precipitates the phallic period.

Children by this time are aware of the physical differences between the sexes and exhibit curiosity about them. The chief source of pleasure is deflected from the anal to the genital region. Masturbation is a common experience. This is primarily narcissistic in character—the child is interested in himself and his own genitalia. There exists considerable confusion in the mind of the child about the use of sexual organs, and he begins to have ideas about sexuality. For the first time comes a sense of a need for others as an object of sexual activity, and the choice naturally falls on the parents. They are closer to the child emotionally than anyone else, and they represent power and prestige. Knowing the difference between sexes, the child wonders why in rather concrete terms. It occurs to the boy that loss of the penis is possible and to the girl that she has lost hers.

The male child was first dependent on his mother, and it is natural when he develops the first ideas of sexuality that he chooses his mother as a love object, the Oedipus complex. He also realizes that his mother belongs to his father and that the latter is a formidable rival. He realizes there would be serious consequences if he should become a real rival for his mother's affections, and, connecting the penis vaguely with the sexual act, he fears its loss. This fear of castration leads to a repression of infantile sexuality, since any sexual expression of his preference for his mother is dangerous. However, since the child loves both parents, he resolves the conflict by identifying with the father and introjecting his standards. This further strengthens the superego, whose appearance was begun during the anal stage of development, through complete acceptance as one's own of the attributes and standards of the parent. Such a solution, ending in identification with the parent of the same sex, is a positive resolution and a normal course of events. The resulting repression of all infantile sexuality brings the child to the latency period.

The Electra complex in the female follows a slightly different sequence of events. Her first love object during the oral and anal stages is the mother. A growing awareness of sexuality during the phallic stage of development causes her to choose her father as her love object, and the mother is seen as the rival for his affections. Since the penis is already lost, she has less immediate fear and goes through the conflicts of this period more slowly than a boy. Finally, however, she may begin to see the possibility of having a child as a compensation for the loss of the penis and may then identify with the mother, whose voice becomes her superego.

Both the male and female may go through the oedipal situation in a negative fashion and identify with the wrong parent or with neither. A successful resolution of the oedipal situation is essential to healthy personality development.

Once infantile sexuality is repressed, the child is not consciously concerned with sexual matters. All such urges are sublimated in education and play. The child spends this time learning how to behave in society.

At the age of puberty, there is a gradual revival of all the infantile sexual stages. The revival of the phallic period dominates, but the phallic interest gradually develops into real genital interests. Oral and anal interests also occur, and bathroom humor is popular. Since the threat of castration is not wholly gone and narcissism is still very evident, the first love object in this stage is usually of the same sex, the normal homosexual period. Interest turns gradually and tentatively to the other sex. The first love affair is usually phallic since, in finding himself as an adult, the individual is concerned primarily with himself as a lover. The final genital stage, true heterosexuality, is reached when the individual is concerned primarily with the love object.

It should be clearly understood that the stages of development shade and merge into successive stages and that interests of each stage persist as permanent parts of the personality. Each stage has its particular frustration and major trauma, and successful resolution of the conflict of each is essential to normal development. The unresolved conflict remains in the unconscious and from there motivates behavior in an unhealthy fashion and in unhealthy directions.

Contributions since Freud. Some of Freud's own pupils and later students of behavior who followed in his path have differed with his theories and have introduced new concepts in the field of psychoanalytic thought. Adler, Jung, and Rank started the neofreudian school of thought, in which new ideas challenged the original freudian theories. There is and has been constant change in ideas and techniques of analytic psychology. To become fixed and dogmatic about any one school would be an act of negating the significance of each new level of knowledge succeeding out of the past and the subsequence of one to the other. Theorists formulate, reformulate, and modify their ideas throughout their professional life spans. This is not a process to perplex the student but is a phenomenon of creative thought. Psychoanalytic theory is constantly undergoing change and modification in the light of new experience and theory. The different theories have contributed immensely to the growing body of knowledge about human behavior. Horney, Sullivan, Klein, and Fromm are also considered here in brief outline.

Alfred Adler, a follower of Freud in the early psychoanalytic movement, broke with the master and founded an independent school known as individual psychology. One of the major tenets of Freud that he discarded was the libido theory based on the importance of infantile sexuality. He turned toward the area of interpersonal interactions, particularly attitudes toward the self and others, as a basis for a theory of personality development.

Beginning with the helplessness of the infant as a primary and influential experience, he conceived personality as beginning from a feeling of inferiority and striving throughout life toward superiority, power, mastery, and perfection. Organic inferiority, or congenital body defect or weakness, determined the areas in which superiority was sought or struggle avoided. The organic inferiority itself was not considered as significant as the individual's and other's attitude toward it. Adler certainly popularized the expression "inferiority complex."

Adler interpreted social feeling and interest, courage, and common sense (reality-testing) as the usual attributes of normal human beings. He also supported the thesis that all behavior is goal directed; the specific personal goal of the individual and his methods of trying to achieve that goal constituted the individual's life-style. Change in a life-style that has resulted in maladaptation could be accomplished by changing the life goal. Adler also emphasized two currently popular concepts—the psychologic unity of man and man's genuine human potential.

Carl Jung, who also was active in the early psychoanalytic movement, differed from Freud on some basic tenets and as a result started his own school known as analytic psychology. His theory of personality seems closer to archaeology, history, literature, and mythology than to psychiatry. He interpreted the libido as a single life energy with many aspects and expressions and with less emphasis on the *central* importance of sexual development for personality growth. The libido tends to follow one of two basic attitudes—introversion (subjective and inner directed) and extroversion (objective and outer directed). Both attitudes are necessary for a full and rich life. The extreme or one-sided development of one attitude results in an unconscious development of the other where the second attitude can, from the unconscious, lead to conflict and maladaptation.

In his presentation of "Patterns of Behavior and Archetypes," Jung postulated that each species of animal, including man, is born with a characteristic mode of behavior. "Archetypes are typical forms of behavior which, once they become conscious, naturally present themselves as ideas and images, like everything else that becomes a content of consciousness."

Jung also identified four functions of personality—sensation, intuition, feeling, and thinking—and thought that behavior could be explained in terms of the balance of attitudes and functions that characterize any given individual's mode of operation. Sensation and intuition are modes of apprehension of the world, sensation representing concern with the here and now and intuition representing concern with what things have been or will be. Feeling and thinking are judgmental in nature, with feeling being concerned with a sense of values and thinking with ideas in the abstract. Again, all functions must be in balance for healthy living. The overdevelopment of any one function results in the unconscious overdevelopment of its opposite, with a consequent threat to mental health.

In studying patients, Jung emphasized a distinction between sign and symbol; the former is an image that represents agreed upon concepts (for example, the flag), and the latter represents a deep personal individual dream or vision. The cross, for example, could be a sign to one person and a symbol to another, depending on its personal meaning. One of the important sources of symbols is the collective unconscious, the sum of the experiences of the human race, which is found in the deep unconscious. Jung believed that his analytic school was more firmly rooted in the present and the future than Freud's school of thought.

Otto Rank was another of the early psychologists who broke with freudian psychology. He had a very close relationship with Freud, who encouraged him as a student and a developing psychologist. It was after Rank had visited the United States for a lecture series that his divergent ideas formed the schism from Freud's psychoanalytic theories.

Rank's theories emphasized interpersonal relationships and explained that internal emotions and thoughts were factors that determined and controlled behavior. He stressed that man was born with response potentialities that include appetites or impulses (hunger, sex, and thirst) and emotional responses (fear, guilt, and love). These response potentialities are expressed in behavior. The individual chooses how he will express particular responses. Man learns to express his responses in relationship to his environment. Rank emphasized the personality as a whole and the will of the individual to make choices. The will is considered as the integrative factor or the active relationship of the person and his world. The will develops as a counterwill toward others in the process of learning to distinguish one's self as an individual separate from others. This rebellion or differentiation arouses guilt, and the successful resolution of such guilt represents both the healthy person and the goal of therapy. The ultimate goal is both separation and union (to live in harmony with others). It implies learning to accept one's own will and the will of others while belonging with and caring for others. Rank's views had more impact on the applied social sciences than on medicine.

Karen Horney has also had considerable influence within the psychoanalytic movement. She has developed a school of thought that utilizes the process of adaptation to life situations as an explanation for personality development. She attributes to man the inherent desire and ability to change, to grow, and to expand, not merely to avoid pain or suffering. A prime motivating factor in behavior is the need for security, which is not a universal factor but one that operates when security is threatened. She does not believe that the infant's sense of helplessness leads to a drive for mastery or power since, with his potential, the infant need not always feel helpless. However, she does consider that the infant's feelings of helplessness, when they do occur, lead to an exaggerated need for security and form the background for a neurotic adjustment. The social orientation of Horney's concepts is evidenced by her belief that one of man's basic needs is to value himself and to be valued by others. She also believes the individual develops an ideal self-image that constitutes an integrating factor in behavior. Horney also treats conflict as essentially pathogenic, with a neurotic reaction involving repression of part of the conflict. The repressed material in the unconscious continues to influence behavior to a great extent. Horney, like others, emphasizes the unity of man and his functioning as a total person.

The name *Harry Stack Sullivan* is associated with the so-called interpersonal school of the William Alanson White Psychiatric Foundation. According to Sullivan, the crucial aspects of personality development are to be found in personal interrelationships; thus grew the substance for the interpersonal theory of psychiatry. Many of Sullivan's ideas are strikingly similar to Freud's basic concepts. The infant has critical body zones around which interaction with significant others takes place. These experiences set up modes of communication with the self and with others. He sees the human infant as helpless and sees that the infant is reliant on significant others to relieve biologic tension, such as in the need for food. The infant begins to adjust his behavior to satisfy these needs to assure security. If satisfaction is unmet or absent, tension and anxiety result. Behavior and motivation toward anxiety-tension reduction become major behavioral goals for the individual. He also suggests empathic communication between the infant and the mothering one. Anxiety in the adult evoked by the infant is relayed back empathically to the infant. From these processes the child's self-concept, self-image, or self-dynamism is developed.

Sullivan calls the earliest mode of the infant's communication "prototaxic." The child at this time has no awareness of himself and has no concept of time or space. The "syntaxic" mode of experience is the thought process that shows logical connections. It is based on language's conveyance of accurate messages. Validation occurs when the right word is fitted to the right situation. "Parataxic" communication, on the other hand, is based on misleading and unintelligible communication. A beginning connection is made between events, but the connection is often illogical. An example is a child who puts on a fireman's hat and becomes a fireman. To him the part becomes the whole. Parataxic distortion analytically suggests the process of transference. The patient's attitude toward the therapist, or in this case the nurse, is based on a fantasized or distorted evaluation of that nurse with other figures from the patient's past life.

In addition the child develops beginning personifications of the self based on interaction with significant others. If the child's securities have been enhanced, he has no anxiety, and if the child is rewarded with tenderness, then he develops the concept of the "good me." On the other hand, if the significant mothering person responds to the child with axiety and tenseness the concept of the "bad me" develops. The child assumes that the response is a reflection of his own lack of personal worth. If these experiences are strong and painful, the child reacts with dissociation experienced as "not me." This evolves gradually, coming from the experience of intense anxiety. "Not me" is based on a primitive parataxic mode and is often the deviation that leads to schizophrenia. In special circumstances, such as occasional dreams, the experience of "not me" can be appreciated by everyone.

Sullivan's theories focus on communication and interpersonal behavior. He explains that communication is a crucial aspect in interpersonal transactions. Since in psychotherapy speech is the major vehicle for a person to express his thoughts and feelings, Sullivan stressed the therapist's awareness of the totality of the communicative acts. He emphasized that in analysis it was important to consider more than the behavior of one individual. It was an interpersonal transaction and the therapist had the role of a participant observer.

Melanie Klein departed from the classic analytic technique in her treatment of children. Since children do not verbalize easily, she utilized the process of play therapy as a means of interpreting their behavior. Her findings suggested that children too have unconscious conflicts, and her analysis of children confirmed Freud's deductions about mental life during childhood.

Erich Fromm, like Sullivan, has focused on the healthy potential for growth and self-realization of man as a central idea in personality development, but he has given this concept a somewhat different emphasis. Man represents the highest order of animal, and one of his most human characteristics is relative freedom from internal and external influences. Man has moved increasingly toward the independent use of rational choice, and it is this historic evolution that is a basic factor in personality development. The major need of a human being is to find meaning in life through the use of his own powers. The basic human conflict lies between the security given by following instincts or rigid social mores and the use of reasoned solutions to the problems of existence. For Fromm, new solutions produce new problems requiring new solutions. It is this progressive movement toward rational living that constitutes growth and development. Since man's experience is basically social, his satisfactions are socially oriented. Fulfillment and the meaning of life are derived from productive work and the loving relationship with others.

Commonalities. Regardless of the specific school, all psychoanalytic groups agree on at least four basic concepts:
1. Behavior has meaning and is not determined by chance.
2. The unconscious plays an active role in determining behavior.
3. All behavior is goal directed.
4. The early years of life are extremely important for personality development.

Needless to say, the acceptance of the four basic concepts is not restricted to psychoanalytic thinking.

In general, the new concepts added to psychoanalysis by those who followed Freud have tended to broaden the basis of personality development beyond a strictly psychosexual one, have introduced a greater emphasis on social and cultural factors in personality development, and have placed a greater emphasis on the drive within the individual to seek health.

AN ECLECTIC APPROACH

Although many approaches to psychiatric therapy rest on the bedrock of freudian psychology, there have been many deletions and additions to the basic concept. The discussion that follows is based on commonalities that cut across theoretic boundaries.

Infancy, or approximately the first 12 to 15 months of life, is filled with rapid physical and developmental transformation. During no other period of life is the organism subjected to such rapid growth changes. At birth the neonate is almost totally helpless and dependent. The infant can do little but suck milk by reflex action, sleep, and signal discomfort or pain by crying. In a relatively short period of time this child turns into an alert toddler, whose spirit, energy, and enthusiasm are fascinating. The toddler actively explores his world and gains mastery over it by incessant experimentation. What exactly happens to a person at this time is lost. It lies beyond the individual's recall, buried in wordless oblivion. The inability to recollect our period of infancy offers limitation to our deep understanding. We depend mainly on observations and presumptions. We do know, however, that these are the months when foundations are laid for future emotional stability, for character traits, and for intellectual development. More than any other life experience, infancy will be solidly incorporated in the individual.

Infant experience. One ability the infant possesses, the unexplained power of communicating tones of emotional feeling or the power of empathy, is highly significant. He is able to sense and respond to feelings of approval or disapproval of the parent or nurse. Feelings of approval increase his sense of well-being, and disapproval causes discomfort. This happens long before he is capable of understanding the meaning of either feeling or before he is capable of any discrimination in regard to experience. Although all experience is planted forever in the personality, at this time the infant simply has a vague comprehension of things as pleasant or unpleasant and a vague association of them in relation to the mother or mother-figure. At this period the world is simply a cosmic universe with no limitations to any single entity, either self or others. Satisfactions are achieved with the first magic tool, the cry, and comfort and discomfort are known but not understood.

Then begins the period of personal habit training, with the deliberate use of approval and disapproval as tools that bend the child's behavior into approved social paths. Restraints on freedom, combined with a steady growth in the ability to differentiate perceptions, lead to the evolution of the sense of self or I, and a very important thing happens. Although the process is not fully understood, the organization of the individual around the self or I or ego results in an entity that henceforth seeks to perpetuate itself and to maintain itself always in the direction and characteristics it acquired in its earliest stages.

What determines the direction and characteristics of the self? It comes about primarily through interaction with significant people in the environment. Approval or disapproval, with the resultant increase and decrease in the sense of well-being, begin to be discriminated in a crude way. The first vague grasp of cause and effect dawns, and the child, his security of paramount concern to him, begins to adapt his behavior to ensure his security. Attention becomes focused on those types of behavior that call forth some response; other types receive no attention since they are not significant to security. It is obvious that the more consistent the parents are, the easier will be the process of learning for the child, and the less confusion and uncertainty will be built into the personality.

Several factors are of sufficient importance at this stage to merit brief discussion. The selective attention mentioned previously—that is, attention paid to *significant* things in the environment—has two results, both springing from the development of self. The experiences or parts of it that are insignificant to the child are not brought into awareness and exist only outside the awareness. These experiences are incorporated into the substratum of the self; however, they can often be integrated into the conscious self-system when attention is called to them if they do not conflict markedly with the perception or direction of the self-system. Unpleasant experiences, especially those that are painful in their threat to security, are actively rejected by the self and denied access to awareness. These parts of experience, which become part of the personality, continue as dissociated parts. It is not that they do not have any influence on personality and behavior. They most certainly do, but without awareness of the self.

Early childhood. As the child emerges from infancy and starts to talk and walk, he enters a phase where he must learn to balance his new motor skills and his verbal and intellectual abilities. The young child also now finds himself in a different relationship with his mother. The nurturing and provision of needs during infancy now change to certain restrictions and limitations. Expectations are now set, and the child is expected to comply. It is a difficult transition for the unreasoning child to make. The child exists in an autistic world, a world that has a highly personal meaning for him, not related at first to the real world. He begins to learn to handle the ambiguous symbols of language, first investing them with his own meaning and learning as he goes to share the meaning others give them. Learning to communicate with others enhances the development of self. The use of empathy need no longer be solely relied on, and the newer use of language conveys approval and disapproval more accurately and easily. The process of acculturation is hastened.

The other occurrence of importance during this period is the child's adoption, wholly and without question, of the attitudes, beliefs, and standards of those persons about him who are significant to him. He has not yet the experience or judgment to question them, nor can he as yet think logically to question them, although the roots of logical thinking are there in his developing ability to see cause-effect relationships. Even more importantly for his future, he accepts the evaluations that others place on him without question. If he is loved and wanted, then the direction of his self will probably be strongly toward loving and wanting. If he is disliked, the direction of his self will probably be toward hostility and dislike. If he is respected, he will probably be able to respect others. His first and most deeply learned perception of himself in relation to other people, the root of his security and his future personality development, is a reflection of how the significant persons around him perceive him.

At this moment, lest a wrong conclusion be drawn, the concept of personality as a dynamic, changing, onward moving process should be thought through again. Early experience is profoundly important for personality evolution, but it is not an absolute determinant. Corrective experience can take place at any stage of development and can often lead to a new definition of goals and a new self-perception. For example, a child who is brought up in a home in which he is unwanted and disliked will have a negative emotional attitude toward himself and others. The same child, if he is removed from his parents at school age and is *consistently* respected and wanted from then on, may and probably will change the direction of his growth to a more positive orientation. This will not occur at once, since the strength of the tendency to perpetuate the original direction of the self is strong. This explains the failure of the light-and-sweetness you-be-kind-to-me-I'll be-kind-to-you approach that baffles the neophyte in his first contacts with so-called mentally ill patients. The direction of personality growth can be altered, but this will occur through an intelligent, consistent, long-drawn-out effort. More positive aspects of the personality that exist in its dissociated part can be integrated into the self, but only slowly, because it involves a major change that will not be readily accepted.

Having learned to discriminate between himself and the rest of the world, the child learns that discomfort exists within himself and is not cosmic. This accompanies the development of the concept of the self or I. He now discriminates the universal experience of anxiety. This ability to feel intensely uncomfortable is both an asset and a liability. It serves as a warning or danger signal, indicating clearly that either satisfaction or security is threatened or that one threatens the other, for it is not unusual for the satisfaction of a need to threaten security.

Anxiety functions either to avoid a threat or to obscure awareness of its true significance. Here the previously determined direction of personality growth is important. A child who respects himself respects others, and his security is less often threatened. Hence his need for and use of anxiety is reduced. The child who is hostile in reacting with others brings forth many threats to his own security and hence tends to need and be dominated by anxiety more extensively.

During this period the child first achieves a fairly firm integration of himself as an individual. He has scarcely ventured beyond home and school and must still accumulate most of the knowledge he will require to guide his life.

Late childhood. Having absorbed and accepted the standards, codes, attitudes, and evaluation of himself held by the significant persons in his infancy and childhood, the growing child shows a new capacity, which his biologic endowment of energy forces him to use. This capacity is the continuing necessity to expand his activities, to reach out, and to interact with widening circles. He needs more companionship of his own age group and seeks it. If playmates do not exist, he creates them in fantasy. Now he learns cooperation, accomplishing things with other personalities. If his attitude toward himself is sound, his progress will be rapid, and his sense of well-being will be enhanced. In a steady forward direction the child is fitted to his culture, and his culture is fitted to him.

The association with other children in play activity is a vital learning experience. The child has already developed social skills of one degree or another, patterns and ways of interacting with others that are designed to meet his needs and promote his security. In play with others he learns new roles, more independent ones. He learns a wider range of roles and develops a greater capacity for give and take. His sense of belonging widens. Old techniques that are unsuccessful in the new milieu may be discarded for better ones or may be reserved for use only in the home situation, where they may continue to be effective. However, even in the home situation there is ordinarily steady pressure toward the use of more mature techniques in social relationships and toward the curbing of immediate satisfactions in the interests of the greater satisfactions of delayed pleasures and the satisfactions of others. If the child is relatively secure, he learns and progresses, exploring with both failure and success, and defines for himself a status and prestige on ever-widening horizons acceptable to himself and to the other persons with whom he establishes relationships. He interchanges roles as necessary with increasing flexibility and ease. If, however, he is insecure, the road is apt to be rocky.

Adolescence. Adolescence can be defined as the period between pubescence and physical maturity. It is biologically concerned with the transition from childhood, originally spurred by the puberty growth spurt and by hormonal changes, effecting rapid changes in secondary sex characteristics. Its goals are the attainment of adult prerogatives, responsibilities, and self-sufficiency. Adolescence is often considered a period of potential crisis. It is a period of physical and emotional metamorphosis during which the youth feels estranged from himself as the child he has known. It is a time of seeking inward to find out who one is and a searching outward to locate one's place in life. During this phase there is also a search for another, a longing for someone with whom to satisfy cravings for intimacy and fulfillment. There is a turbulent awakening to love, to loneliness, and to despair. The adolescent lives with a type of sensitivity that carries him to the heights and depths of his emotions. For those who have had emotional stability and a sense of security during childhood, the course of adolescence can be charted with relatively little difficulty.

The maturing of the sexual drive at this period is accompanied by considerable emotional stress and reorientation of goals in terms of sexual objectives. How much of the emotional stress is biologic in origin and how much culturally induced is a moot point. There exist societies in which adolescence presents no struggle. In American society the adjustment is largely determined by the previous pattern, since this pattern is modeled on past experiences that tend to prevent radical newness in interpersonal situations.

Adolescence is a period rife with conflicts. The drive toward independence is coupled with comparatively immature judgment, which makes it a risk. The desire for independence usually draws conscious or unconscious resistance from parents. The strong need to be exactly like one's peers opposes parental demands. The sensitive need for complete approval is endangered by the uneven physical development that is accompanied by awkwardness and physical peculiarities in appearance. The standards of one's own generation appear so much more modern and worthwhile than the standards of parents, so that family identification becomes a little painful. This phenomenon challenges parents and may produce changes in parent-child relationships. The adolescent needs and wishes both to be alone to develop his own set of values and to be with others to share their values. Usually he has a desire for adult privileges and an apprehension about adult responsibilities. There is a physical readiness for sexual maturity and a cultural block in the way of its achievement. On the whole, adolescence is a period of ambivalence. The secure child can survive it, pass through it, and emerge from it an adult. The insecure child will, of course, find it more painful, although he too may eventually emerge as an adult in more than a physical sense.

Adolescence is a time of particular significance to psychiatry. It is during this period that we witness severe emotional casualties in significant numbers. Even though the "damage" may have occurred earlier in childhood, it is during this period of turmoil that symptoms are likely to develop. Some utilize total rebellion against parental and societal values and seek to live outside the behavior that society considers the norm. This often gets them in trouble with the law, school, and parents. Further restrictions, however, usually lead to further rebellion. Other adolescents attempt withdrawal from social participation and sometimes from the self as a means of coping. They may retreat into fantasy and at times into delusion. Still others may show no specific symptoms or social deviations. They may deal with their stress by passive endurance, in effect by being "good." In any case, however, many adolescents need assistance in dealing with the internal and external stresses of this period. Their ability to accept assistance, or to reach out to it, is a very difficult task because adults and the authority they represent are a major part of the problem.

Maturity. The lengthy developmental process, almost an apprenticeship in living, draws to a close as the individual attains his identity. Adult status is usually granted by chronologic age and by physical maturation. Hopefully the person is sufficiently well integrated and emotionally mature to utilize life's opportunities and accept its accompanying responsibilities.

The ultimate goal of healthy personality development is to become an adult capable of predominantly positive emotional orientation toward others, of initiative, and of responsibility. The final goal is achieved when the individual is capable of accepting the satisfaction and security of another as being of equal importance with his own. He is then capable of mature, adult love. Usually during this period the person asks another to share the journey, as most will give up their sought-after independence to share with another in marriage. Energies at this time begin to shift and are directed beyond one's own personal growth and development. The life cycle continues, but at this point it is as a member of the parental generation. Many adults experience a profound personal reorientation as they become involved in the unfolding of a child's life. This phase ends at a somewhat indefinite time but is usually around the time the adult expects to have attained a stable position in life.

There exists within all of us a strong tendency to achieve mental health. Most persons seek experience that corrects deficiencies in acculturation, sometimes with good results and sometimes with disastrous ones. One rebellious, defiant young student nurse was discovered to have a deep resentment of female authority that grew out of personal experience with her domineering mother. In few vocations could she have come more quickly to grips with her basic problems than in the nursing field, where female authority, truly authoritarian in nature, is all too often the accepted pattern. Unfortunately, the student failed to resolve her conflicts and finally forced her own removal from the school of nursing. Such experiences are not always so unfortunate, especially if positive attitudes exist within the self as resources.

The point to keep in mind is that the personality, conscious and unconscious, is never fixed but always fluid and therefore capable of change. And since the basic orientation is forward and toward health, however devious the present path, no person is ever hopeless.

Middle years. The transition from young adulthood to the middle years involves a state of mind rather than a physiologic change. Although menopause does occur during these middle years, women are usually well into this transitional phase before the "change of life" begins. Often during this period one's children cease to be a major responsibility. Again, it is a time for looking inward and planning for the future. There is a gradual awareness that one's body is slowing down. Not all people reap life's harvest during this phase. For some, there are regrets, disillusionment, and bitter resentment that life has slipped through their fingers. For all, the balance of life is upset by awareness of passing time. Usually a "stock-taking" and reevaluation occur. The problems of ill health are often felt at this time since physical limitations are often imposed on the person. As with the other developmental phases, some individuals pass through middle age with relatively little difficulty. For others it is a crisis situation. A common psychiatric diagnosis is involutional melancholia, which occurs during the involutional period, a time of decrease in bodily vigor. For women this period usually covers the years 40 to 55, for men 50 to 65. It can occur in people who have no previous history of mental illness. The main symptom experienced is depression, at times paranoia. The incidence of this condition is high; it accounts for 5% to 10% of first admissions to mental hospitals.

Old age. Old age is arbitrarily considered to start at about 65 years of age, the time most people retire. Many of the problems of the elderly revolve around how the individual moves into this stage. Is it an unhurried and dignified closure to life or a hollow survival where the person feels useless, unneeded, and burdensome?

An increasing proportion of the population is in the aging group, which has its own crisis problems to face. Since there is decreasing room for such people within the social structure and inadequate institutional facilities to provide the kind of care they need, many wind up in psychiatric facilities where they do not belong. The problems of the elderly are centered in the decreasing physical abilities and the heightened attack upon the self-image and self-respect. This is probably related to the cultural values of society, which place greater importance on youth and achievement.

What causes aging and what aging actually is have not been determined with universally accepted accuracy as yet. Aging, like many other processes, is highly individual. Some persons age faster in one organ or system than others. Problems of reduced achievement and physical ability, retirement, social usefulness, chronic illness, and place in the community confront the elderly. The response of the individual to such challenges will be related to past experience, self-concept, and the preparation for this period of life. Some people enjoy retirement, others are destroyed by it.

As the individual ages there is an increasing dependency on those around him for meeting basic needs. Care often becomes a problem, and it is at this period that family conflicts usually arise. Mentally there is a change toward a more restrictive, conservative, and rigid pattern of living. This is complicated by increasing limitations imposed by the brain cell changes associated with the aging process. The slow loss of cortical cells imposes limitations, but it has a positive influence by protecting the individual against the impact of ultimate death. In a way, this process helps life taper off gently by decreasing ties with important persons.

Elderly persons are known to spend an increasing amount of time thinking and talking about the past. When the future holds little and thoughts about death are painful and frightening, interest will return to earlier years. Gradually the ability to recall recent events becomes more difficult. It is as if a shade were being pulled down on recent happenings until eventually nothing remains except childhood memories. This type of memory failure is the most characteristic feature of senility. If the person lives long enough, he will not only live in the past but will also act as though he were in the past. This is called psychosis, and the person so affected is no longer capable of caring for himself.

Burnside (1976), an outstanding geriatric nurse, notes that in our society there exists a pervasive negative attitude toward the aged. This attitude is often evident among professionals, including nurses and psychiatrists. She refers to Freud and his pessimistic views that people over 50 lack the ability to enter into and use psychotherapy. This has long influenced the care of the elderly in general and psychiatric hospitals.

She cites numerous studies that demonstrate the paucity, if not the absence, of gerontology as a component in nursing curricula. If nurses are to meet their professional responsibilities in maintaining health and preventing illness for the elderly in our society, then programs preparing nurses must include content and experiences that will develop empathy, sensitivity, and understanding of the elderly in health and illness. (A discussion of the aging process can be found in Chapter 14.)

Death and dying. Death is part of man's life cycle. It is the inevitable outcome of life, and our awareness of death influences life profoundly. We in the medical profession have an intimate relationship with death.

Death has different meanings to a person at different periods of life. A child usually becomes aware of death at about age 4 or 5, but he usually relates death to concerns of separation anxiety, with fear of the mother's death. A person's attitude toward death usually changes as he grows older. Death becomes familiar to the aging person as he spends time thinking about it, has some degree of expectation, and eventually deals with it.

An integral part of nursing is to face the dying patient and to offer assistance and support to him and the family. Often an attempt is made to shield the person, to protect him from the truth. It has been suggested that it is the medical professional who needs protecting from this unpleasant and difficult situation.

The care of the dying patient is an important subject. Too often our responses are pathologic in nature. Often efforts to protect the dying person from this knowledge have been unfortunate and sometimes disastrous. A wall of deception separates the person from his family. This is the time that communication and nearness are vitally important. In essence the patient is often denied the right to "set his house in order." Many dying patients have felt that the effort of deception has almost succeeded in depriving them of awareness of this experience. More unfortunately, the insistent denial of the extent of the person's illness leads to confusion, profound distrust, and personality disorganization. The patient is often not permitted to verbalize what he senses is happening. It is a pity that so many people die utterly alone.

Elisabeth Kübler-Ross (1969) has postulated five stages in the process of dying that offer keen insight into their experience. First is the stage of denial and isolation. The patient's initial response to awareness of terminal illness is "No, not me, it can't be true." At times patients go through elaborate stories to support that process of denial. Many patients shop around for a better diagnosis and reassurance. Denial, at least partial denial, is used by most patients to deal with illness. It functions as a buffer after the shocking news. It allows patients time to collect themselves and to develop less radical defenses. Most patients do not utilize denial exclusively, as they briefly talk about the reality of their situation and then indicate their inability to look further.

The second stage is anger. When denial can be no longer maintained, it is replaced by feelings of anger, rage, envy, and resentment. The next logical question is, "Why me? Why couldn't it have been him?" This stage is more difficult to cope with. The anger is displaced in all directions and projected into the environment: "Doctors are no good; they don't know what they're doing." Nurses are even more the target of anger. The moment they leave the room, the call lights go on. When they straighten the bed, they are accused of not leaving the patient alone. The patient may feel anger because of the feeling of the injustice of illness and death. Anger is expressed toward those who are not in the patient's position. A patient who is respected and understood, who is given attention and a little time, will soon lower his voice and reduce the angry demands. The tragedy is that too often nurses do not think out and try to understand the reason for his anger. Too easily nurses become personally offended, and anger is the response returned. This attitude is often demonstrated by curt visits, abrupt care, and short tempers.

The third stage is the stage of bargaining. When denial and anger do not work, the patient tends to think of entering into an agreement that will postpone the inevitable. He believes there is a slim chance of being rewarded for good behavior. There is an implicit promise that the patient will ask for no more. But this promise is never kept. Most bargains are made with God and are usually kept secret. The nurse should not brush these remarks aside, for they have their basis in guilt.

The fourth stage is characterized by depression. When the severity of the illness increases so that denial is no longer possible and physical stress is imminent, the patient is no longer able to smile it off. The numbness, anger, and rage are replaced with the sense of loss. This feeling of loss can be associated with the loss of the actual part or of a body function. This is just one of a series of losses to come. Realistic pressures and burdens increase the feeling of depression. Also, it must be remembered that this state is often a preparatory state for grief. The terminally ill person has to prepare himself for his separation from the world. The initial reaction, to cheer the person up, is useless, and it does not acknowledge the person's state. Statements of this type are often an expression of the needs of health professionals, an inability to tolerate the situation.

In the fifth stage, acceptance, if the person has been helped to work through the previous stages, he is neither depressed nor angry about his state. Many terminally ill patients will contemplate their coming death with a degree of quiet expectation. Often there is more need for sleep and dozing. Acceptance should not be confused with a happy stage. It is a stage almost void of feelings. It is as if all the pain has gone. The struggle is over. At this time the family usually needs more support and understanding than the patient himself. When the person finds some inner peace, his circle of interests diminishes. He often wishes to be left alone, not stirred by the problems of the world. Visitors are not desired, and usually the patient is not talkative. Communication becomes more nonverbal than verbal. The moments of silence together are often the most meaningful communication. It is comforting for a patient to feel he is not forgotten when nothing else can be done for him.

Erikson's eight stages of man. In the process of reaching psychosocial maturity, as pointed out by Erikson (1963), every person goes through certain developmental stages, each featuring a developmental task that must be successfully completed if the succeeding tasks are to be resolved in turn. Although any given developmental task may be successfully completed at its appropriate stage, it is never completed for all time, since regression may occur or stress may arouse again an interplay between the positive and the negative outcomes inherent in the task.

Erikson has identified eight stages of psychologic development of man associated with the stages of physical growth. They are as follows:

1. Basic trust vs. basic mistrust (oral-sensory)
2. Autonomy vs. shame and doubt (muscular-anal)
3. Initiative vs. guilt (locomotor-genital)
4. Industry vs. inferiority (latency)
5. Identity vs. role confusion (puberty and adolescence)
6. Intimacy vs. isolation (young adulthood)
7. Generativity vs. stagnation (adulthood)
8. Ego integrity vs. despair (maturity)

During the period of infancy one of the major tasks confronting the new individual is the development of trust—trust in one self, in the environment and the people in it, and in the meaningfulness of existence. Such a sense of trust is derived through the close and intimate association with parent or parent-surrogate. A continuous and consistent warm and supportive relationship results in a basic and essential sense of trust. The sense of trust rests on a feeling of inner goodness, which is an outgrowth of the relationship. A parent-infant relationship that is inconsistent, cold, or rejecting or that provides little or sporadic support provides experience that builds mistrust into the basic personality of the infant. The relationship is most sensitive at the period when the child experiences a sense of loss as he discriminates himself from his environment and recognizes his parents as separate entities. The inability to trust the self and the environment can cripple personality development and deprive the growing individual of those interpersonal relationships and experiences that are essential to growth and self-realization. In psychopathology the absence of basic trust can best be demonstrated in infantile schizophrenia. In the adult, weakness in basic trust is seen in persons who withdraw into schizoid and depressed states. Reestablishment of basic trust is the key in many forms of psychotherapy.

The second developmental stage occurs in early childhood, and the developmental task at this age is the establishment of a sense of autonomy. Muscular maturation sets this stage for two simultaneous sets of social modalities—holding on and letting go. These basic conflicts can lead in the end to either hostile or benign expectations and attitudes. Thus to hold on can become destructive and cruel by retaining and restraining; it can become a pattern of response "to have and to hold." On the other hand, to let go can be the letting go of destructive forces, or it can become relaxed, to let pass or to be.

The development of the second stage is a result of the need to establish a differentiation between the self and its own will and the pressures of outside influences. It begins with the period of I, we, and no and is a period of concern with self and with resistance to outside pressures. The favorable outcome of this stage is a development of a sense of autonomy on the part of the growing child. The negative outcome is a sense of doubt and shame, usually the result of a consistent loss in the battle of no's with people who are bigger and stronger. This stage becomes decisive in the ratio of love and hate, cooperation and willfulness, and the freedom of self-expression or its suppression.

The third developmental stage is the play age, and the developmental task is the establishment of initiative. The freedom to explore and to reach security in taking the initiative in action comes as the child moves out of the home and family and into his immediate community. The curiosity, the exploration, and the accompanying fantasies can also lead to feelings of guilt with its resulting anxiety. If the guilt rather than the curiosity, exploration, and initiative in action is reinforced, the negative outcome of guilt may result. The growing personality may develop a sense of badness, with restrictions in initiative in later stages of development. This is also the period of the development of conscience. Residual adult conflicts over initiative are expressed as either hysterical denial, including inhibition or impotence, or an overcompensatory showing off. Psychosomatic disease response is also common.

The next developmental stage is the school age. The growing personality confronts the task of developing the trait of industry, which is essential for the capacity to enjoy work. In this stage the world expands again, and the skills and tools in working in and relating to the world are developed. The child learns to work with others and to produce things both individually and with others. It is important for the growing personality that the initiative in action developed in the preceding stage amounts to something—that which results reflects competence and worth. The danger in this period is the development of a sense of inferiority and mediocrity, usually a result of lack of recognition for efforts.

The fifth developmental stage occurs in puberty and adolescence, and the developmental task is the achievement of a sense of identity. Rapid physical development and the advent of sexual maturity precipitate the crisis of concentration or diffusion—the sense of one's own identity or diffusion of identity that results from attempting to be too many things to too many persons.

The emotional integration taking place is more than the sum of one's childhood experiences. It is the accrued experience of the ego's ability to integrate all life's identification. Ego identity, then, is the accrued confidence that one's past is matched by one's meaning for others. Role confusion is the danger of this stage. Doubt as to one's sexual identity can lead to delinquent behavior or to psychotic episodes. The difficulty in choosing an occupational identity disturbs most adolescents. To "keep themselves together," they temporarily overidentify to the point of total loss of their identity, as can be evidenced by hero worship and clique behavior.

The sixth developmental stage is young adulthood. The developmental task is the ability to establish intimate relationships with others. The negative alternate choice is isolation. Having established a sense of his own identity and some degree of harmony within himself, the young adult becomes capable of investing some of himself in others. This means the establishment of friendships and eventually a satisfying and satisfactory marriage. If close relationships with others threaten a weak sense of self-identity, isolation ensues and restricts individual ability to achieve self-realization.

The seventh developmental stage is adulthood, in which the developmental task is generativity and the negative resolution is self-absorption. Generativity is reflected in the individual's establishment and guidance of the next generation. Self-absorption is again a restricted factor in self-realization and results in a sense of stagnation.

The last developmental stage, and the last adult crisis, comes in the late middle or late years of life in which man sums up his personal balance. The result is either a sense of integrity or of despair and disgust. Integrity is achieved when the individual accepts responsibility for what his life has been and finds it has both internal and external worth. This state of mind can be further explained by an experience that conveys some world order and spiritual sense. It is a deep understanding of how one's life is an aspect or segment of history. To become a mature adult, each individual must attain a degree of ego integrity. Each cultural group develops its own particular style of that integrity.

Piaget's developmental stages. Jean Piaget is one of the outstanding child psychologists in the world today. His discoveries of children's philosophies, the construction of reality by the infant, and the stages of mental development have altered our ways of thinking about the intellectual development of the child (Elkind, 1968).

Originally Piaget explored the extent and the depth of children's ideas about the world itself and about their mental processes. He discovered that children differed from adults in their ways of reasoning and their world views. As an example, he found that young children believed anything that moves is alive, that the names of objects reside in the objects themselves, and that dreams come through the window at night. Children also were found to believe that everything has a purpose and that everything in the world is made by and for man. This is why children ask questions such as "Why is the grass green?" and "Why do the stars shine?" The young child's behavior can be explained by his inability to put himself in another person's position or to take another person's point of view.

Later, Piaget investigated the origin of the child's spontaneous mental growth. He found that when young children lost sight of an object, the object not only disappeared but also went entirely out of existence. Thus a 5-month-old infant experiences this feeling when a toy rolls out of sight.

For the past 35 years, Piaget and his colleagues have amassed an outstanding amount of information about the thinking of children and adolescents. His investigations focused on how children acquire the adult versions of the concepts of number, quantity, and speed. He sought to distinguish how the child copes with change and how he distinguishes between permanence and transience and between appearance and reality.

Through the years of research, Piaget has elaborated a general theory of intellectual development. He proposes that intelligence, adaptive thinking, and action develop in stages. Each stage determines the mental abilities, which set the limits and determine the character of what can be learned during that period.

The stages here are offered in brief outline form. The first stage of development (up to 2 years) is called the sensory-motor period and is concerned with the evolution of the abilities needed to construct and reconstruct objects. The second stage (2 to 7 years), the preoperational stage, is concerned with symbolic function. This develops with the acquisition of language and the first indications of dreams. At the end of this stage the child should be able to distinguish between words and symbols. The third stage (8 to 11 years) is called concrete operations. Now the child can do "in his head" things that before he could not do. In the last stage (12 to 15 years), formal operations, adolescents can think about their thoughts, construct ideals, and reason realistically about the future.

REFERENCES

Baker, F.: From community mental health to human service ideology, Am. J. Pub. Health **64:** 576-582, 1974.

Bentz, W. K., and Edgarton, J. W.: The consequences of labelling a person as mentally ill, Soc. Psychol. 6:29-33, 1971.

Bronfenbrenner, U.: Two worlds of childhood, New York, 1970, Russell Sage Foundation, pp. 1-14.

Brown, F. G.: Social linkability, Am. J. Nurs. 71:516-520, 1971.

Burnside, I. M., editor: Nursing and the aged, New York, 1976, McGraw-Hill Book Co., pp. 1-21.

Butler, R. N., and Lewis, M. I.: Aging and mental health; positive psychosocial approaches, St. Louis, 1973, The C. V. Mosby Co.

Caplan, G.: Principles of preventive psychiatry, New York, 1964, Basic Books Inc.

Carstairs, G. M.: Mental health; what is it? World Health, May, 1973, pp. 4-9.

Cattell, R. B.: The nature and measurement of anxiety, Sci. Am. **208:**96-104, 1963.

Dumas, R.: This I believe . . . about nursing and the poor, Nurs. Outlook 19:47-50, 1969.

Elkind, D.: Giant in the nursery—Jean Piaget, New York Times Magazine, May 26, 1968.

Erikson, E. H.: Childhood in society, New York, 1963, W. W. Norton & Co., pp. 247-273.

Erikson, E. H.: Identity: youth and crisis, New York, 1968, W. W. Norton & Co.

Freud, S.: General introduction to psychoanalyses, Garden City, N.Y., 1949, Garden City Publishing Co.

Hollingshead, A. B., and Redich, F. C.: Social class and mental illness, New York, 1958, John Wiley & Sons, Inc.

Jung, C. G.: Patterns of behavior and archetypes. In Lindzey, G., and Hall, C., editors: Theories and personality, New York, 1965, John Wiley & Sons, Inc., pp. 59-93.

Kübler-Ross, E.: On death and dying, New York, 1969, The Macmillan Co.

Kübler-Ross, E.: Questions and answers on death and dying, New York, 1974, The Macmillan Co.

Lambo, T. A.: Innovation, not imitation, World Health, May, 1973, pp. 10-15.

Leininger, M.: Witchcraft practices and psychocultural therapy with urban U.S. families, Human Organizations, Spring, 1973, pp. 73-83.

Lemert, E. M.: Legal commitment and social control, Sociol. Soc. Res. 30:370, 1946.

Lemert, E. M.: Social pathology: a systematic approach to the theory of sociopathic behavior, New York, 1951, McGraw-Hill Book Co.

Lidz, T.: The person: his development throughout the life cycle, New York, 1968, Basic Books, Inc.

May, R.: Love and will, New York, 1969, W. W. Norton & Co.

Osborne, O. H.: Anthropological issues in mental health nursing. In Leininger, M., editor: Contemporary issues in mental health nursing, Boston, 1973, Little, Brown & Co., pp. 39-61.

Peck, H. B.: Psychiatric approaches to the impoverished and underprivileged. In Arieti, S., editor: American handbook of psychiatry, vol. II, New York, 1974, Basic Books, Inc., pp. 524-534.

Reuck, A. V. S., and Porter, R.: Transcultural psychiatry, Boston, 1965, Little, Brown & Co.

Scheff, T. J.: Social conditions for rationality: how urban and rural courts deal with the mentally ill, Am. Behav. Sci. 7:21, 1964.

Scheff, T. J.: Being mentally ill, Chicago, 1967, Aldine-Atherton, Inc.

Scheff, T. J., editor: Mental illness and social processes, New York, 1967, Harper & Row, Publishers.

Selye, H.: The stress of life, Nurs. Forum 4:28-38, 1965.

Selye, H.: The stress syndrome, Am. J. Nurs. 65:97-99, 1965.

Sullivan, H. S.: Conception of modern psychiatry, Washington, D.C., 1947, William Alanson White Psychiatric Foundation, pp. 1-147.

Wittkower, E. D., and Prince, R.: A review of transcultural psychiatry. In Arieti, S., editor: American handbook of psychiatry, vol. II, New York, 1974, Basic Books, Inc., pp. 535-550.

ADDITIONAL READINGS

American Nurses' Association: Standards; psychiatric-mental health nursing practice, 1973, The Association.

Bowlby, J.: Attachment and loss, vol. I: Attachment, New York, 1969, Basic Books, Inc.

Bowlby J.: Attachment and loss, vol. II: Separation; anxiety and anger, New York, 1973, Basic Books, Inc.

Buhler, C.: Values in psychotherapy, New York, 1962, The Free Press of Glencoe.

Coles, R.: Children of crisis, Boston, 1964, Little, Brown & Co.

Davies, K.: The migrations of human populations, Sci. Am. 231:93-105, 1974.

DeVos, G.: Cross-cultural studies of mental disorder; an anthropological perspective. In Arieti, S., editor: American handbook of psychiatry, vol. II, New York, 1974, Basic Books, Inc., pp. 551-571.

Janzen, S. A.: Psychiatric day care in a rural area, Am. J. Nurs. 74:1632-1635, 1974.

Jones, M.: Beyond the therapeutic community, New Haven, 1968, Yale University Press.

Leighton, A. H.: Social disintegration and mental disorder. In Arieti, S., editor: American handbook of psychiatry, vol. II, New York, 1974, Basic Books, Inc., pp. 411-424.

Madden, B. P.: Raising the consciousness of nursing students, Nurs. Outlook 23:292-296, 1975.

Patterson, E. M.: Social system psychotherapy, Am. J. Psychopathol. 17:396-409, 1973.

Stokes, G., and others: The roles of psychiatric nurses in community health practice: a giant step, Brooklyn, N.Y., 1969, Faculty Press, Inc.

CHAPTER 3
Patterns of behavior

From the previous discussion of personality development, it becomes apparent that numerous opportunities exist for the individual to acquire handicaps that will interfere with his ability to adjust to life. Organic lack or destruction, traumatic experience, or the acquisition of unhealthy attitudes can lead to a behavior pattern that can seriously hamper the attainment of satisfactions or security in a manner acceptable to the person or to the society in which that person lives. When this occurs, the degree of personality impairment is a measure of the state of mental health.

For practical purposes, mental health may be defined as the abilities to develop a realistic and accepting self-knowledge, to feel genuine concern for others, to be more inner-directed than outer-directed, to meet the needs of self without hurting others in the process, and to tolerate stress and frustrations. Such abilities are determined by the individual's perception of himself in relation to others and depend on original endowment and past experience. The degree of any person's mental health fluctuates from day to day and from situation to situation, yet mental health tends to have a certain continuity and consistency.

A meaningful concept of mental health is important. A psychiatrically "normal" person is one who is in relative harmony with himself and his environment. He usually is free from symptoms, is unhampered by mental conflict, and is able to maintain a satisfactory relationship with others. There is a general feeling of well-being, but this does not imply the person is always happy. He can deal with the discomforts, disappointments, and sorrows of life and has a capacity for buoyant return. In effect, he has the competence to deal with the environment. The person achieves more than mediocrity; he achieves satisfactions beyond those required for his most basic needs. To attain these characteristics, one must have developed a degree of ego strength. These characteristics enable an individual to deal with stress, thus making it possible for him to deal effectively with a variety of environmental situations. The emotionally healthy person thinks well of himself, has self-esteem. In turn he can think well of, trust, respect, and admire others.

RANGE OF BEHAVIOR

There is a wide range of degrees of mental health shading so subtly into each other that hard and fast lines to distinguish its presence or absence are nearly impossible. In addition, the final judgment as to the existence of mental illness itself is cultural in nature, and certain types of maladjustment are more socially acceptable than others. Types of behavior that are bizarre or strange or that violate cultural standards with strong emotional impact are usually labeled as symptoms of mental illness. Society feels impelled to take action in regard to such conduct. Other types of behavior indicating a lack of mental health may be ignored or accepted. For example, a person who is withdrawn and avoids relationships with others may well be regarded as a little strange but is seldom recognized as being as sick as he is. On the other hand, a person who violates sexual standards flagrantly, perhaps by exposing himself in public, calls for prompt attention. The latter is quickly categorized as mentally ill; the former has to prove it.

The violation of social customs, especially in sensitive areas, draws a punitive reaction from society. The Joint Commission on Mental Illness and Mental Health pointed out the significance of this fact for the mentally ill patient and for the quality of the care he receives. The mentally ill patient does not appeal to the sympathy of the public as does the physically ill patient. Instead, the types of symptoms presented by the mentally ill result in behavior that causes public rejection.

The origin of behavior deviations lies in the motivations that are acquired through experience. Behavior is seldom frankly psychotic as an objective phenomenon; it is behavior as seen in the total situation, its appropriateness and its effectiveness in contributing to security, that is important. A man thoroughly frightened and racing wildly down the street screaming for help is not in the least maladjusted if there happens to be a man-eating tiger at his heels; quite the reverse is true if the flight were precipitated by some vague feeling of anxiety that had no obvious objective stimulus.

Anxiety, that intense sense of personal discomfort, is a profound motivator of behavior. It occurs when an individual's self-esteem is threatened either from the outside or from the inside. The situations that cause anxiety are usually the result of past experience. Some of us are made anxious by love, some by hate, and some by indifference. The method of resolving the conflict produced and reducing the anxiety is largely that of previously learned behavior patterns. The elements of newness or uniqueness in any situation may bring about a change in the behavior pattern. The greater the sense of individual security, however, the more likely this change in behavior will occur.

The behavior of maladjusted persons does not differ in kind from that of so-called normal persons; it differs only in degree. Everyone projects at some time. Some persons project more often than others, and mentally ill patients may project more extensively and use projection as a major technique in adaptation. The rather shy person who seems mentally healthy, generally speaking, but who refuses an invitation because important persons will be present is using the same broad pattern of behavior shown by the patient in a state hospital who sits alone in one position, head down, never speaking, and apparently unaware of his surroundings. This similarity between so-called normal behavior and abnormal behavior may be one of the factors that helps explain, to some degree, the rejection of mentally ill persons.

Rejection of identified mental patients or rejection of people whose behavior is different is a common practice. Many experience abnormal behavior as a threat to their own sense of stability. They might fear their own loss of control. Human behavior potential encompasses an entire range of responses. As Sullivan stated in *The Interpersonal Theory of Psychiatry*, "Everyone is much more simply human than otherwise." All human behavioral responses fit on a sliding scale. At one end the responses are thought to be those of a normal person. On the opposite end the responses are thought to be those of a mentally ill or psychotic person. Human beings usually slide up and down that imaginary scale, depending on their current ability to maintain mastery over internal and external stress. Therefore, there is a similarity between behavior that is considered normal and that which is considered abnormal; it is the degree of behavior that separates normal from abnormal within the norms of a culture or society.

For the sake of convenience, we group behavior into broad patterns that have certain major characteristics in common. However, no two individuals behave *exactly* alike, and no two persons, sick or well, ever duplicate each other. This is a reasonable assumption due to the profound possibilities for variations and differences in the organic endowment and the past experiences of people. No situation is exactly the same for any two people, since the interaction between environment and organism is highly significant; no two people bring the same selective perception to any given situation. With this infinite variety it becomes apparent that behavior interpretation is no easy matter. We cannot easily judge the meaning of an experience for another because we always see it in terms of our own experience. Recognition of this fact is the first step in learning to observe behavior intelligently.

The deviations from the normal range of behavior that indicate sufficient disorganization of the self to render it ineffective in maintaining security in a socially acceptable manner are called mental illnesses. There is beginning to be some disagreement about the use of the term "mental illness." As mentioned previously, the words mental illness imply a physical or biologic orientation. This has been supported by the medical profession as the medical model of psychiatry. To date, however, no other term in common usage conveys a similar meaning to most people. Mental illness is a term used to categorize and describe psychiatrically diagnosed syndromes of personality maladjustment. The term "mental illness" implies that the individual is lacking in mental health. For further differentiation mental illness is split into two major diagnostic categories—neurosis and psychosis. A fine line between the two is indistinct. (It must be noted, however, that there is strong controversy over psychiatric diagnosis itself. The presented classification is offered to assist the student in attaining this more traditional information. It is not the only diagnostic approach.)

As used today, the terms "neurosis" and "psychoneurosis" are interchangeable. Clinically and diagnostically, psychoneurosis is referred to as certain specific disorders including conversion hysteria, hypochondriasis, obsessive-compulsive disorders, perversions, neurasthenia, and anxiety reactions (see Appendix A, p. 414). However, the words "neurosis" and "neurotic" have become household terms. They are used to describe behavior characterized as inappropriate, inadequate, maladaptive, and sometimes infantile. As a result the neurotic person subjectively and objectively exhibits a discrepancy between psychologic potential and actual performance. Analytically, neurosis refers to "core conflicts" around which symptoms are built. Neurosis is considered a *minor* psychiatric disorder. It is true that neurosis is less crippling and less catastrophic than the more lasting psychotic disintegration, but neurotics suffer, and they impose misery on others. Although there is no loss of reality, reality becomes painful and miserable. The familiar is sought, and change is avoided, even though that change would offer relief.

Freud described the neurotic process as having roots in childhood and early developmental conflicts between child and parents. Later Horney (1936) observed that neuroses needed to be considered in the context of modern society and the competitive nature of our culture. The demands of competition and the goal to succeed are often driving and threatening to the individual in his ability to gain a sense of security. The pressures of competition are frequently fraught with hostility and unhappiness.

Psychosis is considered a *major* mental illness. Simply stated, it refers to any severe mental disorder in which functioning in reality is disturbed. Traditionally psychotic disorders are subdivided into two categories, organic brain syndromes and functional psychoses. Functional psychoses, those without known organic basis, include the specific conditions of schizophrenia, affective psychosis, paranoid states, and psychotic depressive reactions. Use of the term "psychosis" has also undergone popularization to include its adjective form, "psychotic." In this usage psychotic indicates the severity of the mental illness. Thus a person with the psychosis schizophrenia may be labeled psychotic only when the symptoms are intense or interfere with mental competency.

The disorders labeled psychosis differ from other groups of psychiatric disorders because of one or more of the following five criteria. First, psychoses are major disorders that are more severe, intense, and disruptive than other psychiatric disorders. They tend to affect all aspects of the person's life. Second, psychoses are associated with withdrawal behavior. The psychotic patient is less able to maintain effective relationships. External objective reality has less meaning for the patient, and reality is often perceived in a distorted way. Third, affectivity of responses is disrupted. The person's emotions are often qualitatively different from the norm, and at other times emotions are so exaggerated quantitatively that they constitute the whole existence for the patient. Fourth, intellectual functioning may be directly disturbed by the psychotic process; language and thinking are disturbed; judgment often fails; and hallucinations and delusions may appear. Fifth, regression is likely to occur. There may be a generalized failure of functioning and a return to earlier levels of behavior. Regression is more than a temporary lapse in maturity and may include a return to primitive patterns of behavior.

The following presents a brief description of behavior patterns that occur. (For more details see subsequent chapters that deal with particular disorders.) It is important to keep in mind that insecurity may dominate the feeling tones of many persons, but the particular situation that arouses insecurity and the method of handling the subsequent anxiety will differ from person to person; the method or pattern will be an expression of the personality.

WITHDRAWAL

One method of handling the problems of interpersonal relationships is by withdrawal, the purpose of which is protection. By withdrawing and avoiding relationships, an individual attempts to avoid further damage to his security. The danger of such a pattern is that it inevitably produces loneliness, thus a vicious cycle often develops. Compensations may be developed, but the pattern of avoidance carries over into the compensatory adjustment and thus effectively limits its usefulness. Regression may occur, and the ultimately unsuccessful outcome may be a retreat to infantile levels. In such a stage, thinking once again becomes autistic, that is, highly personal in meaning and not validated or checked by experience or reality.

Withdrawal is manifested in many degrees and may even be quite spotty in its appearance within the personality. Persons may avoid only types of situations in which security has been previously undermined and yet maintain a positive approach to the rest of their experiences. For example, a student may do extremely well in every subject except history, which he cannot learn. His first history teacher may have been a sarcastic person who constantly belittled him, a fact he may not remember at all or may recall with difficulty. He does not associate this occurrence with his inability to master the particular subject. In the process of first studying history, his security was undermined. So, despite what appears to be outward efforts to conform, the unconscious block he set up operates to keep him from grasping the fundamentals that would make history easy for him. He avoids coming to grips with it and simply laughs, explaining that the subject is too much for him. Most of us have exactly such blind spots.

Withdrawal has many degrees of expression. It may occur only as a temporary or seldom used pattern through various phases to the withdrawn psychotic patient, who seems completely indifferent to his environment. Patients never completely lose all contact with reality or all relationships with others, however inadequate these relationships may be. Withdrawal may be expressed through avoidance of contact with others on every possible occasion or through frequent contact with many different people with all relationships kept on a superficial level. It may be expressed through quick, violent friendships that come to an early and abrupt end. The cynical rejection of people as worthless may also be an expression of withdrawal.

When withdrawal begins to dominate the pattern of behavior, loneliness ensues. The organization of the self is directed toward rejection, and self-rejection is reflected in rejection of others. The cycle set in motion is hard to break. The potentialities for complete regression are always present, and a crisis in living may precipitate it. The ultimate outcome depends on the positive attitudes integrated into the self, on the balance of positive attitudes and powerful motivations in the unconscious and dissociated self, and on further experience.

AGGRESSION

Aggression is another method of handling the problems of interpersonal relationships. Aggression is angry, hateful, or destructive ideas or behavior. It is a frequent pattern for those whose self-perception and hence perception of others are predominantly hostile. The expression of aggression, either open or symbolic, is common to all of us, since hostility is a universal experience. When it dominates the personality and the direction of its development, difficulties inevitably ensue. Open aggression may discharge energy, but it calls forth retaliation that is a threat to security. Again the problem becomes one of a vicious cycle.

The extent and form of expression of aggression may vary markedly. The sarcastic remark, the unfavorable comments relayed "for your own good," the memory lapse concerning names and appointments, and the constant ridicule of others may all be expressions of hostility.

Hostility may be expressed frankly and openly toward certain persons, and the hostile individual makes sure that they are aware of the dislike he feels. It may also be expressed as a general contempt for people and for their aspirations, their ambitions, and their opinions. The individual who always concentrates on the weakness of other persons in his perception of them is expressing his hostility toward people in general and himself in particular. This is often seen in the "I love you dearly, *but*—" pattern in which the discussion of the "but" is elaborated with a treatise of one's faults. The "I love you dearly" that prefaces the approach is a screening attempt to prevent retaliation and expresses some fear of reprisal. Hostility is frequently disguised because the person who feels and indirectly expresses it often does suffer from the fear of retribution.

One of the more subtle forms of hostility results from reaction formation or the development of the exact opposite trait as a compensatory protective device. This is the person who is exclusively thoughtful and courteous. Interestingly enough, such people usually make one thoroughly uncomfortable and with good reason, because such is their exact unconscious intention. Another serious outcome is that a strongly hostile perception of existence may arouse so much fear and anxiety within the self that the hostile perception is turned on the self lest it find outward expression. Such an inward direction for deep hostility underlies genuine suicidal attempts. Harshly punitive experiences in situations that arouse deep hostility may induce such a pattern. Aggression may also be displaced onto the environment, and an individual may be quite destructive with material objects, consciously or unconsciously. This is usually accompanied, however, by a subtle expression of hostility in interpersonal relations.

The pattern of hostility may relate only to certain types of situations. A staff nurse may get along quite well with students, auxiliary workers, and other staff nurses but make life difficult for those in authority. The pattern of hostility may even be limited to female authority. This is related to previous experiences of circumscribed occurrence that have undermined security and called forth hostility as a response. If sufficient positive attitudes are part of the self, corrective experiences are likely to be fruitful for personality growth. On the other hand, consistently unfortunate experiences in other areas may lead to a spread of the pattern of hostile perceptions.

The most serious manifestation of this pattern is mental illness in which impulsive, uncontrolled, aggressive behavior explodes and is usually accompanied by a speeding up of the entire activity of the personality. Verbal and physical aggression are open and frank, interrupted often by a raucous humor, which is an indication of the enjoyment of such expression. Even in this syndrome, however, the fear of retribution is indicated by flashes of depression or self-punishment, probably in an attempt to avoid punishment from others.

Depression. A serious manifestation of the aggressive drive turned inward is depression. These two syndromes, aggression and depression, are likely to occur in combination or with depression following aggression. The ultimate expression of the aggressive drive turned on the self is suicide. Depression is a destructive process. The self punishes itself, and the total person, body and mind, suffers. The emotion of guilt is present. In depression there is a lowering of mood, sometimes described as painful dejection. It is associated with sadness, gloominess, despair, and despondency. There is difficulty in thinking, and psychomotor retardation is present. In general, this retardation or slowness often masks anxiety and agitation. The person fears retaliation for these aggressive drives. The person feels he has gone too far; therefore the aggression is turned inward to avoid the consequences and to pay retribution for his "sins."

Depressions are at times reactive in nature. They are precipitated by external stress resulting from a loss. The loss has specific meaning to that person; hence different losses to different people can precipitate a depression. They range from loss of a significant person, through death or absence; to loss of material possessions, such as money or property; to loss of status, by being fired or through scandal. Depression can also be representative of a more severe mental illness. Some depressions are considered psychotic, since they include gross misinterpretation of reality. Severe depressions are at times internally based, spontaneously occurring without external stress.

The state of depression is generally considered pathologic in nature, but grief and mourning are the normal responses to loss, and initially depression may appear. The differentiation, however, lies mainly in that the feelings and responses in deep depression are disproportionate and prolonged.

PROJECTION

The third pattern of handling the problem of attaining security in interpersonal relationships is projection. As has been pointed out before, this is a common mechanism and one that is used frequently by all of us. The protection function here is obvious. The sense of security is protected by attributing one's own personal faults or failures to others. Listen to the postmortems over a heated disagreement. In ninety cases out of a hundred the other fellow is wrong. We seldom fail on our own merits but because someone else makes it impossible for us to succeed. This list of traits that arouse a sharply disagreeable reaction in us is usually a list of our own traits of which we are almost always unaware.

Projection is perhaps more easily identifiable than the two previously discussed behavior patterns, withdrawal and aggression. It is a little harder to disguise on close acquaintance. An example of projection is excusing failures through blaming the interference of others. A more serious form of projection develops as a result of certain compensatory conceits to help rebuild the shattered sense of security. These conceits are manifested through an inflated sense of one's own importance and are expressed by referring all environmental happenings as being significant to the self. The pen left carelessly by the secretary on the left side of the desk instead of its usual place on the right has meaning. The secretary is saying, "I'll do as I please; you can't boss me" or "Your character is changing." This process can continue in development until the environmental forces appear to combine into an organized conspiracy against the patient; "The FBI is out to get me." Here we see both the basic self-perception, a negative and hostile self-organization, and the compensatory reaction it produced, an inflated self-conception not founded on reality but on a self important enough to be of concern to the Federal Bureau of Investigation.

Clinically this false belief is referred to as a delusion. The belief exists without appropriate external stimulation. It is usually maintained in spite of reality and in spite of "plain-as-day" proof. Delusions are condensations of perceptions, thoughts, and memories. They are misjudgments of reality based on the mechanism of projection. In delusions of a persecutory nature, for example, the delusion is a projection of the patient's "bad" conscience. The imagined persecutors are not only threatening and punishing the patient but also are often perceived as tempters who lead the patient to sin.

The use of projection rests on a fundamentally derogatory self-estimate, combined with a tendency to seek security insistently. The personality carries within itself the seed of its own defeat, since it selectively perceives and integrates those parts of experience that are consistent with the self-organization. The derogatory or critical attitude toward the self is expressed in a superior manner. The critical attitude toward self is also expressed in constantly critical attitudes toward others, often in so-called normal behavior. The individual whose central characteristic is criticism is always present. The ultimate disorganization is found in the state hospital patient with elaborate ideas about being a very important person who is persecuted and held prisoner in the hospital by the combined forces of the army, navy, marines, and the air force.

Hallucinations are sensory perceptions in which there are no external stimuli. They are frequently auditory in nature, but they also include the visual, tactile, olfactory, and gustatory senses. Hallucinations are often motivated by the need to reduce anxiety, and they may help the patient to adjust to a reality that appears frightening. Hallucinations appear to reflect internal conflict. They not only warn, scold, and defend the patient but also direct him to act. Hallucinations offer chastising remarks or give approval. Most patients respond to the hallucinations in episodes, with a shift from outside events to inside ones.

Hallucinations are often noted in nonpsychiatric patients. They can be a consequence of neural or chemical conditions. The alcoholic in delirium tremens is well known for visual hallucinatory activity. Elevated body temperature, fatigue, isolation, and other toxic conditions, as well as intense desire or fear, provide conditions in which sensory discrimination is impaired.

USE OF PHYSICAL DISABILITY

Another devious method of attempting to attain security is by concentration on the physical aspects of existence with the development of certain physical defects or ailments. Here a double purpose is usually accomplished. The individual develops physical infirmities that force him to avoid anxiety-producing situations; this also reduces the demands likely to be made on him by society. In addition, he secures a certain amount of sympathy because of the physical illness itself. It is also a weapon with which to demand the attention of others. If one physician finally reaches a limit with the patient when he can find no organic cause for the presenting complaint, there are always others. Such a pattern of behavior is evasive in nature. Its selection as a means of resolving conflicts and protecting the self is usually related closely to early experience. If physical aches and pains were the only method of gaining any sign of affection from parents, that is the pattern likely to be followed in any crisis thereafter. If experience outside the home has confirmed the parents' original evaluation of the child as important only when sick, the pattern becomes fixed. If the stress a developing personality undergoes is severe, the more likely the pattern is to be used. A severe and prolonged physical illness early in life may also serve to focus attention on the workings of the body and may result in a tendency to react to severe stress with the development of some ailment. The process of accruing advantages from an illness is referred to as secondary gain. This form of attention-seeking is a means of gratification of dependency needs. It can be found in both physical and mental illness.

"Psychophysiologic" or "psychosomatic" are terms often used to label conditions manifesting physical symptoms with a basis in emotional disturbances. We find this type of behavior in a wide range of expressions from normal to abnormal. Strong emotions have a physical accompaniment. Anxiety is both a physical and an emotional phenomenon. A headache before an examination is easy to explain, as is a feeling of nausea at some unpleasant experience. In addition most of us, at some time or another and sometimes more often than others, use physical complaints as a means of evasion. Once in a while it is pure malingering, consciously and with malice aforethought, as when we avoid a dinner we do not want to attend with the excuse of a nonexistent headache. This simulated illness or injury reaches various extremes. It may occur in criminal cases or in compensation cases, or it may be used to dodge hazardous situations, such as military service. There are, however, many times when we use the alibi unconsciously. We *do* have a headache, yet it miraculously disappears when the hour for the party to begin has passed. Quite virtuously, we go elsewhere and have a good time.

A more severe instance is the person with a chronic complaint who has it to rely on when any situation that may carry a threat to security arises. Degrees of such behavior exist all the way from the slightly incapacitated person to the bedridden, paralyzed individual who forces the entire household to organize itself around his needs.

It is an amusing commentary on our culture that one of its major preoccupations in personal life is with the function of the gastrointestinal tract. Nausea and vomiting, diarrhea, constipation, hyperacidity, and hemorrhoids are common occurrences, important topics for conversation, and accepted alibis for almost anything.

Some substitute processes for physical ailments do occur, such as the circumscribed memory loss that we call amnesia. Besides its frequent physical onset, memory loss can be related to psychic trauma, the loss of a loved one as an example. In function and purpose it is similar to the use of physical ailments to evade and excuse.

As can readily be seen, this behavior pattern has coherence only through its method of action and the limited aims it sets for satisfactions. Everything is subordinated to the achievement of a precarious security. Its forms of expression can range through the entire manual of medicine. Unfortunately, however, security is often more strained and can be lost since the behavior needed to maintain this elaborate system often alienates those in the environment. In some instances, prolonged use of physical complaints for psychologic purposes may actually produce somatic illnesses. This usually manages to completely confuse the organic-minded member of the health team.

RITUALISTIC BEHAVIOR

Another method of handling the problems of interpersonal relationships is through rigidly ritualistic behavior designed to retain control over the situation and to keep anxiety at a minimum. This appears most obviously as compulsive acts that *must* be done regardless of how foolish they may seem intellectually to the doer. This repetitive, stereotyped motor action is often performed against the individual's wishes. Because of a profound sense of inferiority, the individual responds to an anxious situation with a compulsive act. This is built into a sort of magic operation that gives him security; that is, it gives him the sense of control over a situation and at least a temporary decrease in tension. Usually, compulsive behavior is extremely difficult for others in the environment, and the patient subtly expresses his self-judgment and contempt toward others.

This compulsive-obsessive type of behavior has many forms of expression. Usually preceding the compulsive act are obsessive ideas; the normal person shows evidences of both. The song that keeps running through the mind until it becomes annoying is an example. An obsession is characterized as an idea, an emotion, or an impulse that repetitively and insistently forces itself into consciousness. A conscious effort to change the preoccupation usually comes to naught the moment attention is distracted, and one finds oneself humming or singing the recurring song again. After the apartment is locked, some persons *must* go back to make sure the last cigarette was put out or the gas turned off, although the trip back proves unnecessary. The toothbrush *must* be hung up to dry, or sleep is elusive. Ash trays *must* be emptied, or anxiety and worry occur. Fundamentally, these are magical operations that dispel a threat by keeping the situation in a certain known sequence, which is a form of control over the environment. One is thereby in control and therefore secure.

Compulsive-obsessive behavior may occur simply as an occasional episode in normal experience or as a constantly recurring episode in relation to one act or one situation. It may progress to a severe and prolonged ritual that actually severely handicaps a person in his adjustment. One of the best examples is the elaborate handwashing ritual of the compulsive patient. Every time his hands touch something, he must wash them. It is believed this represents a cleansing in a symbolic sense, that handwashing controls anxiety aroused by a sense of guilt that exists in the dissociated self or unconscious. Anxiety is controlled by a symbolic act or by magic. The individual who must wash his hands every time they touch something has not enough time left to live his life in a regular fashion.

CLOUDING OF REALITY

Another method of handling personal problems is to blur or cloud reality with some outside influence that either changes the nature of reality or enhances one's sense of the ability to deal with it. Morphine, for example, produces a delightful sense of well-being that can only be matched by the attainment of complete biologic satisfaction with a maximum of social approval. For those whose attainment of security is difficult because of problems in personality development, various types of artificial attainment may well become a prop on which they can lean. Alcohol and various other drugs may offer the same false security. Recovery from their effects enhances the lack of security and leads to a renewal of and dependence on their use; hence a cycle is established and reinforced. This resolution of conflicts seems to be typical of persons whose tolerance for anxiety and frustration is very low.

ABSENCE OF INTEGRATIVE FACTORS

The final method is probably the least understood of all. We can do no more than describe it. This consists of failing to integrate past experience as an indication of the future; the past and future have little significance for the individual. He neither profits from past experience nor takes account of future consequences. Verbally, he is fluent and often superficially charming, but depth and duration of emotion are alien to him. He lives purely for the moment, reaching out to satisfy predominantly biologic satisfactions with little concern for enduring personal security. There is no modification of actions by the person's conscience, since there seems to be little regard for the demands of society. This is demonstrated by behavior that violates the established laws, mores, and customs. The failure to follow rules is thought to be a result of an unsocialized id and not psychosis, mental deficiency, ignorance, or confusion. Many theories exist as to the cause of the antisocial behavior. Most suggest the influence of social, environmental, experiential, and constitutional factors.

DEVIATIONS OF ORGANIC ORIGIN

The techniques of behavior previously discussed are at the present time considered functional in origin, although recent discoveries in biochemistry raise some questions about this. There are no organic or somatic changes that seem to account for their appearance. Other types of maladjustment severe enough to be considered mental illness do originate in damage to the central nervous system, which is the system most influential in the coordination of human behavior into a unitary response. When such damage does occur, specific symptoms usually indicate the area involved. There is also an uncontrolled accentuation of the individual's basic personality. For example, the gray cells are destroyed by syphilitic invasion of the cerebral cortex. The powers of association, fine muscular coordination, the ability to calculate, and the ability to remember accurately depend on cortex cells and are destroyed. In addition to these symptoms, a breakdown in personality may occur; its direction will be determined by the direction of the personality previous to the organic damage. For example, a hostile person will show a disorder characterized by hostility, and a withdrawn person will show a disorder characterized by withdrawal. The end result is always a fusion of organic, intellectual, and emotional components.

• • •

This chapter has shown some of the ways in which behavior can deviate from the accepted social pattern and has given brief indications of the sources of such deviations. Early experience, as has been indicated, is extremely important for the direction and growth of personality and the attainment of mental health. If experience builds a healthy respect for the self, permitting the more powerful motivational systems direct access to consciousness and providing satisfaction without serious threat to security, the chances of mental illness are low. The more powerful the motivational systems that are forced by painful or traumatic experience into the dissociated or unconscious part of the self, the greater will be the danger of acute disruptions of the personality. The degree of mental health is related closely to the individual's awareness of his own motivations as balanced by the depth of stresses to which he is exposed. By this is meant not only intellectual insight but also emotional acceptance of that insight. The motivations recognized must be acceptable to the individual's self-perception. The individual must be able to live comfortably with his weaknesses, and his strengths must be well assessed.

REFERENCES

Bettelheim, B.: Truants from life: the rehabilitation of emotionally disturbed children, New York, 1955, The Free Press.

Cleckley, H.: The mask of sanity, ed. 5, St. Louis, 1976, The C. V. Mosby Co.

Cullen, A. A.: Labeling theory and social deviance, Perspect. Psychiatr. Care 12:3, 1974.

Davidites, R. M.: A social systems approach to deviant behavior, Am. J. Nurs. 71:1588-1589, 1971.

Deutsch, H.: Neuroses and character types, New York, 1965, Universities International Press.

Fagin, C. M.: Nursing in child psychiatry, St. Louis, 1972, The C. V. Mosby Co.

Frazier, S., and Carr, A. C.: Introduction to psychopathology, New York, 1964, The Macmillan Co.

Hinsie, L. E., and Campbell, R. J.: Psychiatric dictionary, ed. 4, New York, 1970, Oxford University Press, pp. 22, 34, 148, 191, 316, 333, 445, 599-601, 619-620.

Horney, K.: Cultural neurosis, Am. Soc. Rev. 1:221-230, 1936.

Peplau, H. E.: Interpersonal relationships and the process of adaptation, Nurs. Sci. 1:272-279, 1963.

Ploy, S. C., and Edgerton, R. B.: Changing perspectives in mental illness, New York, 1969, Holt, Rinehart and Winston, Inc., pp. 1-7.

Roncoli, M.: Bantering: a therapeutic strategy in obsessional patients, Perspect. Psychiatr. Care 12:171-175, 1974.

Rappeport, J. R.: Antisocial behavior. In Arieti, S., editor: American handbook of psychiatry, vol. III, New York, 1974, Basic Books, Inc., pp. 255-269.

Sullivan, H. S.: Conceptions of modern psychiatry, Washington, D.C., 1947, William Alanson White Psychiatric Foundation, pp. 43-86.

Sullivan, H. S.: The interpersonal theory of psychiatry, New York, 1953, W. W. Norton & Co., p. 32.

ADDITIONAL READINGS

Aichorn, A.: Wayward youth, New York, 1955, Viking Press.

Brown, M. I.: Socialization—a social theory of adaptation, Nurs. Sci. **1**:280-294, 1963.

Davitz, L.: Where did you grow up? Am. J. Nurs. **71**:1974-1979, 1971.

Goldfarb, W., Mintz, I., and Stroock, K. W.: A time to heal: corrective socialization, New York, 1969, International Universities Press, Inc.

Leininger, M.: Nursing and anthropology: two worlds to blend, New York, 1970, John Wiley & Sons, Inc.

CHAPTER 4

Theoretical approaches to psychopathology

Psychopathology is the branch of scientific inquiry that deals with the morbidity, or pathology, of the psyche, or mind. Psychopathology is a very complex phenomenon and can be viewed from many angles and approached at different levels. For example, behaviorly, mental disorders are conceived of as a complicated pattern of responses to environmental stress. Phenomenologically, mental disorders are seen as expressions of personal discomfort. From a physiologic point of view these disorders are interpreted as sequences of complex neural and chemical activity; intrapsychically, mental disorders are seen as unconscious processes that defend against anxiety and conflict. These specific approaches to understanding psychopathology lend themselves to a number of specific theories and concepts. Each approach has a legitimate and fruitful contribution to make. They serve to organize experience in a logical manner and to offer explanations by which experiences may be analyzed.

No one theory on psychopathology is accepted by even a nominal majority of professionals in the field. Although there are many books and articles on the subject, numerous contradictions on definition and consequently on indicated therapy exist. Many factors influence thinking on the subject and, as a result, on the conclusions reached. It has been pointed out before that precision tools and tests in the field of psychiatry are not available.

The study of man as a person with the potential for improvement, not as the victim of outside forces that control his destiny, is only a couple of centuries old. Beginning with Freud the study of man has been approached through many avenues. It is important to remember that different approaches start from different assumptions and ask different questions, which often produce different answers. So we have more than one theory on what constitutes psychopathology and correct therapy. These theories may well be more complementary than contradictory.

Factors that influence the definition of psychopathology and therapy are the value system of the definer, the experience of the definer, and the philosophic and political climate of the age. What any given individual will see as pathologic behavior will depend on what he sees as the good life and the ultimate goals of man and what supports or interferes with the achievement of either. If control of basic biologic drives (if there is such a thing) in conformance with socially acceptable expression is seen as the ultimate goal, then behavior will be interpreted in such terms and therapy will be directed accordingly. If self-growth and individual self-direction with expansion into the environment are seen as the ultimate goal, then behavior will be judged in a different light and therapy will be differently directed.

It is interesting to note that psychiatrists, psychologists, and psychiatric nurses are apparently influenced by the types of persons with whom they work. Rogers developed the nondirective approach to personality problems with college students. Freud did most of his work with so-called neurotic patients. Sullivan developed his interpersonal theories in work with young schizophrenics. The contrast between the writings of a psychiatrist in private practice and the writings of a psychiatrist who has worked most of his professional life in a state hospital is obvious.

A 1968 discussion pf psychiatric nursing* produced differences in opinion that were a reflection of the different types of patients with whom the discussion participants worked. No agreement as to what constituted psychiatric nursing could be reached among a psychiatric nurse who worked with young adolescents diagnosed as acute schizophrenics, one who worked with patients in a state hospital setting, a dean who worked with students and faculty, and a director of a nursing service and nursing school who worked primarily with nursing service personnel and student nurses. The nurse who worked with adolescents emphasized the nurse's role in the development of a symbiotic but healthy relationship that becomes, in essence, a weaning phase. The nurse working with the larger group of patients in a community-supported hospital emphasized detachment, neutrality, and intellectual competency. The dean dwelt on the need for ability in family group therapy. The nursing director saw the nurse's role within the framework of the old medical model, with the doctor prescribing treatment and the nurse helping the patient with his reaction to the treatment so as to derive the most from it.

The definition of psychopathology and therapy is also influenced by the climate of the society in which one lives. We are moving toward a state of contradiction that should lead to interesting results. On the one hand, there is a

---

Perspectives in Psychiatric Care, vol. 6, no. 6, 1968.

widespread acceptance of the concept that individuals have the need and the capacity for growth and the acceptance at ever higher levels for rational responsibility for behavior. On the other hand, there are greater pressures for social conformity as interdependence grows in a complex technologic society. At the present moment there appears to be a divided trend toward greater emphasis on individual responsibility and on individual conditioning into socially acceptable forms of behavior.

Millon (1973) has classified the theories of psychopathology into six broad categories—biophysical, intrapsychic, phenomenologic, behaviorial, sociocultural, and integrative. These represent old and new approaches to the field of psychiatry. They come and go in waves as first one and then the other becomes more popular. We are currently in the midst of a period of resistance to the more psychoanalytic and traditional approaches and of a search for more effective therapeutic measures. How long this search will continue is uncertain.

BIOPHYSICAL THEORIES

In biophysical theories of psychopathology, biologic deficiencies are considered to be the cause of behavior disorders. Although there is not yet proof that such cause exists, the search for underlying factors continues, and the growing body of knowledge contains enough evidence to support further research in this area. The deficiency may be in the anatomic structure (as in mental deficiency), physiologic function (as in hysteria), or biochemical (as in drug intoxication). The analogy to physical illness is stressed by this group of theorists, who believe that physical insult to organs or organ systems produces physical symptoms, and insult to the central nervous system produces behavioral and social as well as physical symptoms. As would be logical in such an approach, biophysical methods of therapy are the treatment of choice and are considered to be the ultimate goal in psychotherapy.

Some of the knowledge that tends to support the biophysical theories is evidence that heredity and environment are more closely interwoven than had been suspected. Heredity plays an important role in psychopathology. Genetic factors, however, can be modified substantially by learning and experience. Heredity operates not as a fixed constant but is subject to the circumstances of the individual's upbringing. Psychologic development at the various crisis stages depends on biologic maturation. If the task to be accomplished is not presented at the correct time of maturation, it is never learned. The tendency to consider biologic factors as setting limits to behavior but not explaining its variance has been disturbed by the establishment of the fact that the chance of two siblings in the same family having the same genetic endowment is one in 64 trillion. In addition, the sequential development of genetic patterns allows for a variety of manifestations that may or may not determine behavior. In both physical and mental problems, the idea that single causative factors exist is disputed. Overt disease patterns of any type may not reveal the causative factors, and internal or external environmental forces may play varying roles in causation.

Another bit of evidence is found in the wide range of biochemical differences among so-called normal persons. The normal curve concept accounts for the wide range of difference but does not explain it. When the normal limits of any biochemical response are arbitrarily set by the inclusion of 67% of the population, there is a wide range within the normal and no recognition of what that range might mean to the individual as a total functioning person. For example, the normal range for blood sugar is 80 to 120 mg per 100 ml of blood. A person with a usual blood sugar of 80 mg might be in for more trouble if it rises to 120 mg (still normal) than a person whose usual blood sugar is 120 mg but rises to 125 mg (abnormal). Also, a consideration of the biochemical differences among normal individuals is the number of factors that may influence any response or any aspect of biochemical existence. The wide variation is illustrated by the fact that at least nine gene-controlled substances are involved in the mechanization of blood-clotting, thus allowing room for many factors to influence blood-clotting time. What is true of blood-clotting is true of many other physiologic manifestations, including behavior.

There is also an increasing recognition that physical and mental disorders can result from inborn metabolic errors, although the establishment of undeniable cause-effect relationships is not yet high. However, increasingly sophisticated research methods add to the number. One of the most dramatic discoveries in recent history is that phenylpyruvic oligophrenia (phenylkentonuria, or PKU, one form of feeble-mindedness) results from an inborn error of metabolism, the absence of an enzyme that normally would cause phenylpyruvic acid to be transformed into tyrosine. In the absence of the enzyme, the acid is excreted in the urine. As knowledge increases, more disorders of both physical and mental types are understood in terms of biology. The supporters of biophysical theories of psychopathology expect increasing numbers of behavioral problems to be explained in such terms.

It has been fairly well demonstrated that growth, biologic and otherwise, is individual. As one proceeds at his individual rate, there occur periods at which one is more sensitive to certain kinds of stimuli. Such occurrences are biologic as well as psychologic, and the biologists even suggest that there may be some relationship between the two. Psychologically, there are considered to be special periods in development when certain types of behavior appear. Stimuli are necessary to elicit the behavior. Difficulty in preceding stages of development may interfere with subsequent development.

Parallel to this are the individual differences in biologic maturation, so different metabolic needs for different tissues occur at different times. At certain periods the metabolic processes are sensitive to reactions to which they would not respond at other times. Regardless of whether the psychologic or biologic influence is predominant, both sides agree fundamentally that certain kinds of behavior are ripe for appearance at certain times in development. The failure to learn those behaviors at the appropriate times leads to serious difficulties in later developmental stages. The biologists believe that further understanding of the biologic facts of life will be found in the realm of the biophysical.

The more psychologically oriented theorists attribute a great deal of behavior to early conditioning, while the biologically oriented theorists agree that early experience is important but attribute this to hereditary factors and to the interaction with the environment of these factors. They point out that no two individuals have the same biologic combination and that this fact could account for the variations in behavior. No two people have identical central nervous systems, gastrointestinal systems, cardiac systems, or any other systems. Within the variations of individual systems, there exists the opportunity for limitless combinations that could biologically account for the uniqueness of the person and his behavioral responses. While the importance of early experience is acknowledged by all, biologists emphasize the importance of the genetic equipment that the individual brings to the task of maturation as a determining factor in the ability to accomplish the task.

As would be expected, the biophysical theorists lean toward somatic forms of therapy. So far they have not had a history of successful treatment that stood the test of time and put sound foundations under their theories. While brain surgery, shock therapy, hydrotherapy, and chemotherapy have all had their successes, all such approaches have been based on empirical rather than theoretic grounds. They seem to work, but the reason why they work is uncertain. There can be no question that the use of drugs has markedly reduced the control problem with hospitalized patients and that patients who in the recent past would have been hospitalized are able to remain in the community. There can be no doubt that with the advent of the chemotherapeutic era, the number of patients hospitalized has decreased. However, other factors may be involved, such as change in attitude, the development of clinics and care centers, better education of health personnel, and the movement of treatment closer to medical centers. The only logical thing to be done at the moment is to keep an open mind. The theories may eventually converge.

Prominent exponents of biophysical theories are Emil Kraepelin, Eugen

Bleuler, Roger Williams, Franz Kallman, Bernice and Samuel Eiduson, Edward Geller, William Sheldon, Paul Meehl, Lothar Kalinowsky, and Paul Hoch.

INTRAPSYCHIC THEORIES

In the intrapsychic theory the key to the development of psychopathology can be found in faulty experiences in early life. Every child is born with a variety of drives or instincts that require nourishment and stimulation. When there is conflict or deprivation of these needs, anxiety and insecurity develop. A variety of defensive maneuvers is adopted to handle this stress, ultimately leading to maladaptive behavior. Defenses operate at an unconscious level and continue into adulthood, so that the person, although unaware of it, acts in the present as though he lived in the past. Childhood anxieties and the defenses erected against them are thus considered to be the main causative factors in behavior disorders.

Such thinking has dominated the psychiatric scene for quite a while and has just recently come under severe attack. While not accepting the freudian concepts as originally presented, many psychiatrists and psychologists have been influenced by them. These freudian concepts are the foundation on which all other intrapsychic theories are based. Psychiatrists and psychologists have made intrapsychic conflict within the individual the cornerstone of their theories of psychopathology and consequently the basis of their therapeutic plans and methods. In any therapy resting on such basic concepts, the goal is to uncover and to understand the original circumstances of the conflict and, armed with understanding and acceptance, to become better able to deal with the self and the environment. As would be expected under the circumstances, the intrapsychic group, especially Harry Stack Sullivan, has had a strong influence on psychiatric nursing.

In the process of therapy the intrapsychic school of thought concentrates on the historic development of behavior disorders and uses certain classic methods. The therapist employs a passive and neutral approach, using free association, interpretation of resistances, focus on internal rather than external reality, dream analysis, and frequent contact with the patient. The phenomenon of transference is a central concept in the use of psychoanalytic techniques; the patient transfers past attitudes and feelings to the therapist, strengthens his own ego through the therapist, and eventually becomes able to stand on his own feet and do without the therapist through healthy resolution of the transference.

Outstanding names associated with the intrapsychic school are Erik Erikson, Karen Horney, Erich Fromm, Heinz Hartman, Lewis Wolberg, and Carl J. Jung.

PHENOMENOLOGIC THEORIES

Phenomenologic theories of psychopathology take a different approach to the study of man in difficulty. There is no special interest in the historic development of the difficulties in the early childhood experiences and their influence on adult behavior. Instead, emphasis is placed on the emerging person as the central focus of therapy. Every individual reacts to the world and to reality in terms of the way *he* perceives it, a way that is uniquely his own. No matter how distorted this perception may be, it is the person's way of perceiving events that determines behavior. Reality is, according to phenomenologic theorists, what the individual says he perceives it to be. That consciousness or awareness is central to understanding man or being able to help him is obvious.

Experiencing, as seen from the point of view of the person involved, becomes a central issue in therapy. Such experiencing includes all levels of being, and only such truth as includes experiencing of all levels has the power to induce one to change his behavior. Only the acceptance of conscious decision and responsibility can lead to change. Thus the therapist is less concerned with techniques than with attitudes toward therapy; these attitudes are directed toward understanding of the person involved and of how experience appears to him.

Each individual has his own unique patterns of potentialities (here there is agreement with the biophysical theorists). With respect to potentialities, the basic responsibility for how much will be achieved is the responsibility of the person concerned. The goal of therapy becomes not to understand the development or to remove the symptoms of behavior disorders but to free the patient to become all that he is capable of becoming. This would in no way relieve the patient of responsibility for his own behavior. In addition, the final judgment of the value of therapy would be made by the extent to which the patient could feel that he fulfilled himself and not by the extent to which he conformed to the outer-directed norms of socially acceptable behavior.

The phenomenologic theories are based on the concepts that the individual experiences reality in a unique way and that every individual has inherent potential for growing and increasing the use of personal potential in an ever-expanding interaction with the environment, including the people in it.

The infant's response to reality is positive and negative in terms of whether the infant advances or negates the achievement of self-realization as determined by reality as it appears to him. Like other theories, this one acknowledges the need for positive self-evaluation, though it may disagree somewhat on the method of its achievement. There may develop a discrepancy between self-image and experiences, which is the source of discrepancies in behavior. If behaviors are inconsistent with the self and the self-image, they become threatening. Distortion of experience to protect the self becomes necessary. If the divergence between experience and the perception of experience (self-protection) becomes wide enough, disorganization of the self results with consequent behavior disorders. The process of therapy becomes one of accurate perception of reality that enhances the feeling of self-worth. Therapy is thus the "freeing" of the individual in the direction of greater self-direction based on a feeling of self-worth and achievement of potential.

Adler is attributed with developing the first phenomenologic therapy system. He emphasized the importance of studying how a person sees, thinks, and feels about situations and recognized that goal-directed behavior had significance. Other well-known advocates of phenomenologic theories of psychopathology are Carl Rogers, Abraham Maslow, Rollo May, Ludwig Binswanger, F. J. J. Buytenduk, R. D. Laing, and Albert Ellis.

BEHAVIORAL THEORIES

Behavioral theories of psychopathology rest on the belief that all behavior, normal as well as abnormal, develops in the same manner and can be understood only by the scientific and careful observation of overt behavior. Behaviorism originated with the view that subjective introspection was unscientific. The measurable properties of behavior constitute the data from which all behavior is explicable. Behavior in the sick person differs from so-called normal behavior only in social adaptiveness in extremes of magnitude and frequency and not in kind. While not a wholly new approach to the explanation of normal and abnormal behavior (Wundt and Watson are their predecessors), the behaviorists have more recently founded their approach directly in theories of learning.

One of the most popular of the present disciples is B. F. Skinner. Operant conditioning methods based on his theories are being more widely used. Such theories reject introspection, hypothetical inner states, and the unconscious as constructive grounds for assisting persons with behavior disorders; Skinner's theories insist on the adequacy of stimulus and response reinforcement as being effective theoretic backgrounds for treatment. Behavior develops according to laws of learning theory, and the same laws apply to adaptive as well as maladaptive behavior. The kind of behavior developed is determined by the reinforcement pattern to which the person is exposed.

Therapy with the behaviorist is not concerned with removing the underlying cause of behavior as it is with psychoanalytically oriented therapists. Instead, the relevant data are considered to be the patient's behavior, and the goals of therapy are the elimination of maladaptive behavior by nonreinforcement and the encouragement of the development of new behavior through reinforcement of adaptive responses. The patient has learned his behavior; he therefore can unlearn the old behavior and learn new. In other words, work directly with the symptom (behavior), and the underlying condition (supposed) will no longer exist.

Although conditioning is explicitly used, such as the term "operant conditioning" describing the therapeutic approach, it is not to be confused with the classic conditioning concerned with reflexes that are usually autonomic in nature. The behaviorists are concerned with the total performance of the individual in which social agencies or social control are major factors in behavior, and they therefore deal with matters much more complex than the classic concept of pavlovian conditioning.

Since behavior is ultimately determined by peer response, the use of peer group response to behavior is the major technique used in therapy by the behaviorists. Reinforcement of desirable behavior and nonreinforcement of undesirable behavior are consciously used. The progressive differentiation of complex behavior is supported by reinforcing the more simple elements involved and by proceeding by small steps toward the more complex desired behavior. Intermittent reinforcement is employed since normal social response is characterized by it, behavior is learned that way, and the performance must be sustained under intermittent reinforcement. Reinforcement is based primarily on approval, reward, or the removal of disapproval or pain. Nonreinforcement rests on ignoring, punishing, or removing the stimulus that produces the behavior. Such a therapeutic approach is being more widely used with the mentally ill and the mentally retarded. Many ethical and moral questions have been raised and debated concerning the use of these treatment methods.

Some of the better known names in the field of behavioral theories are B. F. Skinner, John Dollard, Neal Miller, Albert Bandura, Richard Walthers, Joseph Wolpe, H. J. Eysenck, and C. B. Ferster.

SOCIOCULTURAL THEORIES

In this approach society and culture—the environment—are seen as the factors that cause the individual to react with disturbed behavior. In other words, the cause originates outside the self and the decision that mental illness is present is directly related to what is considered normal and acceptable within that society. The focus of sociocultural therapy is holistic and brings to bear the nature of the person's problems as he perceives them with reference to home and family, ethnic and socioeconomic factors, as well as psychobiologic components. This is a public health model of approach as compared to the traditional clinical or medical model.

Hospital therapy has been influenced by this approach in that patients are encouraged to assume an active role in their treatment regime and in the social functioning of the unit through patient government. Where the staffs incorporate this focus, rehabilitation is a prime concern in order to avoid the tendency toward chronic institutionalization.

In community mental health there is demonstrated concern and strengthening of programs in the prevention of mental illness. This movement gained considerable impetus in the 1960s and 1970s. Governmental agencies provided support funds for the development of comprehensive community mental health centers. There are increasing members of agencies and programs to assist people in trouble as soon as possible. These include suicide prevention, crisis intervention, walk-in clinics, and storefront clinics. It becomes obvious that these groups recognize that community factors contribute to the individual's problems. The attempt is to provide assistance from that vantage point—the understanding of community factors that cause behavior disturbances.

Some well-known advocates of this approach are Alexander H. Leighton, Erving Goffman, Maxwell Jones, Thomas J. Scheff, Erich Lindemann, Melvin Sobshin, Ernest M. Greenberg, and Howard S. Becker.

INTEGRATIVE THEORIES

The integrative theories of psychopathology suggest that psychologic processes are multidetermined and multidimensional. The theories that focus their attention on only one line of data are criticized. At the turn of the century Adolf Meyer spoke out for the principle of man's intrinsic biologic and psychologic unity.

Some of the better known names associated with this approach include Theodore Millon, Paul E. Mechl, and Roy R. Crinker, Sr.

OTHER THEORETIC APPROACHES AND TREATMENT

There are many new and developing ideas and trends in the conception of psychopathology and in its modes of intervention and treatment. The following theoretic approaches and treatment modalities offer the reader a brief survey of the diverse movement in the field.

Szasz (1960) created considerable controversy by the publication of his views some time ago in *The Myth of Mental Illness*. He raises the question "Is there such a thing as mental illness?" Szasz argues that there is not and believes that the notion of mental illness has outlived whatever usefulness it might have had. He suggests our adversaries are not demons, witches, fate, or mental illness. We cannot "cure" these. What we do have are problems in living, which may be of biologic, economic, political, or sociopsychologic origin. His argument suggests that mental illness is a myth whose function is to disguise the bitter pill of moral conflicts in human relations.

The reality therapy of William Glasser (1965) is based on the premise that people in all cultures possess a need for identity throughout their lives. No person thinks, looks, acts, and talks exactly like another. Reality therapy differs from psychoanalysis and operant conditioning in that it is applied to the problems of irresponsibility, incompetence, and daily living.

Like Szasz, Glasser says mental illness does not exist. All persons have two basic psychologic needs, the needs to love and be loved and to feel worthwhile to the self and others. The ability to meet such needs varies widely. To meet these needs without trampling on the needs of others is the ultimate goal of existence. To do so there must be involvement with others, and there must be a state of being in touch with reality. Those who are having problems with living share in common the loss of touch with reality. The goals of therapy include helping the patient face reality and meeting his unfulfilled needs within its framework. To do so the therapist must become involved with the patient, since involvement with others is essential for the patient. The therapist must reject unrealistic behavior while accepting the patient and remaining involved with him. The therapist also needs to teach the patient better ways to meet his needs within the framework of reality.

At times, mental illness or the schizophrenic experience has been regarded as a positive and creative experience. In 1959 Karl Menninger stated, "Some patients have mental illness, and then get well and then they get weller! I mean they get better than they ever were" (Silverman, 1970). There is mounting evidence that some of the most profound schizophrenic disorganization is a prelude to impressive personal growth, not so much a breakdown as a breakthrough. Boisen (in Silverman, 1970) considered schizophrenic reactions as follows:

> . . . not in themselves evils but problem solving experience. They are attempts at reorganization in which the entire personality, to its bottom-most depths, is aroused and its forces marshaled to meet the danger of personal failure and isolation. . . . The acute disturbances tend either to make or break. They may send the patient to the back wards, there to remain a hopeless wreck, or they may send him back to the community in better shape than he had been for years.

Jay Haley (1969) looks at the process somewhat differently. He believes that diagnostic procedure has become slipshod and lackadaisical in identifying schizophrenia. At one time it was relatively clear that a person was either schizophrenic or was not. Today we find that the label of schizophrenic can be applied to anyone. An adolescent temper tantrum can earn that diagnosis. He also takes an interesting, somewhat satirical look at its etiology. In the *The Power Tactics of Jesus Christ*, he postulates the possibility of the process of working at being "crazy." It is suggested that people who attempt schizophrenia without the correct family background have miserably failed. They can erupt into psychotic-like behavior in difficult situations but are unable to sustain that behavior when the environmental stimuli decreases. In summary Haley states:

> The schizophrenic must have come from the right sort of family, with appropriate parents as models. He must have learned to manipulate and balance complicated, conflicting family triangles, and he must be perceptive enough to keep his feet in a morass of trickery and despair. . . . As a consequence he must become skilled in concealing his emotions, he must learn to indicate that whatever he did just happened and he is not responsible for it. . . . It should be immediately evident that few people can meet the complicated requirements of the world of the average schizophrenic. There is one final requirement which eliminates most contenders. . . . He has to devote his life to an absolute and stubborn crusade. His crusade is this: Never to let his family off the hook. The hundred million affronts he has suffered are never to be forgiven to the end of his days.*

Haley sees the traditional hospital setting as fostering the situation. He suggests:

> Only in the mental hospital can schizophrenia achieve its full flowering. Just as a plant reaches its greatest growth in well manured ground, so does the schizophrenic achieve his full range on the closed wards of mental institutions. . . . Only when he has been incarcerated for a period of time does he recognize the merit of the establishment. Then he is almost impossible to remove. Nowhere in the world can he find an environment so similar to life at home and yet with opponents so much less skilled than the members of his family.*

John Rosen founded direct analysis, another method of psychotherapy for psychopathology. It was originally developed for psychotic individuals and focuses on the recreation of that person's early maternal environment. Unlike conventional analysis, the therapist accepts the parental role as a foster parent. He becomes a loving, omnipotent protector and provider for the patient. He must become the idealized parent. The interaction between the patient and therapist is complicated as the role of good parent is deliberately assumed. The goal is for the patient to gradually move toward maturity and grow up again psychologically.

The origins of family therapy are attributable to the child guidance clinics popular in the 1920s and 1930s, when the mother was included in the analysis and treatment of the child's problem. Later, as children were hospitalized in

---

*From The power tactics of Jesus Christ by Jay Haley, pp. 129-130. Copyright © 1969 by Jay Haley. Reprinted by permission of Grossman Publishers.

children's wards, involvement of parents and families became more prominent in the exploration of the child's problem. These led to the basic tenet of family therapy: that the mental problem or disturbance of one member of a family could be a sign of problems within the total family group. Several therapists who were involved in the one-to-one relationship with clients observed that events occurring within a family could precipitate a relapse for the treated member or, in some instances, improvement of the client caused symptoms to develop in other members of the family. Ackerman (1958) described this mechanism as emotional contagion.

Further consideration of the needs of clients in family therapy led to the realization of the complexities involved. The systems theory, as the theoretical framework, is often used. Jackson (1968) used the word "conjoint" to describe the therapy sessions, which included various members of the same family. The nuclear family consists of the primary members of the family group living to-gether. The extended family includes significant persons related to the nuclear family—grandparents, cousins, uncles, aunts, and so on. Fleck (1966) recog-nized that the abnormalities of family functions were difficult to define. Con-sequently, the knowledge and methodology of dealing with family disturbances require skill and a holistic approach. Smoyak (1975) states, "Operationalizing family dynamics allows the nurse to generate family therapy and to develop operational strategies. These theories and strategies need testing for cross-cultural relevance." Family therapy involves responsibility for the individuals and the sum of the family group. Psychiatric nursing knowledge and skills are a foundation for the additional competencies that need to be developed for family therapy. The relationships of individuals and families to nurses has al-ways been natural and one of ease. The role of family therapist is a reaffirmation of the nurse's potential in helping a family group.

Psychoanalytically oriented group therapy is another important treatment modality to outline. It is psychoanalysis in groups. The goal of treatment is the alleviation and cure of mental illness through the interaction of patients in groups. The therapist is seen as an interested, rational, but permissive author-ity figure with whom the patient feels free to reenact his distorted and irrational behavior. Once out in the open, the behavior can be analyzed, and behavior patterns can thereby be changed.

Eric Berne has introduced transactional analysis. It is a system of therapy based on personality theory utilizing three ego states called Parent, Adult, and Child. In this method there is an attempt to diagnose which ego state gives rise to the stimulus and which ego state controls the response. This process takes place through game analysis. Game analysis exposes the unconscious life plan or script, which forms the basis of ongoing patterns of behavior. Berne sees games as people's methods of relating or transacting with each other. A game is an ongoing series of complementary transactions of an ulterior nature. Games progress to a well-defined, predictable outcome. The main concern focuses on unconscious games, which are plagued by negative effects and play havock with interpersonal relations.

Thomas A. Harris has developed the book *I'm OK—You're OK* out of basic transactional analysis. He suggests that there are four life positions underlying people's behavior. First, and most important, is the "I'm not OK—you're OK" construct. It is suggested that most people still unconsciously operate from this construct; it is characterized by the anxious dependency of the insecure. Second, "I'm not OK—you're not OK" represents the giving up and despair position. Third, "I'm OK—you're not OK" is seen as the criminal position. Fourth, "I'm OK—you're OK" is the mature response of the adult who is at peace with himself and others. Harris sees psychosis as a condition in which a person has blocked out the Adult ego state. When the Adult is not functioning, the person is out of touch with reality. The Parent and Child becomes frequently a jumbled mixture of past data. Treatments consist of developing "I'm OK—you're OK" encounters, so that the Adult can begin processing data, listening, learning, and helping in decisions. Thus the healing process begins.

R. D. Laing is a psychiatrist and a psychotherapist. Recently, his theories and work have been looked at in detail, since they offer different insights into the cause and treatment of mental illness. Laing first made his reputation by writing about his experiences treating schizophrenic patients. He was able to extract fertile insights from the psychotic state of mind and made madness comprehensible. Madness became comprehensible in view of the family matrix that sent the patient mad and in view of the system of psychiatry that kept him there. Laing believes that psychiatry can be a technique of brainwashing, inducing behavior that is "normal" and "adjusted." Are the bars placed inside the patient in a more subtle way than the chains and lobotomies of the past and the tranquilizers of the present? Does this "normal" state deny us ecstasy and betray our true potentialities for a false self? Gradually his theories evolved to the study of the nonpathologic fundamental situation of the human experience. Laing provides us with a stunning demonstration of what it really means to understand patients as human beings rather than just detecting the signs and symptoms of mental illness. One of the characteristic themes to arise from his work is the extended analysis of the family of the identified patient. At this point Laing is skeptical about the very existence of schizophrenia. If anything, he believes so-called schizophrenia is really a communication disorder of the whole family.

Laing's role seems to be evolving into that of a culture critic. In his most recent writings, he combines the examination of severe mental disorders with a general assault on the foundations of Western civilization. Thus, his following consists of not only medical doctors but also philosophers, sociologists, literary people, religionists, and practically any group interested in the history of ideas and the dimensions of contemporary cultures.

IMPLICATIONS FOR THE NURSE

The implications of theories of psychopathology for the psychiatric nurse or the nurse in psychiatry are confusing, to say the least. No one method of therapeutic approach is comprehensive and total. Each exerts selective and differential effects on different components of human disturbance. Each approach or method should not be set in competition with the other; this is naive and unsound. One must begin to recognize that these different theoretic approaches are characterized by specific strengths and weaknesses. How nurses function will be influenced by their basic beliefs about the origin of psychopathology and about the methods used in restoring mental health. There is obvious disagreement concerning these concepts. There is, in fact, disagreement as to whether mental illness and mental health are acceptable concepts in themselves. In any case, it becomes important for nurses to know the theory subscribed to by the institution in which they are employed. It might also be a deciding factor in seeking employment. No one could be expected to be especially happy in a setting where the basic philosophy of therapy was in conflict with the personal value system of the employee.

The ability of nurses to function as therapeutic agents with mentally ill persons is directly related to their nursing preparation and their own initiative in continuing to add to their knowledge and skills. In most basic programs preparing for R.N. licensure the psychiatric–mental health component prepares nurses with beginning competencies and understanding of the factors contributing to the person's disturbance. It is intended that this background also lend itself to the needs of persons in the general hospital who experience emotional responses to illness and other traumatic situations. Nurses must learn to be supportive to the patient and to participate with the other members of the psychiatric team to serve the needs of the patient or client.

More than 25 years ago Peplau (1952) stated, "What each nurse becomes—as a functioning personality—determines the manner in which she will perform in each interpersonal contact in every nursing situation."

In baccalaureate nursing preparation, the beginning competencies may be expanded to include a greater emphasis on the family unit as a component in the person's care plan. The nurse's ability to integrate concepts and principles gained from related disciplines such as anthropology, sociology, psysiology, and psychology to the practice of nursing is directly related to the curriculum design of the particular program.

Community health nurses are often confronted with the emotional pressures and problems within the family setting that need immediate attention. This type of case-finding is an important part of primary prevention. The nurse's role in helping to maintain people who have had a previous mental illness within the community is becoming a more common involvement.

With additional formal preparation on the master's and doctoral degree levels, nurses move into roles and positions for which they assume more independent functioning and responsibility. These include family therapist, group therapist, clinical specialist, psychiatric nursing instructor, and researcher. The leadership role of psychiatric nurses is often determined by the needs of a particular situation or agency and their ability to identify these needs and to work out mechanisms and strategies to meet them.

As early as the 1950s the independent functions and responsibilities of professional nurses were clearly indicated by Peplau (1952) as the domain of nursing. "The nursing profession has legal responsibility for the effective use of nursing and for its consequences to patients. Nursing is a function. It is one of the many functions of a professional health team."

NONSPECIFIC THERAPEUTIC APPROACHES

The therapeutic approaches discussed in the previous sections represent theoretic bases on which intensive individual or group psychotherapy are practiced. Even today many hospitalized psychiatric patients do not receive such psychotherapy but exist in settings where certain practices are considered to be generally therapeutic, regardless of the patient's particular problem, age, sex, or any other factor that would be taken into consideration in individual therapy. Such broad therapeutic assumptions influence hospital setting, organization, and function.

One of the basic therapeutic assumptions is that activity at least prevents regression and at best helps promote recovery. In the latter, activity provides both reality contact and an opportunity to practice or to develop social skills. This concept accounts for the numerous activity programs found in most psychiatric hospitals. It has led to the utilization of a number of departments or programs—occupational therapy, recreational therapy, social therapy (such as dances and movies), work details, art therapy, and workshops, for example. The pervasive influence of the idea that activity is of therapeutic value is easy to recognize in most institutional psychiatric settings.

Somewhat harder to recognize in most large institutional mental hospitals, but easily recognizable in new psychiatric hospitals, is the therapeutic assumption that the physical environment contributes to patient therapy. Cheerful surroundings approximating social settings outside the hospital are at present considered desirable. Many efforts at improving the physical appearance of patient care units have been accompanied by improved patient behavior. Whether this results from improved patient morale or improved staff morale remains a moot point. In either case, it is a generally accepted belief that the physical environment is a therapeutic instrument.

Another generally accepted assumption, although one not always acted on, is that nonrestraint is therapeutic. History would appear to support this thesis. When Dr. Philippe Pinel of France struck the chains from patients, patient behavior improved. The spreading open-door policy in psychiatric hospitals is a resurgence of an old idea. New variations in treatment go somewhat beyond nonrestraint and include giving the patient more responsibility for his behavior, as in patient government.

Aspects of the basic helping relationship can be constructively assumed by all personnel who come in contact with patients. This concept, too, is not a new one, but it is being revived with greater emphasis. Physicians spend more time working with and through other team members, and physicians and nurses spend more time working with attendants or aides, helping them toward greater understanding of the patients for whom they provide care. Nursing education is trying to prepare its practitioners at all levels and in all areas for more effective use of the helping relationship.

An assumption that is only beginning to receive real attention is that the working relationship among the personnel who care for patients is also a therapeutic tool. It has been conclusively demonstrated that covert conflict among personnel leads to regressed behavior on the part of patients. It has not been as clearly demonstrated that cooperative working relationships are a therapeutic tool.

That the social structure, and especially the implicit social goals, of the setting in which a patient finds himself is a therapeutic tool is another basic assumption. If the personnel group goal is centered on patient control, the patient suffers. If the personnel group goal is focused on patient recovery or improvement, patient behavior improves.

Patient interaction with other people—staff, other patients, or visitors—contributes to recovery possibilities. This assumption underlies the many efforts in and outside the patient care unit to provide the opportunity for and to encourage patient interaction with others. One of the major responsibilities of the nurse in the psychiatric hospital is to promote patient socialization.

Through all of the nonspecific therapeutic approaches, current trends are emphasizing active patient participation and increased patient responsibility for himself. Another current trend of significance is an increased understanding of the impact of expectations on patient behavior and, consequently, conscious efforts to improve personnel expectations of patient behavior.

REFERENCES

Ackerman, N. W.: Psychodynamics of family life, New York, 1958, Basic Books, Inc., p. 101.

Beavers, S. V.: Music therapy, Am. J. Nurs. 69:89-92, 1969.

Berni, R., Dressler, J., and Baxter, J. C.: Reinforcing behavior, Am. J. Nurs. 71:2180-2183, 1971.

Burch, J. W., and Meredith, J. L.: Nurses as the core of a psychiatric team, Am. J. Nurs. 74:2037-2038, 1974.

Cacciatore, E. W.: Conjoint therapy as an adjunct to individual therapy, J. Psych. Nurs. 11:19-24, 1973.

Fleck, S.: An approach to family pathology, Comp. Psychiatr. 7(5):307-320, 1966.

Ford, D. H., and Urban, H. B.: Systems of psychotherapy, New York, 1965, John Wiley & Sons, Inc.

Glasser, W.: Reality therapy, New York, 1965, Harper & Row, Publishers.

Grace, M. J.: The psychiatric nurse specialist and medical-surgical patients, Am. J. Nurs. 74:481-483, 1974.

Haley, J.: The power tactics of Jesus Christ, New York, 1969, Grossman Publishers, pp. 119-146.

Harris, T. A.: I'm OK—you're OK, New York, 1969, Grossman Publishers, pp. 104-111.

Jackson, D. D.: Therapy, communication and change, vol. 2, Palo Alto, Calif., 1968, Science and Behavior Books, pp. 222-248.

Jones, M.: Beyond the therapeutic community, New Haven, Conn., 1968, Yale University Press.

Kolb, L. C.: Modern clinical psychiatry, ed. 8, Philadelphia, 1973, W. B. Saunders Co., pp. 87-122.

Laing, R. D.: The divided self, Baltimore, 1965, Penguin Books, Inc.

Laing, R. D.: The politics of experience, New York, 1967, Ballantine Books, Inc.

Larkin, M., and Crowdes, N. E.: A systems approach to private practice, J. Psych. Nurs. 13:5-9, 1975.

Millon, T., editor: Theories of psychopathology and personality, Philadelphia, 1973, W. B. Saunders Co.

Peplau, H. E.: Interpersonal relations in nursing, New York, 1952, G. P. Putman's Sons, pp. ix-xviii.

Schaefer, H. H., and Martin, P. L.: Behavioral therapy, ed. 2, New York, 1975, McGraw-Hill Book Co.

Silverman, J.: When schizophrenia helps, Psychology Today, Sept., 1970, pp. 63-66.

Smoyak, S., editor: The psychiatric nurse as a family therapist, New York, 1975, John Wiley & Sons, Inc.

Szasz, T.: The myth of mental illness, Am. Psychol. 15:113-118, 1960.

Wise, T. W.: Developing psychiatric consultation unit in a community hospital, Maryland Med. J. 24:41-43, 1975.

ADDITIONAL READINGS

Armacost, B., Turner, E., Marten, M., and Hott, E.: A group of "problem" patients, Am. J. Nurs. 74:289-892, 1974.

Berne, E.: Games people play, New York, 1964, Grove Press, Inc., pp. 13-20.

Bourgeois, T. L.: Reinforcement theory in teaching the mentally retarded, Perspect. Psychiatr. Care 6:116-126, 1968.

Nelson, P.: Involvement with Betty: an experience in reality therapy, Am. J. Nurs. 74:1440-1441, 1974.

PRINCIPLES OF NURSING

CHAPTER 5

A perspective for understanding

The interactions of personal lives, the nature and ways of a people, the character of a nation, the interrelationships of a world are all touched and shaped by behavior perceived and the understanding communicated. How any one person will behave toward another will depend on his interpretation of the second person's behavior. Although we acknowledge commonalities among individuals, we would be remiss if we did not recognize the concomitant differences. Different cultural values and customs are elements that influence one's behavior as well as one's interpretation of behavior. The United States has long been a melting pot of peoples from foreign lands. Today we are witnesses to cultural changes and to revolutions of groups in rapid transition. The process of understanding is more than a scholarly inquiry into the concepts and determinants of a culture. It is a living, breathing, evolving process. Leininger (1973) points out:

> Biology and heredity provide the physical limits within which man will function. But his culture determines how he will function. A culture is an organized system of behavior that provides the content for human interactional development. Through a continuing socialization process man learns how he is expected to act, what language he is to speak, what gestures he is to use, what norms he is to obey, what values he is to hold, and what attitudes he is to express. . . . Culture defines situations.

It is a difficult process to gain acceptance and develop a working relationship with a cultural group that has different values, but it is an important task to accomplish. For nurses it is a necessary and meaningful challenge. The qualities of sincere interest, compassion, patience, respect, and acceptance of each other's differences are prerequisites to success. If one accepts the holistic ap-

105

proach to nursing, attention to the cultural makeup of patients is important; for the mentally ill, it is imperative.

To offer health care to individuals of other cultures does not suggest that nurses must change that culture. More than ever, the health professions have become knowledgeable and have accepted the fact that the curative practices of the Chinese, the American Indian, and other cultural groups have much to offer modern medicine. Attitudes, behavior, and practices that are different from the "American way" must not be rejected outright; one must inquire, study, and analyze these differences in keeping with the cultural values and customs of particular groups or individuals. Among U.S. citizens there are many subgroups of different social, ethnic, and religious backgrounds. Are they not the components of the American culture?

The experiential background of nurses influences their self-concept in relation to other people. For example, when young nurses meet their first mentally ill patient, a patient who is complaining bitterly about the persecutions he is undergoing, they react personally. They will, in all probability, experience some fear, uncertainty, discomfort, and curiosity or fascination; they are also apt to retreat from the situation. These are typical attitudes toward mental illness, attitudes that are fortunately undergoing change. If they were nurses in a culture in which mental illness was considered evidence of divinity, their reaction would probably be one of awe and reverence. On the other hand, if they were experienced and competent psychiatric nurses, they would probably identify the patient's symptom, understand its expression, and move to meet the need expressed. In each of these instances the nurse's response would vary because of the differences in interpretation of the patient's behavior. In other words, what the nurse believes to be the reason for the patient's behavior is an important factor in the response made to it.

The nurse's behavior is one of the most important therapeutic tools. In order to maximize the nurse's effectiveness, careful and candid examination of one's feelings, attitudes, and aspirations is important. This process of introspection and assessment is not an easy task. The sincere effort and hoped-for success in analyzing and understanding one's feelings and motives are interwoven with the ability to cope with the feelings and behavior of others. As nurses see their own areas of strengths and weaknesses and accept these for what they are, they gain an understanding of others and their right to be human, also. With the emotionally disturbed person nurses will look for the reason for his anger, criticism, resentment, or need for warmth and closeness before they react to the behavior. They must differentiate between patient responses displaced from events in their past and patient responses aroused because of behavior of the moment. Only then will they be free to see the patient as he really is, to understand and tolerate his behavior, and to work constructively with him in a therapeutic relationship.

In a therapeutic relationship nurses assume responsibility for the conscious direction of their own behavior. Nurses are expected to continually examine and reexamine their behavior. They are expected to seek guidance and clarification in analyzing that behavior to evaluate its effect on the patient and to become aware of their own personal response to these interpersonal situations. Perhaps for nurses it is more important because of the cumulative effects of the minute-by-minute, hour-by-hour, and day-by-day demands that they face. The nurse should not be afraid to ask, "What is it that makes me feel inferior, inadequate, unworthy, or unsure of myself?" They should consider honestly how these feelings interfere with their work. Then, it is possible to effect a change in response. Knowing one's emotional needs is a most challenging, yet personally rewarding, experience.

In the care of patients with emotional problems, it is extremely important for nurses to keep seeking the why behind the patient's behavior without projecting their own reaction to the patient. The important why is the one seen from the patient's point of view, rather than from the nurse's. It is a why that must necessarily be sought objectively and with understanding of the cultural as well as the psychologic factors involved. Nurses must constantly assess their own attitudes and actions in order to avoid imposing their own values on others. The ability to meet the emotional needs of a patient with a personality disorder depends largely on the ability to understand why he behaves as he does and what he is trying to accomplish, without clouding the conclusion with one's own feelings or values. The goals in nursing care are defined through an analysis of the patient's behavior as an expression of his needs. The eternal "why" must be applied again and again until the pattern of a patient's behavior spells out the kind of corrective experience he needs to help him achieve mental health.

Interpersonal relationships with patients are a definite therapeutic tool and have a real effect on the course of a patient's illness. They can be as efficacious as morphine in the treatment of pain, or they can be sand and salt rubbed on open wounds. Nurses' behavior toward a patient must be directed by an intelligent understanding of why he behaves as he does and what purposes his behavior may accomplish. Nurses must therefore develop skill in objectively identifying the why of patient behavior.

Nurses are often told to use themselves—that is, their personality—in relating therapeutically to their patients. Empathy, the ability to feel the feelings of others, is an important tool with which to make meaningful contacts with patients. Empathy is an understanding of the other person as if one were that other person. In one's own fantasy it is possible to imagine what someone else is feeling at a particular moment. When a person empathizes, there is a momentary abandonment of self and a reliving in oneself the emotions and responses of another person. Empathy is often confused with sympathy. Sympathy, however, contains the elements of condolence and pity and suggests a parallel feeling between the person and self. Because with sympathy the feeling between the person and self is so close, there is a loss of objectivity, hence an inaccurate understanding of the other person.

Nurses are usually in the position of having frequent opportunities to observe and interact with their patients. Through these many contacts and with careful listening, nurses can offer individual responses without losing part of their own identity. Empathic understanding serves to increase knowledge of the patient's difficulties as well as to enable the nurse to offer feedback to the patient. Through this process the patient may receive clues as to how he is being perceived by others. Thus there are countless opportunities to give the patient a feeling of being understood. It is through this process of being understood that the patient becomes freer to realize some of his potential, and from that to develop his abilities and strengths.

A common error is the acceptance of superficial reasons for behavior that really tell us little about another person. A patient refuses to cooperate "because he is mean." Granted—but *why* is he mean? Does he need to hurt others, and if so, why? Does he see all other persons as a threat to himself and need to strike first, and if so, why? Is he bitter and cynical, expecting little from others and willing to give less, and if so, why? How deeply and how objectively we reach for that all-important *why* will govern, to some extent, how we will define the patient's needs and how we will treat him as a person. If we accept him as mean, then we may go no further. Unfortunately, many patients experience rejection because their outward behavior is negative. If we reject the rejecting person, how will he be reached, how will trust in interpersonal relationships be established? We may try to reach him as one who has been deeply hurt; we may realize the necessity of avoiding further hurt and of offering him a relationship that is safe and secure; and at the same time we may realize that by the very depth of his hurt he will need this relationship for a long time in order to trust it. The delayed development of a sense of trust is a difficult area to correct. Either approach, rejection or establishment of trust, will have a very definite effect upon the patient, but one will be detrimental and the other may be helpful. The following case study demonstrates the point.

One patient spends his entire time sitting quietly with his head bowed, showing little interest in anything or anyone. He does as he is told, slowly and without interest. In response to requests for him to do something and in attempts to engage him in conversation, he often responds with annoyance. He is completely indifferent to personal appearance, although he will passively allow someone to dress him and comb his hair.

Why? What purpose can such behavior serve? What does it accomplish? Why is that particular purpose important to the patient? How does a patient's response affect the nurse and his nursing care?

The most obvious effect of the patient's behavior is to reduce to the lowest possible level any relationships with other persons. He seeks no one. He may passively accept others in a fashion that gets rid of them as quickly as possible, show annoyance designed to drive them away, or alienate them by unacceptable behavior. His indifference to appearance or poor physical hygiene are construed consciously or unconsciously as a means to alienate people. If this is true, then the behavior, no matter how intolerable by our standards, is purposeful to the patient. He may be living comfortably in a fantasy world of his own, or he may be quietly and miserably living alone, preferring his lonely misery to the greater one of association with others. What his behavior accomplishes (his purpose) is isolation from other persons, even though it is this intolerable isolation that has often created the symptoms. The important need for human contact is further denied.

Man is a social being, and his social needs are deep-seated and powerful motivating factors in behavior. Security in social relationships is a need that influences all that we are and all that we do. Yet here is a person who, while seemingly quite passive and indifferent, uses those very traits to keep himself away from other people and to keep people away from him. We know then that the patient's insecurity in interpersonal relations is so severe that it has overwhelmed him. He feels safer turning his back on real life and real people. In other words, he is defending himself by blocking off any experience that could possibly threaten his self-esteem or that could hurt him in any way. If he doesn't take a chance, then he can't be hurt. He has forgotten, however, that he will be hurt if he doesn't take that chance. Obviously, the challenge of emotional relationships of any kind with others is something to be feared. This is a phenomenon very commonly seen in normal life. Many sensitive persons refuse to compete for fear of losing, because the prospective loss will hurt sufficiently to make the gamble and the chance of winning not worth the effort. The self-effacing person who is afraid to voice an opinion is no stranger to any of us. The patient, however, has carried the reaction to extremes. He is an individual so deeply insecure in interpersonal relationships that he defends himself by completely rejecting them.

What does the patient's behavior pattern tell us of his perception of himself in relation to others? We know that his self-confidence is practically nonexistent and can surmise, therefore, that he feels extremely inferior in comparison to others, or he may see others in some sense as a very definite threat to himself and his self-esteem. This may be as far as we can go in general terms from what the patient has shown us in his behavior. Much more specific estimates in terms of how the patient perceives himself can be made when the patient's social history is known and more time has been spent with him. The basic information to begin planning his nursing care, however, is at hand through understanding what the patient's behavior tells us about him. The previously described behavior tells us these significant facts; the patient needs relationships that reassure him as to his worth, that carry absolutely no threat, judgment, or criticism of him, and that will be present long enough and consistently enough to give him an opportunity to accept others. We know he will make it difficult for anyone who tries to help him by rejecting them, by looking for incidents that confirm his fear, and by not knowing how to respond if he wishes to do so. Allowances for the patient's inability to accept help quickly must be made in planning to bolster his weakened ego. This analytical process should be used by the nurse in initial encounters with patients.

A second case study describes a different mode of behavior.

> A patient is extremely restless, physically overactive, and irritable. He is easily distracted by persons and events in his environment and expends a great deal of energy flitting from activity to activity. He takes over for other patients and is quite interfering. Waiting on other patients, instructing them in what to do and when to do it, and fighting their battles against personnel are frequent occurrences. His assaultive episodes, which are usually verbal, occur most often when he intervenes for other patients. He cares little for personnel and is very sarcastic and supercilious toward them. Placing physicians, nurses, or other staff members in an embarrassing position gives the patient great pleasure, and he exploits such occasions to the fullest and without mercy. In addition to the constant activity, the patient frequently shows periods of mounting tension that culminate with a loud verbal outburst, almost invariably directed toward personnel. At such times the patient may be markedly crude and profane.

What does this behavior accomplish? The constant activity serves as an outlet for tension to some extent, but its restlessly changing focus and shifting interest make it seem as though the patient were afraid to stay with or come to grips with any real problem or purpose. It is a screen, a block, that keeps other things submerged. In much the same way, hard physical activity can be used by the so-called normal person to keep from thinking about unpleasant matters. One thing the patient's behavior certainly accomplishes is to keep him so active and distracted that he is diverted from the normal course of events. It protects him from some situation or emotion that he fears. That the fear is not wholly relieved is indicated by the patient's obvious continued tension. The threat, whatever it may be, is still present.

Another purpose of the patient's behavior is to make personnel as uncomfortable as possible. Hostility is frankly expressed. On exactly what grounds the patient's hostility is aroused may not be clear, but there are several possible reasons for it. In a hospital situation, personnel represent authority, and the patient's feeling may stem from hostility toward authority. Or perhaps the fact that personnel are "sane" may make the patient feel uncomfortable enough to arouse his resentment. His sarcasm, ridicule, and superciliousness may be directed toward reducing personnel to or below the patient's own status. Whatever the basic reason, the patient's behavior expresses his need to strike at the persons who control his environment. The personnel pose a threat to him, a threat strong enough to call for attack.

The patient's attitude and behavior toward other patients are also of significance. Although he does not attack or express hostility toward them, he does not accept them as being on the same level as himself. He takes care of them, he directs them, and he defends them. He relates himself to other patients by showing an interest in them in a condescending manner. He assumes a superior-inferior status with himself always in the superior role.

The patient's behavior then has two purposes that can be deciphered simply on the basis of observation. He is first of all actively engaged in keeping at bay something that threatens him. In addition, his behavior contributes to his own self-esteem through attacks on personnel that reduce them in stature and through placing himself in a superior relationship to others in the environment. The patient is frantically and consistently trying to increase his sense of importance in his own eyes and in the eyes of others.

The patient's behavior tells us, then, that his self-perception is that of an individual threatened by everyone with whom he comes in contact. His greatest threat, calling forth open hostility, is from persons in authority or persons who are higher in the social hierarchy than himself. The patient needs to develop sufficient self-confidence to enable him to be comfortable with other people.

Retaliation against the patient's expressed hostility will confirm his fear of danger and strengthen his need for the elaborate defense he has built. Frequently, this type of patient becomes the scapegoat of many situations. He is easily pinpointed as the cause of group difficulties owing to his obvious behavior. Jokes and giggling, to the extreme of hostility and rejection, are often noticed. The problem is in building the patient's self-confidence slowly and steadily and in avoiding any threat, psychologic or physical, directed at him. Fundamentally, the objective in caring for this patient is the same as for the first patient discussed. The nursing care of the two patients varies considering the type of obstacles the patient's behavior places on the road to achievement of the nursing goal.

A third case study presents some different behavior.

> The patient is completely preoccupied with heart trouble where no physiologic evidence is demonstrated. He is frequently observed taking his pulse. He suffers from palpitations and complains of heart pain, inability to breathe, poor circulation, and many other difficulties. He objects to and resists strenuously any activity because of his illness. His thoughts, his time, his energies, and his interest are focused only on his illness. His conversation is on nothing but his illness. A thorough physical workup has ruled out any organic pathologic condition. This fact only convinces him of the incompetence of the medical staff and justifies his wish to be transferred to another hospital.

What does this behavior accomplish? Why do people tend to sympathize with physical illness? They do so because it is physically uncomfortable and because physical illness cuts one off from the usual pleasures and pains of everyday existence. These are the important reasons for sympathy. The chronic invalid is limited in his participation in social experience, and this is his greatest tragedy.

The physical complaints without adequate somatic cause accomplish one thing—they limit the range of the patient's experience. If one is ill, there are not only reasons why one cannot do many things ordinarily expected of the average person but also reasons that are socially acceptable. A person with poor health cannot be expected to work hard for a living. The patient's behavior is then defensive in purpose. It provides him with a means of evading many situations, and when one evades, it is usually because of fear of failure. The patient's concentration on his heart disease permits him to think well of himself despite the fact that he is not accomplishing anything very constructive to win the approval of his fellow men. He cannot be expected to do much since he is ill.

A person who evades is a person afraid of the consequences. Preoccupied with his own health, the patient is unable to establish and maintain adequate interpersonal relationships with others. He lacks confidence in himself in relation to others to such a degree that he avoids the thing he fears. He compromises with life and settles for temporary sympathy. He perceives himself as an individual incapable of success and as inferior to others and defends himself from the same opinion by others through evasion and alibi. His difficulty is his lack of confidence in himself; his restoration to health is congruent with a growth in his opinion of himself.

A fourth case study presents a patient who is found in a general hospital setting.

This patient is admitted to a general hospital for abdominal surgery. He complains that the hospital bed is hard and that the sheets are not clean enough. He demands to see his physician immediately and is annoyed when the physician is not promptly produced. He criticizes his surgical preparation. He wants water; he wants a bed pan; he wants to go to the bathroom; he wants the head of the bed raised/lowered; he wants the window opened/closed; and so on, ad infinitum.

What on earth can such behavior accomplish except to drive hospital personnel to the contemplation of justifiable homicide? The resultant effect on the nursing staff often is a covert response. This type of demanding patient is often ignored. The night calls are answered slowly, and staff members avoid being seen by the patient so that they will not need to respond to his numerous requests. Unfortunately less contact increases the patient's need and the demands increase; hence a vicious cycle begins and is reinforced. Once he is labeled demanding, the patient finds it almost impossible to change that image or be allowed to respond differently. In such instances, nurses, doctors, and staff reinforce the image and behavior patterns.

Two accomplishments stand out when such behavior is viewed objectively. First, and most important, the behavior brings other persons to the patient's side. The patient is reaching with poor technique but fervent need for reassurance. The patient is frightened but unable to acknowledge fear out loud, and he is in need of understanding, tolerance, and reassurance that do not brush aside his fears as unimportant or unnecessary.

Second, criticism of everything in the hospital indicates the patient's uneasiness and makes him feel a little more comfortable by attacking his environment. The criticism indicates the patient's fear and his feeling that the hospital is not a place where he is safe and secure. He is not a nasty dispositioned nuisance—he is a very frightened person. His perception of himself is the perception of a person in deadly danger.

The ability to understand patient behavior is essential if the nurse's response is to contribute to the patient's recovery. Nursing care with understanding is the heart of psychiatric nursing—it is the core of nursing itself for that matter. It is a skill developed only through discipline and constant practice. With every patient the pertinent questions should be asked and reasonable answers sought. What does the patient's behavior accomplish? Why is this purpose important to the patient? How does the patient judge himself as a person? Having reached a tentative conclusion on these important points, the nurse should then try as tactfully as possible to help the patient help himself toward the accomplishment of his purposes in a healthier manner. The nurse must begin to assess *what experience means to the patient, not to the nurse.* For example, a promotion can be a source of satisfaction to one person, a stimulating challenge to another, a threat to a third, and a precipitating factor in a mental illness to a fourth. Intelligent nursing requires not merely that nurses be able to imagine themselves in another person's situation and visualize how they would feel there, but also that nurses be able to imagine themselves in another person's situation and visualize how *he* feels. This ability is called empathy.

Constant practice and the readiness and willingness to revise conclusions can help in developing the art of understanding the meaning of experience to others. Judgments should not be based on isolated instances but on the patient's pattern of behavior as revealed in many situations. Judgments should also not be based on hearsay, rumor, or someone else's opinion. This is a common occurrence in hospital settings. Little of what actually happens matters, since both parties follow their role expectations of behavior. The patient who is expected to act demanding or nasty does so because he has nothing to lose. The nurse then plays the harried, intolerant, but trying-to-be-tolerant helper. Superficial explanations of behavior should not be accepted, and the why of the patient's behavior should always be sought. If he lies, why is it important for him to lie? If he hates, why is it important for him to hate? If he is destructive, why is it important for him to destroy?

Interpersonal relationships, the give-and-take between patient and nurse, are tools of nursing care used in promoting patient health. The ability to use interpersonal relationships as a tool in therapy depends on developing skill in understanding behavior and on understanding the significance of that behavior.

SELF-UNDERSTANDING USED AS A THERAPEUTIC TOOL

In developing skills needed to participate effectively in the care of patients with personality disorders, nurses must know how to realistically approach the problem of bringing about change within themselves. They will become comfortable enough in their relationships with patients to be helpful only when they feel some security about their ability to respond appropriately to patient behavior. The method of approaching this problem is important because it will probably determine how effective the nurse will eventually become. It is not enough to identify the attitude or feeling the nurse *ought* to assume toward specific patients. Knowing how one ought to feel or act does not necessarily change feelings or behavior. In fact, knowing only how one ought to feel can produce real feelings of guilt.

It is necessary to be realistic and to face the difficulties involved in adjusting the responses of the nurse to patient needs. The behavior of mentally ill patients has a high potential for producing anxiety in the persons who work with them. Anxiety calls forth defenses. It is easy to let our response to patients be determined by the need to protect ourselves from the anxiety aroused. It is perfectly natural to feel anger, resentment, pity, and dislike as well as liking for mentally ill patients. These responses are among those we feel toward people who are not mentally ill. Our first step is to learn as much about behavior as we can, so that we can increase our understanding of what is actually happening. This in itself is helpful, but it is not enough. We must apply what we learn to our own behavior and feelings as well as to the behavior and feelings of others.

Nurses who feel they ought to be kind and understanding, while they are actually irritated with a patient, are caught on the horns of a dilemma. The possibility of developing feelings of guilt is good. Feelings are not turned on and off at command. Nurses need to learn to accept themselves as part of learning how to accept others. They can try to identify what they actually feel and think as the first step in bringing about change in themselves, since this will identify what is to be changed. Next they need to face the fact that simply telling themselves *not* to feel that way is wasted time. Nurses need to analyze the why's both in their own behavior and in their patients' behavior. It is often helpful to do this with someone else in the situation rather than to try to do it alone. Exchanging experiences frankly with classmates may have some value, since it is reassuring to find one's own reactions shared by others. Discussing personal reactions with more experienced persons in the situation is almost a necessity. Participating in group conferences about patient care is another source of help. Such experiences, with increasing knowledge brought to bear on them, contribute to the development of skills in interpersonal relationships through increased self-understanding and through increased understanding of others.

Nurses must become more realistic about the limitations of their role. Any one nurse cannot meet the total needs of the patients. Nurses cannot relate effectively with every person. But more importantly, they should not pretend interest if they do not feel it. Most people are sensitive to clues about someone saying they are interested when in reality they are not. People suffering from mental illness often tend to be more sensitive to such clues. Denying an emotion that the patient senses is untherapeutic. If a patient asks the nurse, "Are you angry with me?" and the nurse responds, "No, it's OK" and does not mean it, then the patient's feeling is invalidated. This conflict systematically reinforces to the patient the split between what he senses and what he is told. If real impressions are constantly invalidated, then unreal impulses begin to emerge and take hold.

Orlando (1972) suggests that nurses discuss frankly with the patient their own reactions to him when those feelings or reactions are a source of difficulty in providing nursing care, as, for example, when nurses are angered by the patient's behavior. This should be done only if *nurses give the patient the reason for their reaction and invite the patient to react.* Such an approach assumes that nurses first know why they feel what they feel and can correctly identify the feeling.

Nurses have the right to make mistakes with their patients. In establishing meaningful relationships, making mistakes, reassessing, and trying again are part of the process. This trial-and-error process is better than having one set path of approach and sticking to it, regardless of what is happening. Psychiatric nursing practice can be seen as a process of mutual self-disclosure. The nurse and the patient reveal the emotions they are experiencing and discuss what is happening currently in their relationship. This opening up of self in the therapeutic relationship demonstrates the naturalness of having and sharing thoughts and feelings. The situation becomes therapeutic because the feelings and their responses can be validated and clarified, thus healthier patterns can be learned.

A UNIQUE CONTRIBUTION BY EACH NURSE

What each nurse brings to a therapeutic relationship is a unique contribution—what the nurse is as a person, which is different from what any other person is. This is one of the reasons why there are no standard replies to patient questions and no standard pattern of behavior for any situation in a psychiatric setting. The same words used by two different nurses may well have two different meanings to the same patient. There are no magic words, and stereotyped behavior responses to types of situations are potentially dangerous.

It is generally accepted that the consistency of nurses' feelings and thoughts with their behavior constitutes a therapeutic asset. This is why self-understanding of how nurses really feel is so important and why stereotyped behavior responses to situations and patients are potentially dangerous. The resulting inconsistency between feelings and actions lessens nurses' effectiveness in a relationship. This is why nurses who try to coax a patient when they would like to swat him are practically never successful. The first problem that needs attention in such a situation is the nurse's own feeling.

The degree of congruence or consistency in feeling, thoughts, and behavior exhibited by the nurses affects their therapeutic potential. The extent to which their behavior reflects what they really are as unique individuals affects their therapeutic potential as well. It is not usually possible to develop a helping relationship unless one really wants to. How the helping relationship does develop is an expression of the uniqueness of both the patient and the nurse.

REFERENCES

Aichlmayer, R. H.: Cultural understanding: a key to acceptance, Nurs. Outlook 17:20-23, 1969.

Brockmeir, M. J.: Who are the significant others? Nurs. Outlook 17:34-37, 1969.

Burnside, I. M.: The patient I didn't want, Am. J. Nurs. 68:1666-1669, 1968.

Johnson, M. A.: Developing the art of understanding, New York, 1967, Springer Publishing Co., Inc.

Leininger, M. M., editor: Contemporary issues in mental health nursing, Boston, 1973, Little Brown & Co., p. 25.

Orlando, I. J.: The discipline and teaching of nursing process, New York, 1972, G. P. Putnam's Sons, pp. 1-43.

Santopietro, M. C., and Rozendal, N. A.: Teaching primary prevention in mental health, Nurs. Outlook 23:774-777, 1975.

Velazquez, J. M.: Alienation, Am. J. Nurs. 69:301-304, 1969.

ADDITIONAL REFERENCES

Gillis, M., Sr.: Attitudes of nursing personnel toward the aged, Nurs. Res. 22:517-520, 1973.

Goldsborough, J.: Involvement, Am. J. Nurs. 69:66-68, 1969.

MacGregor, F. C.: Uncooperative patients: some cultural interpretations, Am. J. Nurs. 67:88-91, 1967.

Mansfield, E.: Empathy: concept and identified psychiatric nursing behavior, Nurs. Res. 22:525-529, 1973.

Stoll, K.: A patient's humiliation, Am. J. Nurs. 65:95, 1965.

Taylor, C. D.: The hospital patient's social dilemma, Am. J. Nurs. 65:96-99, 1965.

CHAPTER 6

The nurse, the patient, and the community

Everyone has certain basic needs that must be met, no matter how different the surface behavior may be. Glasser (1965) proposes that everyone who needs psychiatric treatment suffers from one basic inadequacy: he is unable to fulfill his essential needs. The severity of the symptom reflects the degree to which the individual is unable to fulfill these needs. He states it is important that "we must have at least one person who cares about us and whom we care for ourselves. If we do not have this essential person, we will not be able to fulfill our basic needs. . . . Psychiatry must be concerned with two basic psychological needs: the need to love and be loved and the need to feel that we are worthwhile to ourselves and to others."

All of us need a fairly comfortable self-opinion with which to live. One person may attempt to achieve it by excelling as an athlete and another by excelling as an intellectual. Still another may attempt to bolster his self-opinion by constant criticism of others, making himself appear superior in comparison. An individual may also imagine himself quite outstanding and retain that opinion by refusing to participate in any experience in which there is the slightest chance that his sterling traits may be challenged. All of these persons are striving to maintain a good opinion of themselves even though their behavior differs.

Regardless of the behavior pattern that may characterize a patient's behavioral disorder, there are certain care principles that may be applied to all persons who show such disorders. Generalizations regarding nursing care must be accompanied by certain cautions. We have no generally accepted theory on the cause or cure of mental illness. Therefore, based on this, we have no single, solid theoretic base for psychiatric nursing. The generalizations that follow are guidelines developed through experience, research, and the developing concepts of nursing. Graduate study and research on the question of What nursing is are beginning to identify a defined body of nursing knowledge and practice. Leininger states that "caring is the essence of nursing and is the most central and unifying focus for nursing decisions, practices, and goals."

ACCEPTING PATIENTS AS THEY ARE

The average person has certain standards of conduct that he demands of other persons with whom he associates. Failure of others in meeting those standards calls forth retaliatory measures of varying degrees. Strict attitudes about eating habits are typical. The person whose table manners are not impeccable may well expect to be punished for his behavior if he enters social circles in which impeccable table manners are a criterion for social acceptance. He may be ignored, he may be criticized, or he may be isolated from group relationships by complete rejection. These measures are punitive in nature and are designed to make obvious that certain types of behavior are not acceptable and that acceptance depends on an alteration or correction of the offensive habit. With a reasonable degree of security and self-confidence, the average person can interpret what is happening and alter his behavior to gain approval and acceptance even though his feelings may be hurt in the process. For those who can learn, this is a lifelong process. In addition to correcting behavior in response to the feedback from persons in the environment, the average individual may also be capable of pursuing a course of action he believes to be right despite pressure from others.

When we react to a person who is suffering from an emotional disorder, an entirely different problem is presented. The problem is not one of educating through reason. The patient has already acquired inefficient methods of handling his life problems; these methods are usually defensive in nature and based on strong emotional needs. Reeducation of deep-seated values and of attitudes toward others and the self with resultant behavior change is the heart of therapy, and this involves a major personality reorganization. The patient needs to unlearn much before he can learn again. He has already been exposed to reason and to the ineffective use of punishment and reward in society, and such measures have failed. He needs something different, something that gives him an opportunity to see and to accept what he must unlearn first, before he can bend his energies toward learning again. He needs a low-pressure social environment in which he can learn to live again with others in much the same manner as a person with paralysis must learn to walk again. A paralyzed patient, newly recovered, is not expected to get out of bed and do a 100-yard sprint. An emotionally ill patient is not expected to meet normal standards of behavior at all times. He needs, first and foremost, to be accepted as a person.

To accept a patient as a person does not mean we sanction or approve his behavior. We simply acknowledge the fact, by our attitude and behavior, that the patient is as he is and has a reason for his behavior. Conveying acceptance of a patient is not to be confused with resignation or drifting with the situation. Acceptance is an active process, a series of positive behaviors designed to convey to the patient a respect for him as an individual human being who possesses worth and dignity. We use empathy and compassion, interest and concern, attention and assistance for the patient as a means of establishing a trusting relationship that the patient can accept. Accepting the person means caring about him, for what he is, thinks, feels, and needs. It means giving the best of ourselves as persons and professionals.

Human beings have to learn ways of being accepting toward others. It is important to learn that our own attitudes, overt or covert, expressed or suppressed, have a strong bearing on how we accept others. It has been suggested that love for self and love for others are two sides of the same coin. Experimental evidence exists suggesting the hypothesis that acceptance of others rests on self-acceptance. If our aim is toward a more tolerant attitude of self, especially the not-too-acceptable side of our personalities, we will soon feel greater acceptance of others. It is through this struggle for self-acceptance that we develop more tolerance and empathy for the setbacks of others and for our patients. This approach does away with the condescending attitude of *them* for a more realistic awareness of a shared human condition.

Acceptance is expressed in many ways: relating with the patient in a nonjudgmental and nonpunitive manner, expressing direct and indirect interest in the patient, recognizing and reflecting the patient's feelings, talking (with understanding) to the patient, listening to the patient, and permitting the patient to express strongly held feelings. In accepting patients through a nonjudgmental approach, we avoid all moral judgment and its expression—a patient's behavior is no more right or wrong, good or bad, than the pain that accompanies an ulcer is right or wrong. In both instances, symptoms are presented. The danger is that the symptoms of a mentally ill patient often occur in an area in which the average person is accustomed to making value or moral judgments. This danger should be faced, and any person working with emotional disorders should be alert to and guard against its appearance in personal feeling about patients. The feeling of shock when a patient is crude or vulgar is not wrong, but it is wrong to make the patient feel that he is offending and that he must be punished.

Being nonjudgmental is hard work. We are never free of judgmental feelings that arise from our evolving values. We cannot will these feelings away, and we cannot split ourselves in two, forbidding these feelings to interfere with our professional half. Our responsibility is to keep these ideas conscious; through this consciousness clarification and change occur. Unconscious beliefs emerge in many different ways, distorting perception and behavior. Slamming doors, blaming the wrong person, acting aloof and uptight, and developing physical symptoms, such as headache and stomach ache, are examples of disguised feelings. Stereotyping people or behavior is another habit that keeps us away from others and ourselves. By stereotyping we respond to personalities or situations in ways we have been taught to see and hear, rather than through our own actual experience. There are suggested guidelines that can be used in developing a nonjudgmental personality. To recognize and to acknowledge our judgmental feelings is the first, and most important, step. Progress stops until that honest, courageous, and sometimes painful self-evaluation is made. Next we must accept our judgmental feelings. Judgmental feelings are not removed by being judgmental about ourselves. Having negative feelings about someone else is not terrible. It becomes *bad* when we submerge attitudes and give lip service to ideals that we cannot follow, displacing these attitudes on others. The next step is analyzing the origin of the attitude. Where did this attitude come from? This may require outside guidance, as we admit our need for assistance in understanding this process. The final step is realizing that feelings are generated in every new interpersonal process. Therefore, the process of trying to develop nonjudgmental attitudes never ends. It is an evolving, creative, challenging process. We should refocus our effort on exploring and acknowledging our own feelings; through this approach change takes place.

In a nonpunitive approach, although the patient is encouraged to express his feelings and although his behavior may not meet social standards, the patient is punished neither directly nor indirectly for his expressions or behavior. Such behavior may be ignored. The avoidance of retaliation sounds too easy. It is doubtful whether nurses exist who know they punish their patients, yet the actual occurrence is quite frequent. To be able to avoid retaliation, nurses must develop skill in realizing how retaliation can be expressed. The means of punishment are many and varied. They consist of such measures as avoiding a patient except when something must be done for him, telling him something unpleasant "for his own good," calling attention to his defects by talking about them, reducing him to a diagnosis, failing to explain what is being done to him, laughing at his fears, being condescending and superior to him, expecting him to know and behave as though hospital routine were more important than he, demanding that he respect physicians and nurses, and saying the right thing in words but letting the facial expression and body posture convey annoyance and disapproval.

With the advent of tranquilizers, the opportunity for actual physical punishment and abuse of hospitalized patients has decreased. Still, there are isolated reports of such occurrences. More frequently, however, covert and subtle punitive approaches are exerted on the acting-out patient as a means of behavior control. These acts are easily justified under the false assumption of behavior control. Examples of punitive approaches still operating today include threat of getting medication, threat of increasing medications, threat of telling the physician to cancel the pass, threat of withholding cigarettes or other privileges, and threat of being put into seclusion. We must be very careful not to give the patient conflicting messages as to our intent. For example, we cannot verbally encourage the patient to express his positive and negative feelings, then behaviorally and emotionally punish him for that action. This describes the double bind theory. It involves more than conflicting communication; it also implies that either response (positive or negative) is met with rejection, disapproval, and punishment. In other words, "You're damned if you do, and damned if you don't." This concept is extremely important, since repeated double bind situations throughout life are considered as having possible etiologic significance in mental illness. Exposing the patient to this type of communication will not lead the patient to health and recovery. It reinforces the preestablished pattern, thus setting the person back further. In this situation it becomes almost impossible for the patient to respond and relate in a healthy fashion.

Another method of accepting patients is to show interest in the patient as a person, not as a case or a clinical problem. The interest shown in reading the patient's chart and in studying textbooks for increased understanding of the development of the behavior pattern is only the first step. Interest in the patient as a person must be shown in the presence of the patient, or where the patient can see evidence of such interest, for it to be brought to the patient's awareness and to have any effect on his feelings or behavior. Interest can be shown by seeking out the patient, by using time spent with him on those things in which he is interested, and by developing an awareness of his likes and dislikes. His requests can be met, or the reason for their not being met can be explained in terms that make sense to him. His comments, complaints, and expressions of approval can be dealt with realistically, not brushed aside. His fears can be accepted as real to him, not treated lightly. Subjects about which he is sensitive can be sought out and avoided. In other words, there must first be patient-nurse contact that is not always dictated by absolute necessity, and the nurse must be aware of what kind of person the patient is. This knowledge should guide the nurse's behavior so that respect for the patient is there for him to see when he is able.

A much neglected method for conveying acceptance to a patient is the simple act of staying with the patient. There are many opportunities for doing this, even if the period of time involved is not long. Staying with a patient seems relatively simple, but it is apparently an art that needs cultivation and is well worth practice. An essential element in nursing situations is professional closeness. It can be viewed on different levels. Some nursing functions center on actual physical contact with patients, especially in the context of physical care. The nonverbal gesture of touching a patient or patting a patient's shoulder, for example, expresses a feeling of concern or mutual regard. These nonverbal gestures are best used when they accurately convey the intentions of the nurse. Physical touch can be an emotionally expressive way of making deep, human contact with the patient. However, because of the intensity of this approach and because of the chances of physical touch becoming miscommunicated, it becomes of the utmost importance that the nurse be aware of personal motivations and the possible patient responses. To some, touch conveys a message of concern, to others it means sexuality, to others it carries a feeling of threat, and still to others it may convey the message of being put down. A well-meaning nurse who assesses a situation poorly may upset a patient by this response. Professional closeness focuses exclusively on the interests, concerns, and needs of the patient. It is guided by what is considered good for the patient. The determination of good is not left to chance but is assessed through knowledge, judgment, and experience.

Acceptance can be conveyed to patients by recognizing the feelings they *do* express. This presents several problems, one of which is that certain cultural segments avoid the expression of strong emotions. Another is the uncertainty on the part of many persons as to what to do when strong emotions are expressed; this also is a cultural problem for some. If one can learn to accept, nonjudgmentally and nonpunitively, the expression of emotions and feelings and then one can learn to accept one's self as a realistic sounding board for the patient, the first step will have been made. This reinforces the concept that nurses must deal with their own emotions. If they cannot deal with their own anger, then they cannot effectively deal with the patient's anger. One approach that helps in learning to accept the expression of emotions is to focus attention on understanding what that feeling means to the patient. This requires the development of skill in identifying the feelings actually expressed. The patient's statement, "I'd like to break someone's neck," means that he is angry. Such expressions should be met by the reflection of the *feeling* expressed, not the words. Another method of dealing with such expressions is by the use of an open-end question that leaves the patient free to go in any direction he chooses, that is, it does not direct the patient's answer in any specific direction. "Would you care to tell me about it?" is an example of such a question. It is first necessary to practice identifying the feelings expressed by the words and the behavior of the patient. In case of doubt, paraphrasing *what* the patient has said may lead to further patient expression that will clarify the feeling being expressed.

It is suggested that nursing care in such situations occurs within the interpersonal relationship of nurse to patient. There is a necessity for nurses to observe their own needs and patterns of activity as well as their inferences regarding the needs of the patient. Nurses should not manage patients. Instead they should have an awareness and control of their participation in this nurse-patient situation. The nurse's behavior calls forth responses in the patient. Nurses cannot change the patient's responses, nor can they demand that he act differently. What nurses can do is manage their own behavior to stimulate change in the patient's behavior in a healthier, more productive fashion. This approach differs totally from the custodial, control-oriented care of the past. This truly is a therapeutic nursing relationship.

One difficulty in identifying attitudes and feelings may arise because these important emotions may be confused with the intellectual content of the patient's conversation. The feelings revealed are more significant than the content. Most of us can throw up a verbal screen around our emotions, but it can be penetrated by skilled observers who keep asking "Why? Why? Why?" An example of confusion over the significance of content and feeling and of the effect this confusion can have on the response is given in the following instance. A patient explained that, although he was chairman of his department in a university, he was not trusted by the chancellor. The actual content of this statement would indicate that the patient probably was trusted; otherwise he would not be likely to have held the position he did. A direct response on this basis would be to point that out to the patient. The significant fact in the patient's statement is that *he felt he was not trusted.* This is the feeling expressed. With practice considerable skill can be developed in recognizing feelings and attitudes.

Talking provides a means of conveying acceptance to patients. It can convey to the patient interest, concern, and caring and can be a means of establishing rapport. It can, without doubt, also be misused in the sense that talking can be a means of rejecting patients very effectively. Chattering or social chitchat can be used by nurses to avoid becoming too deeply involved. This often occurs as a defense to anxiety or out of an actual unawareness of this behavior. For example, we can all identify with the overly cheerful nurse who buzzes around saying, "Good morning, how are you today?" Before the patient responds or just as they are getting into something, the nurse either leaves or changes the subject to "Gee, it's a beautiful day today" or "Got to go now, I'll see you later." These responses, although friendly in nature, tend to limit or prevent communication of a therapeutic nature. It closes the door to any meaningful conversation. The patient soon gets the message not to say what is on his mind. Many patients feel frustrated, as they may have a need to express their feelings about what is happening to them. If a patient chances expressing himself and this is met with levity, inattention, or another improper response, the resulting reaction is likely to be withdrawal. Each time this sequence occurs, it becomes reinforced; hence it becomes increasingly difficult to reach the patient.

Bernstein, Brophy, McCarthy, and Roepe (1954) classified types of verbal responses as evaluative, hostile, supportive, probing, or understanding. Evaluative responses are those in which the nurse makes a judgment (good or bad) about the patient's feelings and may go on to imply what he ought to feel or do. An example would be a response to a patient's complaint about nursing care in this manner, "Most patients seem to think the nursing care around here is pretty good. You will get better faster if you have a little more faith in us." Here the nurse implies that the patient is wrong and that he ought to change his attitude for his own sake. Such a response contributes little to patient care.

A hostile response is one that rejects the patient through ridicule or blame or denies him the right to have any feelings on the subject at all. An example would be a nurse responding to a patient's complaint about an aide with, "You have no right to complain about her. She's underpaid and overworked, and you take up too much of her time with your constant demands." This type of response can hardly help even an irritated nurse feel better.

In the supportive response, based on a misguided conception of what constitutes reassurance, the nurse denies that the patient really has a problem and implies that his concerns or worries are unnecessary. An example would be a nurse telling a patient who has expressed fear about a forthcoming operation that "Everybody is afraid of operations, but you have a good doctor, and we have a good staff, and everything will be all right." This would accomplish little except to shut off any opportunity for the patient to face and deal with his fear.

A probing response is one in which the nurse seeks further information and implies having the correct answers, if only enough information is made available. An example would be a nurse who, in response to a female patient's complaint that her husband was unfaithful, says, "Let us find out about this. What makes you sure he is?" This probing approach is ineffective in dealing with patient feelings.

An understanding response is one in which the nurse tries to understand what the patient is saying from his point of view. An example would be a nurse who replies to a patient's expressed concern over a pending operation with, "You are worried about your operation." This leaves the door open for the patient to explore his feelings further in an atmosphere in which it is safe to feel. He is understood. Students need to learn how to analyze their own verbal responses, to recognize what they are really saying to patients, and, especially, to develop skill in using the understanding response. Understanding, reflection, and open-end questions are talking skills that convey acceptance to patients.

Listening to patients is another means of conveying acceptance. The art of listening means more than keeping quiet—it includes opening the ears to hear what is said and using the intellect to understand the meaning of what is said. Encouraging patients to do the talking through brief, nondirective comments and through interest in what the patient is saying can be a rewarding experience. Many patients who begin with superficial comments when conversing with a good listener soon get past the superficial stage with acceptance from the nurse and will reveal much that is of real significance to them. Effective listening is an art or skill that has been underestimated. It requires a concentration on the person talking and not a concentration on how the listener will respond, a fairly common error. Listening requires hearing, interpretating, and selectively responding. Although the listener appears quiet, within him something stirs. During this time span, stress and strain can be released, trust can be increased, and the patient has the opportunity to formulate and express his thoughts and feelings. The true act of listening has often been equated with caring. If nurses really care, then they will take the time to listen attentively and patiently. One must listen not only for the actual words but also for the varied inferences of their meaning.

In establishing a therapeutic nurse-patient relationship, there must be balanced communication, with time for general conversation, therapeutic conversation, and silence. We must evaluate each situation carefully to know when to talk and when to be silent. Many people feel uncomfortable during quiet periods. This is, in part, cultural, as conversation no matter how empty and meaningless is fostered. Many people nervously fill in quiet periods with chatter, and no one really listens; hence meaningful communication is lost. Silence is important because it allows other nonverbal behavior to emerge. Silence should not be immediately judged as hostile, withdrawn, and rejecting. We must learn to utilize the value of silence as a therapeutic tool. It can allow time for the patient to organize thoughts, to experience feelings before verbalizing them, to gather courage to expose some ideas, to recover from what he just said, to work through feelings, and possibly to draw constructive conclusions.

Permitting patients to express emotions is another means of expressing acceptance. Patients are often overwhelmed by negative emotions and need the opportunity to express such emotions without psychologic or physical danger to themselves and others. Perhaps they have never learned constructive ways to deal with these emotions. The expression of these emotions is in direct contrast to accepted patterns in society. The direct expression of strong negative emotion tends to call for suppression; symbolic expression is much better tolerated. It is not safe under normal social conditions to go about striking everyone who is annoying, but it is all right to go to a boxing or wrestling match and to work off the emotion vicariously. Strong emotions, bottled up and kept out of awareness, are potentially explosive and dangerous. Patients with personality disorders are plagued with negative emotional responses that they have not been able to handle successfully, so these emotions are in need of an outlet. Repressed emotional responses are also related to the development of certain psychosomatic illnesses. Anxiety, fear, hostility, hatred, and anger should be expected, tolerated, and allowed expression. In fact, the ability of the patient to express a negative emotion is often a very healthy sign. For this reason, the evidences of fear, dislike, and hostility should be encouraged rather than discouraged.

Strange as it may seem, nurses can sometimes be more help to a psychiatric patient if they are the object of his hostility rather than the object of his affections. Their quiet acceptance of the patient's dislike permits him to discharge an emotion that might otherwise be bottled up, and it also permits the patient to express his negative emotion without the retaliation he expects. One of the dangers of hatred and hostility to the person who feels them is the fear of retribution they carry. Their expression, without punitive return, makes it easier for the patient to learn to be objective about his emotions and to then go on to a more healthy attitude about them.

Vicarious and symbolic methods of releasing negative emotions should be provided until the patient is able to bring his anxiety or hatred out into the open. Metal hammering, punching bags, tennis, badminton, golf, movies, and other activities should be available. The nurse must always keep in mind, however, that any frank expression of strong negative emotions is healthy for patients and that it is most healthy when it is calmly accepted.

If the patient has certain attitudes to unlearn, he must first be able to see them in himself. His behavior is defensive, and any criticism of it strengthens the need for it. Therefore the patient needs an atmosphere in which his behavior is calmly accepted and no threat is present for him. Only when his behavior is viewed objectively will he be able to see it objectively himself. The first step in helping a patient in the painful process of reeducation is to make him as nondefensive with his illness as possible. The nurse should accept him as he is.

Accepting people as they are involves understanding that limits are placed not on the patient's feelings but on the patient's ideas and actions. Psychotic ideas are not accepted as real nor is destructive behavior accepted as though it were all right in the circumstances. The *person* is accepted.

MAINTAINING CONTACT WITH REALITY

Most persons who have developed or who are susceptible to developing behavioral disorders have difficulties with their reality-checking mechanisms. From a psychoanalytic point of view, the ego is the mediator between the person and reality. The ego's most important function is to perceive and adapt to reality; thus it is a reality-checking mechanism.

Most normal persons have some difficulties in perceiving reality; they tend to see reality as they want to see it rather than as it is; this elaborates again the concept of continuity of health. When such reality problems overwhelm individual functioning and interfere markedly with social adjustment they become a major factor in behavior disorders. When caring for such patients, there must not be support of unreality or of the patient's unrealistic ideas, assumptions, or behavior. Supporting these behaviors only reinforces the unreality, thus separating the patient further from the real world. The real world is often too painful for the patient and is the reason he developed his inner world. Going along with a person's blatant unreal ideas, such as "I am the Virgin Mary," intensifies the separation of the two worlds.

Much of what has been said in the previous paragraphs applies to conveying acceptance of the person. Although acceptance of the patient does not include the acceptance of ideas or behavior that is obviously unreal, the patient is not rejected or punished for *either*; the nurse simply does not agree with them. In addition, reality may be called to the patient's attention without demanding that he immediately accept it; it may often be used as an alternative explanation for the patient to consider.

SEEKING VALIDATION FROM PATIENT

It is the meaning of feelings and behavior *from the patient's point of view* that is of primary importance, and only the patient knows how experience looks to him. Therefore, the logical procedure is to seek validation from the patient to check against the nurse's interpretation of how the patient sees things. If, for example, the nurse's observations lead the nurse to conclude that the patient is avoiding him, the nurse can so state and check with the patient whether his feeling is right or wrong. The matter-of-fact presentation of the nurse's conclusion and the request for validation provide the patient with an opportunity to correct or to confirm the conclusion, as only he can do.

Underlying the effectiveness of the process of seeking validation from the patient is one fact on which all schools of psychiatric thought agree. The essence of the helping relationship is the ability to convey to the patient the sense of trying to understand him and his feelings as they appear to him. Seeking validation conveys this effort and may show the patient the first step to mental health.

Orlando (1961) reports that patient difficulties arise from misinterpretation and misinformation about a real-life situation. Knowing the real situation and knowing the patient frequently do not add up to the correct conclusions as to what nursing action should be. The nursing element confirms the meaning of the situation with the patient, and this confirmation is the essential step that often provides the clue to effective action on the part of the nurse. Effective action is that which relieves distress and enhances means for adaptation.

INFLUENCE OF EXPECTATIONS ON BEHAVIOR

We are only beginning to recognize the importance of the influence of expectations on actual behavior. Although what is expected of a patient is not the final determinant of what he will do, it often has an important impact. In the initial phases of the chemotherapeutic use of tranquilizers, one well-known psychiatrist indicated he was not sure whether the results obtained were the result of the chemical properties of the drug or the psychologic result of the staff reaction to being able to give the patient a pill that they were sure would help him. The question remains unanswered.

It has been demonstrated in a wide variety of school situations that when failure is expected, a high number of failures occurs. When the expectation is held that students can succeed, a high percentage do succeed. More is involved than mere expectations, of course. Expectations are influenced by values, concepts of methods, assessment of the potential as well as achievement of people, the willingness to help, the level at which help is offered, and, ultimately, the depth of the belief in human worth and dignity. All of these factors influence the expectation of behavior on the part of others.

We are now certain that expectations have an influence on the behavior of others. This fact may provide a possible explanation of the success of remotivation therapies in psychiatric hospitals. Personnel who became active in getting patients interested in behavior improvement (at whatever level they worked) began by instituting an active program for patients. Since they were involved in a positive, active program, they expected results. And they got them to a surprising degree. For the nurse this expectation is an awareness of what he expects patient behavior to be and why. The importance of seeing the potential for growth in every patient and of actively seeking his strengths and resources becomes obvious.

Glasser's reality therapy stresses responsibility as being one of the important factors to be learned by individuals in the growth and development process. For the mentally ill this is one of their problems; therefore, therapy is directed toward helping the patient to learn to meet this standard of behavior. Glasser points out that meeting responsibility, standards, values, and morals "are all intimately related to the fulfillment of our need for self worth. . . ." He describes therapy as a special kind of teaching or training, akin to behaviors learned in the normal growing-up process. Reality therapy comprises a specialized learning situation of three intimately interwoven procedures:

1. *Involvement.* The therapist becomes so involved with the patient that the patient is helped to face reality and thus recognize his behavior as unrealistic.
2. *Rejection of unrealistic behavior.* The therapist must convey acceptance of the patient and maintain involvement with him in order for the patient to distinguish the significance of rejection of behavior (as in parental discipline) and the supportive caring for the individual.
3. *Replacement of learned patterns for previous behavior.* The process requires the therapist to teach the patient, through the therapist's involvement within the patient's situation, how to fulfill his needs within the parameters of reality.

Glasser (1965) states:

> The guiding principles of Reality Therapy are directed toward achieving the proper involvement, a completely honest, human relationship in which the patient, for perhaps the first time in his life, realizes that someone cares enough about him not only to accept him but to help him fulfill his needs in the real world.

CONSISTENCY AND PATIENT SECURITY

It is axiomatic that all mentally ill patients are insecure and uncertain, no matter what their behavior may appear to be on the surface. Therefore, attention to the small and large details that contribute to security is necessary. One of the most effective measures to promote a sense of security is consistency in experiences.

All persons are more comfortable working in a place with which they are familiar than they are beginning a new job. Not knowing what to expect produces anxiety. Few things so firmly implant safety in expectation as consistent experiences. Consistency in all areas of experience is valuable to the psychiatric patient, for it builds in his environment something on which he can depend.

The use of consistency is of value in routine, in attitudes, and in limitations placed on the patient. Consistency in the attitude of personnel toward the patient is profoundly important. Other people are not an expected source of comfort and consolation to the psychiatric patient. Consistency in attitude, if it is positive, helps him if he learns through day-to-day contact exactly what he can expect. It is even more helpful if he is constantly and continuously exposed to an atmosphere of quiet acceptance. This is not unusual since people are more comfortable with someone who is friendly on all occasions and yet not disturbed by faults. Occasional lapses will be excused by the patient but not enjoyed. Consistency in attitude on the part of the individual members of personnel is important, but consistency from person to person and shift to shift should be deliberately planned. The necessity for teamwork is obvious.

Although the acceptance of patient behavior and the permissive therapeutic atmosphere have been stressed, this permissiveness is limited. Patients cannot be allowed to do exactly as they please for obvious reasons. The homicidal patient is not permitted to kill others, the suicidal patient is not permitted to kill himself, the overactive patient is not permitted to completely exhaust himself, nor is the suspicious patient permitted to starve himself. That the patient *feels* and has a right to feel that way is accepted, but limitations are drawn beyond which his behavior is not allowed to go. The definition of limits and their enforcement are tasks that require a great deal of tact and understanding, since the potential psychologic threat to the patient can be handled in such a way as to place him on the defensive in his relationships with personnel. Consistency in quiet, matter-of-fact enforcement of limitations is one of the most effective methods of using the limits as a contribution to the patient's security. These limitations must be something on which the patient can rely. The attempt to win a patient's liking by being more permissive with him than other members of personnel is disastrous for the patient. While it may earn his personal liking (even though this is doubtful), it contributes to his confusion and insecurity. Limitations on a patient's behavior should be determined by the team, and those limitations should be *consistently* enforced by everyone who comes in contact with the patient.

REASSURANCE

All people need reassurance at one time or another, and psychiatric patients need it constantly. However, here again it is profoundly important for nurses to understand the meaning of experience to the patient, rather than to act on the premise of how *they* would feel in the same circumstances. One of the most reassuring experiences for a patient is the professional competence of nurses. In the care of emotionally maladjusted patients, a large part of this competence will depend on the ability to see how situations appear to the patient. Reassurance is a great deal more subtle than telling the patient that he will get well, that his fears are groundless, that he is a nice person, and that all will end well.

It is impossible for nurses to offer such glib statements. They do not know how a situation will end. This type of interaction usually turns the patient off since it demonstrates nurses' underlying anxiety or lack of concern.

Verbal reassurance is effective only when it does not contradict a false concept the patient needs. The patient punishing himself with the firm idea that he will die at midnight is not likely to be very receptive to reassurance that he will be alive and healthy when the nurse comes on duty the next day. The patient who is sure he is crippled for life by heart disease is not likely to be made very happy by the assurance that there is nothing wrong with his heart. Instead, he will probably cling more strongly to his belief. The value of the idea to the patient and his emotional need for it should be carefully assessed before it is used as a point for verbal reassurance.

Reassurance can best be given to the patient by showing interest in him as a person, by giving attention to matters that are important to him, and by allowing him to be as sick as he needs to be. Reassurance can be given through awareness and acceptance of how the patient really feels. Reassurance is also given by doing all these things without asking anything of the patient in return. It is unwise and emotionally harmful to bargain for behavior with reassurance.

CHANGE IN PATIENT BEHAVIOR THROUGH EMOTIONAL EXPERIENCE

The major focus in psychiatric therapy and in psychiatric nursing is on the feeling aspect of the personality, not on the intellectual aspects. One of the more difficult problems in working with mentally ill patients is a problem relevant to any field of nursing. The problem centers around the naive faith that change in behavior is easily produced by the use of reason. If we tell a patient what he ought to do and why he ought to do it, we expect him to change his way because "he now knows better." We then wash our hands of any further responsibility. The frequency with which we are disappointed in this expectation is sufficient proof that *telling people* is not an effective method of changing behavior. (To personally illustrate this point, consider your own reactions when you are told to do something.) This is especially true when the patient has emotional difficulties.

If a patient could be reasoned out of his psychotic ideas, he would never need treatment in a hospital. The patient would simply need to sit down with some very bright soul who would point out the fallacies in the patient's thinking, and all would be well. The patient's pattern of behavior has been developed to defend himself from anxiety-producing stress, and in building the defensive pattern, reason has been used as one of the tools to support the psychotic or neurotic structure. The patient cannot, therefore, be reasoned into a better state of adjustment.

Any attempt to reason a person out of a belief based on strong emotional needs is doomed, no matter how well adjusted the person may be. Although it is true that false beliefs based on inadequate or inaccurate information can be changed when the correct information is made available, this does not apply to false beliefs that have a strong emotional component, such as the false beliefs of the delusional individual.

All of us have our blind spots in which a cherished belief overrules all facts and all reason. The more such beliefs are challenged, the more vigorously they are defended. Knowledge and reason are not panaceas for the cure of emotional problems. Corrective *emotional* experience, however, can bring about behavior changes in such situations.

Any effort to use intellect and reason in dealing with a patient's ideas that have a strong emotional component must be avoided. From the outside looking in, it sometimes seems as though the patient simply *must* be able to see the reason for his behavior and to correct it. This is from the outside—it is necessary to try to see it from the inside. The patient's emotional need for his beliefs will resist any intellectual challenge brought by others. Reason is not an effective weapon in changing patient behavior.

The interpretation of the patient's manifest behavior should be avoided until the nurse or therapist has background information, and observations of a number of situations. An assessment of the patient's receptivity and ability to handle this is critical. Interpretation is telling the patient about the meaning of his behavior or explaining his unconscious motivations. The ideal goal of therapy is to help the patient to achieve such a degree of emotional security that he can develop and use an understanding of his behavior. Such understanding cannot be forced on him from outside, nor can he use this knowledge until he can emotionally accept it.

Insight, or the understanding of one's own motivation and behavior, can be an extremely painful experience. Its development in a patient with an emotional disorder must necessarily be slow, and support must be present to enable him to tolerate the knowledge that his behavior is not always altruistically motivated. Interpretation can be done only when the patient is ready for it, is secure enough to tolerate it, and is able to apply it to alter his behavior. It is useless in terms of improvement before the patient is ready for it. The only thing it can accomplish under such circumstances is to increase the pressure on the patient and make him feel more uncomfortable. Therefore interpretation of behavior is to be avoided.

It is helpful to remember that attitudes the patient himself does not recognize should not be identified for him. If he were able to tolerate such attitudes in himself, then he would be likely to identify them himself. For example, a patient may criticize the hospital personnel sharply, calling them incompetent and a disgrace to the profession they represent. With information gained from previous observation, the nurse may be fully aware that the patient is showing an attitude of rebellion toward authority. The patient has not expressed rebellion toward authority, but he has expressed an attitude of contempt toward personnel. To reflect the latter is acceptable since the patient has said it; to reflect the rebellion toward authority, revealed indirectly, would be a threat to the patient. He has not recognized and accepted his feeling toward authority as part of himself. Insight can be a threat or a help, depending on the course of the patient's illness, and its danger as well as its value should be kept in mind.

Corrective emotional experience results from healthy interpersonal relationships with others that meet the patient's basic needs for an acceptable self-opinion and a sense of worth to self and others. This involves the use of acceptance, discrimination in listening, focus of relationships on the patient, and involvement with the patient.

AVOIDING INCREASED PATIENT ANXIETY

Fear and anxiety are already problems with which the patient has been unable to cope. Careful study of situations, topics, or approaches that seem to indicate a resultant increase in anxiety in the patient should be made. The knowledge gained should be used to contribute to the patient's comfort.

Certain general types of situations can be avoided since an increase in anxiety can almost safely be predicted if the situation arises. Direct contradiction of psychotic ideas is almost certain to produce anxiety in patients since such ideas are always based on deep emotional needs. The effect is approximately the same as threatening to take crutches away from a person who cannot walk without them. Demands on the patient that he obviously cannot meet are also certain anxiety producers. To insist that a depressed patient cheer up, that an overactive patient go sit down and be quiet, or that a withdrawn patient initiate and carry through group activities simply places the patient in the position of having failed again. Failure causes anxiety in persons already insecure. The level of activity required of the patient should be adjusted with regard to the limitations his symptoms place on him.

The indiscriminate use of medical and psychiatric terminology in front of patients can often produce anxiety. Such terminology identifies a person as a member of a select group and shuts out those who do not belong. It is a thoughtless rejection of patients. In the same sense, careless conversation where patients can overhear may produce anxiety. A psychiatric diagnosis is often seen as a label from which the patient finds it difficult to escape.

Attention should not be called to a patient's defects, failing abilities, peculiarities, or failures. If a patient wishes to mention them, the nurse should accept them calmly and without criticism. To focus attention on weaknesses increases anxiety. In any personal relationship it is a wise rule to concentrate on the individual's strengths.

Insincerity can also produce anxiety since insincerity leaves the patient uneasy as to what to expect and uncertain as to where he stands. Since patients tend to integrate those elements of experience that confirm their poor opinion of themselves, they are most likely to interpret the nurse's obvious insincerity as an attempt to conceal an unpleasant opinion of themselves.

The initial experience in the hospital, with its differences and its newness, is fraught with anxiety-producing potentials. Careful orientation to the hospital, explanation of and preparation for what is about to happen, and a sensitivity for the patient's feelings concerning his admission are necessary. Too often admission procedures are carried out as routine chores, with little time relegated to helping the patient adjust to his new situation. Some patients may be very distressed about having to come or having been forced into the hospital. Often before the actual admission they have had terrible and difficult experiences. To many patients hospitalization itself is the end or the most terrible thing that could happen. To others it may mean relief and safety at last. However hospitalization is experienced, it is a new experience filled with different sights, smells, and sounds. Other disturbed patients can be frightening to a newly admitted patient, threatening to their physical security, or threatening of what may happen to them. The initial emotional experience of admission can influence the effectiveness of the therapy and the course of his improvement. Treatment begins with the admission procedure.

Threats, sharp commands, and indifference to a patient's reactions have no place in the care of psychiatric patients or in the care of any persons; they cause anxiety. These responses are often the result of nurses' anxiety or their inability to deal with the situation in a therapeutic way. They are used in an attempt to keep control over the situation. Eric Berne, author of *Games People Play*, has interpreted his theory of transactional analysis to the hospital setting (Levin and Berne, 1972). He suggests that instead of recognizing a problem and trying to find a solution, we often play games instead. He suggests that there are three possible roles a player can take in any game: victim, rescuer, or persecutor. When a patient is admitted to the hospital, he is usually seen as the victim, and all staff members are seen as the rescuers. Games begin when the staff members jockey with the patient for that position of rescuer. One game common to nurses is "I'm only trying to help you." In the use of this game, unfortunately, many nontherapeutic techniques are justified to reach the position of rescuer. Another game played is "Let's pull a fast one on the patient." This implies the staff's decision—not to tell the patient important information about his condition, because the patient will become too upset. These games diminish the quality of care in a therapeutic nursing approach. The game itself becomes the justification for a problem, rather than a solution to it. Once acknowledged, these games are no longer useful, and work can begin in identifying and solving the patient's problems.

In ordinary social relationships, family, friends, home, and occupation are frequent sources of conversational feelers used to bridge the initial gap between not knowing and knowing other people. In working with psychiatric patients, we again find a contrast to usual social practice. Questions about family, friends, home, and occupation are not very good areas for conversational efforts during the exploratory stages of establishing relationships with patients. The source of the patient's difficulties may arise from and are always related to his interrelationships with those who are closest to him. Feelings of hostility for family members may be the source of a patient's feelings of guilt, and conversation in which the patient admits his hostility may cause anxiety. In regard to family, occupations, and likes and dislikes, we must always listen when a patient talks but be careful to avoid judgments or comments that may add to a patient's anxiety. All of these are touchy subjects and should be carefully handled. We should follow the patient's lead in selecting areas of conversation, at least until we know the patient.

When a patient does burst forth with a confession of some feeling or experience about which he obviously feels strongly, his response following the confession is not always predictable. The patient may or may not be comfortable about the revelation. If discomfort ensues, the subject of the discomfort is probably best brought into the open and resolved between the patient and the nurse.

The immediate data of observation of all patients are often called the "A-B-C's." A refers to appearance, B to behavior, and C to conversation. All aspects of patient appearance, behavior, and conversation should be carefully noted and patterns detected before interpretation is brought to bear.

CONSIDERATION OF REASON FOR BEHAVIOR

Everything the patient says and does should be observed, recorded, and reported for the information of those directing and participating in the patient's therapeutic program. In addition, for the nurse's own information in planning the patient's care, the nurse should learn to recognize the attitudes expressed by the patient, the attitudes he does not recognize in himself, and the attitudes he has toward himself. The patient's behavior should be analyzed to seek its motivation and to understand what the patient is attempting to accomplish. The observation of patient behavior should contribute to the understanding that is basic to good care.

One way to improve skill in understanding why the patient behaves as he does is continuous practice in predicting patient behavior in certain situations. Of course, it is helpful first to learn as much about a patient as possible and, armed with understanding of the patient's basic problems, to then make an intelligent guess as to what he will do. When the prediction is right, analyze why it was right and consider what other action the patient might reasonably have taken. When the prediction is wrong, analyze why it was wrong and seek the logical reason for the patient's actual behavior. In any instance of patient behavior, seek answers to the following questions. What is the goal of the behavior? Why did the patient behave as he did?

Understanding why patients behave as they do is much easier if nurses can view behavior objectively. Objectivity is the ability to evaluate a situation, in this case the patient's behavior, on the basis of what is actually happening, rather than on the basis of one's personal feelings. Complete objectivity would be possible only in a vacuum. Reasonable objectivity is capable of being reached and is a practical goal. This supports the belief that nurses should have a good working knowledge of themselves, their reactions, and their attitudes.

There are several things that objectivity is not—it is not coldness, indifference, or absence of feeling. It is rather the ability to not let one's judgment be confused by the presence of warmth or resentment when the patient is concerned. Emotionally reached conclusions can be detrimental to the patient's welfare.

To be objective it is necessary to indulge, to some extent at least, in introspection to recognize one's own feelings and to guard against their influence on judgment. A real danger, one hard to detect, is the exploitation of patients to meet the emotional needs of nurses. Nurses are human beings, too, and they need to be liked, to be respected as persons, and to be important to others. They need recognition, appreciation, and reassurance. However, nurses are expected to meet these emotional needs other than through patients. With mentally ill patients, nurses must be prepared to give and to expect no return other than the pleasure of seeing patients recover or further debilitation prevented. Above all, nurses must lead balanced lives and have genuine sources of emotional satisfaction other than patients. Whenever nurses find themselves being critical of patients, defending or justifying themselves, demanding that patients treat them in a certain manner, or evaluating patients' behavior in terms of right or wrong, they are then in danger of letting their own emotional needs take precedence over those of patients. Working with psychiatric patients requires a certain hard-headed and frequently painful honesty. The ability to accept the faults they cannot change and the personal limitations within themselves is as important for nurses as their ability to accept patients. One is difficult without the other.

NECESSITY OF MOTOR AND SENSORY STIMULATION

Recent animal and human studies have stressed the importance of adequate motor and sensory stimulation in the performance of developmental tasks and behavior in general. The maintenance of sensory stimulation is also necessary to reinforce reality and to maintain contact with reality. People require sensory input from their surroundings; a sharp reduction of stimuli can lead to panic and confusion. With experimental isolation procedures there are frequent occurrences of fantasies, illusions, and hallucinations. These reactions have been characterized as regression, with a need to replace lost reality with fantasy. This information leads us to reconsider hospital practices that reinforce sensory deprivation. Placing a patient in seclusion because he is acting out may in fact increase the split between fantasy and reality. More important is the problem of allowing the patient to get to the point where this approach seems necessary. Patients show signs and give signals of impending stress before it is acted out. Again this points to accurate assessment and intervention early enough to prevent this situation from occurring. Unfortunately, threat of isolation or seclusion is often used as a means of controlling patient behavior. "If you're 'bad', we'll lock you up" is a powerful message that is more often nonverbal than verbal.

Isolation and sensory deprivation also occur outside the seclusion room in general hospital situations. Picture a large state hospital dayroom where patients are deposited for the day; chairs line the walls with some facing the television set that plays endlessly. The room is large and bare, with few homey touches. Patients stare into space or in the general direction of the television, where the picture is often unfocused or rolling. Now and then a groan is heard and names are called. Mealtimes seem to provide the only break in monotony. The food is bland, served in a routinized manner, chopped, and unrecognizable. Meaningful conversation is absent, hence social isolation and sensory deprivation are imminent. How long has it been since some patients felt fur, sandpaper, or silk; tasted a fresh pepper or peach; or smelled scents of popcorn or freshly cut grass? Long-term hospitalization is thought to increase the chronicity of the original problem by these methods. This fact raises some question as to the efficacy of many existing psychiatric hospitals where the opportunity for patients to hide behind a deadly dull series of routines is limitless. The opportunity to relate with other people, to perform tasks that have some challenge, and to see, hear, and touch things all have their place in the care of patients and in the prevention of mental illness. Input from the environment becomes part of the nurse's function.

REALISTIC NURSE-PATIENT RELATIONSHIP

It is essential that the relationship the nurse offers the patient be founded on a realistic basis. Much as one might like to be all things to all people or all things to some people, it is hardly possible in any situation. The warm and understanding therapeutic relationship of nurse and patient can help greatly in establishing the kind of environment patients need to give them an opportunity to get well. A person must crawl before he walks, and the patient can begin with a relationship that crawls in the sense that its demands on him are few and that he is not expected to live up to the demands of closer and more intimate situations. In addition, a therapeutic relationship protects the patient from demanding more than he can possibly receive and from feeling betrayed as a consequence. What the patient can expect from a close friend is different from what he can expect from a nurse, no matter how friendly the nurse may be. The basis of the nursing relationship is as a support to the patient and is therapeutically goal directed.

THE THERAPEUTIC MILIEU

There has been an increasing realization of the importance and need to consider the social structure of the hospital and ward units on the progress of therapeutic efforts for mentally ill patients. Although since the time of Florence Nightingale the environment and its effect on the patient's progress have been an integral part of nursing care, the focus and emphasis have become more important of late. The frequent reports in newspapers of patient abuse and the persistence of custodial care have stirred the public to demand more than routine care for the mentally ill. Goffman (1961) in his book *Asylums* deals with the pervasive effect of the labeling process, which results in derogatory labels applied to mentally ill patients by the caretakers of the environment in which patients are confined. He also skillfully demonstrates the inappropriateness of the medical model for psychotherapy. Scheff (1967), in his concern for the rights of hospitalized and committed mentally ill patients, indicates that adequate and systematic studies are lacking to support the propositions that patients get worse without treatment and that commitment is necessary for effective psychiatric treatment of most cases. His concern for the effect of the psychiatrist and the psychosocial environment on the patient is examined in his writings.

In the Standards of Psychiatric Mental Health Nursing (ANA, 1973), Standard VII commits the nurse to responsibility for: "The environment is structured to establish and maintain a therapeutic milieu" (Appendix B). There is little doubt that the responsibility for the milieu of the unit falls on the shoulders of the psychiatric nurse. The therapeutic milieu is the intentional use of the environment in the treatment modality for the patients. The milieu includes the persons living in that particular social setting—the unit. The patients, the physicians, the nurses, the aides, and others who are part of a unit are included. The staff members—psychiatrists, nurses, aides, and others—are the resource people who participate and interact with patients for the purpose of helping them to help themselves toward improvement. In this complex the interaction of significant individuals requires attention to attitudes of acceptance among all levels of staff and between staff and patients. The patient enters into a participatory role in his therapy and is encouraged to bring his thoughts and talents to the social interaction within the unit. In this way the patient is given recognition for things he is able to do and is given assistance and support in areas he domonstrates need. A social environment that provides participation, contribution, and cooperation goes far in reflecting the worth and trust for an individual. The therapeutic team within this milieu must be sensitive to and knowledgeable of the individual needs of patients and should judicially work with the patient on the level at which he is able to participate. To demand too much can be overwhelming and discouraging to the patient. To lack stimulation, encouragement, and support for what the patient can do is to revert to aspects of custodial care.

The team relationship of the staff needs to demonstrate recognition for each person's ideas and activities and respect for each as significant to the purposes of the team. The patient enters into this relationship to the degree that he is able and learns and develops his ability in social interaction and/or responsibility. Problems are dealt with as part of the process of living together as it is being lived.

Within the broad area of therapeutic milieu there are often included special patterns or subsystems that are intended to facilitate patients' interaction with reality factors. These include patient self-government, total-push therapy, the open-door policy, home care programs, daycare or nightcare centers, halfway houses, and community mental health centers and services.

Patient self-government is a plan whereby a patient group is formed to make plans and decisions for daily activities on a ward or unit. In cooperation and consultation with the staff, the patients run their own routine activities. The group structure usually provides for the selection of a spokesman or leader.

Other team members volunteer or may be selected to take on duties or concerns of the group, such as assisting other patients with tasks they cannot do for themselves or teaching other patients how to perform certain tasks. Usually these tasks relate to activities of daily living. Nurses and staff are used as resource people to assist in self-government rather than as decision makers. Patients consult with physicians and nurses with respect to how they may assist a fellow patient or to get some help for themselves in understanding their own feelings or problems in this social setting. Matters of discipline or control become part of the social interaction and thus diminish the authority role of the staff. Often peer pressure is significant enough to keep a unit running smoothly. It provides patients with a means of reality-testing by planning, following through, and fostering independence and responsibility. It also provides avenues for ego satisfaction.

Another organization of unit procedures, based on the improvement of patient behavior, has been tried with patients on many levels of adjustment. Depending on the level of patient behavior when the reorganization is undertaken, several patterns have emerged. At the lowest level is the habit-training program designed to improve patient habits in regard to basic physical needs. These include toilet-training, eating habits, personal hygiene, and personal appearance. Patients who are beyond this stage are placed on more active programs involving occupational therapy, recreational therapy, music therapy, and group therapy. This is sometimes called a *total-push program.*

The use of a community-based social approach to the care of the mentally ill has a classic illustration in the town of Gheel, Belgium. This town has provided community care for mentally ill persons since the Middle Ages. Here approximately 2,500 patients are cared for in the homes of the townspeople. The patients participate in the life of the families with whom they are placed. They have meaningful responsibilities as well as privileges in such home life. Although seen by physicians only about once a month, they are visited frequently by district nurses who get to know them well and who are in a position to seek the aid of a physician when need is evident. Patients do not lose social status but are treated as persons with limitations like any other handicapped group. Patients are respected as individuals and assume considerable responsibility for themselves, something that would arouse consternation in less progressive mental institutions. An important aspect of the attitude toward mental illness and mentally ill patients is revealed by the fact that personnel and families in Gheel believe that every patient can be placed in a home that will be helpful to him, even though four or five or more placements may be required before the right family is found. The feeling that a patient, regardless of his condition, can be helped is an essential component of care.

In the 1960s and 1970s the United States has shown greater attention to community-centered care. The Community Mental Health Centers Act of 1963 provide states with federal funds for the construction of comprehensive community mental health facilities. The emphasis on prevention and rehabilitation was given greater impetus.

Prevention, according to Caplan (1961), is defined under three major headings.

1. Primary prevention is concerned with the processes that reduce the risk of people in the community becoming ill with mental disorders. This level examines the community for factors contributing to stresses and causes of mental illness and the direct intervention to correct or remove these factors. Action of community groups and leaders is essential to these tasks.

2. Secondary prevention involves the prevention of disability by case-finding and early diagnosis leading to effective treatment. The purposes are to reduce the duration of known cases of mental disorder and to reduce their prevalence in the community. Early identification of patients with symptoms and immediate treatment are vital to this level. Community services are preferentially used and inpatient care is avoided wherever possible.

3. Tertiary prevention involves the consideration of the return of the patient to the community by preventing the defect and the crippling possibilities of the illness. Rehabilitation of the individual is essential to maintain him at the maximum level of function and as a means of returning the patient to the community.

There are a number of programs or agencies that support the tertiary prevention concept. These include daycare and nightcare services, halfway houses, home care programs, foster home care, and community chapters of former patient groups.

Daycare and nightcare centers have been established as units within general hospitals offering psychiatric care, in comprehensive community mental health centers, and as satellite units of some state hospital complexes. These facilities provide treatment similar in extent and intensity to the full-time inpatient hospital, but they allow the patient to function outside the hospital for up to half the day. This method often decreases the emotional and monetary cost of mental illness for the patient, the family, and the community. It also supports the person in the reality sense, thus reducing his dependency on the hospital and staff. The patient maintains his self-esteem and independence by continuing ordinary activities through part of the day. Where shame is attached to mental illness and hospitalization, this method of treatment helps to reduce this attitude.

Halfway houses are growing institutions in the area of transitional agencies for psychiatric patients. Their purpose is to facilitate the patient's progress as he makes the transition from total hospital care to his normal place in the community. For others, experience in the halfway house may prevent hospitalization altogether. Halfway houses offer the patient an opportunity to test adaptive capacities at his own pace. Halfway houses offer living services ranging from residential, family group living to apartment living. They also offer employment services, such as vocational rehabilitation programs through job training, outside supervised employment experiences, and sheltered workshop experiences. Medical management is regulated to community mental health center facilities. Many of these houses function in a democratic manner and offer a vital service in helping the discharged mental patient regain a place in society.

Home care or the placement of patients in *foster homes* is being used to a greater extent. Follow-up care by hospital staffs or by public health nursing personnel, combined with more careful preparation for the patient's return to the community, is being provided in greater measure. Foster home care may be used as an interim step to living with one's own family. In some institutions, family group sessions are offered to parents and relatives of a patient during his hospitalization as part of the therapeutic and rehabilitative plan.

In all of these movements there are certain common elements that may be major factors in their therapeutic results. First, all of these movements are based on a more clear-cut expression through the use of social environment with respect for the individual patient as a person of worth and dignity. Second, all express genuine expectation that the patient can improve. Third, all reduce the social distance between patients and staff. Fourth, all provide a more realistic social setting for therapy. Fifth, all emphasize and provide meaningful tasks for patients.

Four trends are apparent in these recent developments. One trend is the impact of higher expectations of patient behavior on the part of personnel; as nurses and others expect patient improvement, it occurs. Thus the use of personnel attitudes toward changed patient behavior is recognized as a therapeutic tool. A second trend is the recognition and use of the value system of the social setting in which patients are treated. The implicit and explicit goals of patients and staff have their impact on the extent to which the environment is actually therapeutic. The study of such goals and values and the resulting change, if needed and if possible, also constitute therapeutic tools. A third trend is the greater emphasis upon how personnel handle their own problems and meet their own needs and the impact of this solution on patient therapy. Undoubtedly, there is an increasing emphasis on the ability of staff members to openly express and explore their feelings, not only among themselves but with patients as well. The traditional pattern of repressing emotional responses and denying their existence is under fire from all sides. Emotional honesty and emotional maturity are considered musts for nurses as well as for others, not only in the care of mentally ill patients but in the care of all patients. The fourth trend is the increasing recognition of the importance of involvement on the part of patients and personnel. Decision-making, as it involves both, needs the active participation of both if it is to be successful.

GROUP THERAPY

Group therapy has had a widespread effect since World War II. The original group session in 1905 was used with patients who had tuberculosis. Since that time many varied purposes have been identified as possible uses for the group therapy structure. Armstrong and Rouslin (1963) identified the importance of group therapy methods in nursing practice. Yalom (1970) has made a comprehensive review of the types and purposes of group structures ranging from inspirational (Alcoholics Anonymous) and analytical, to testing and identification.

The role of the group leader requires knowledge of the dynamics of group process, establishes the identity of each individual (such as knowing each patient by name), provides consistency for the group through nonjudgmental and dependable management of the group, accepts disclosures, sets the theme or purposes, and renders support to sustain the group.

Characteristics of groups. The nurse in a psychiatric setting deals to a large extent with situations that concern groups even more than individual one-to-one relationships, although this does not negate in any way the importance of the latter. Unfortunately, as far as patients are concerned, this involves relatively large groups rather than small groups, about which there is more known. Luft (1963) defines group dynamics as "the study of individuals interacting in small groups." Group dynamics and group processes are somewhat less than an exact science, although that is no excuse for not using what appears to be helpful and testing possible hypotheses that are suggested. Group dynamics share with medicine and nursing the common problem of drawing on the facts found in many other branches of sciences, both biologic and social.

One of the major problems in defining, studying, and using effective group processes lies in the differing purposes for which groups exist. In the psychiatric hospital, for example, the patient in a group has no choice as far as the daily activities of living are concerned. On the other hand, participation in group therapy (to be distinguished from group activities) is largely voluntary and depends on the patient's choice. Even though he may be forced (hopefully not) into group therapy sessions, the decision as to the degree of participation remains his. Groups have different goals, but the common element running through all groups having to do with existing or threatening behavior disorders is a change of behavior resulting in better adaptation. In such groups, the process is more important than the content.

The climate of the group has a definite influence on how the group functions to make the achievement of individual or group goals possible or healthy, if achieved. One very important factor is the extent to which all are aware of what is really going on. The more feelings are submerged like the major portion of an iceberg, the less therapeutic is the environment and the less effectively do reality-checking mechanisms work. This is not necessarily true of other groups with other purposes. However, even the group concerned with the acquisition of knowledge may run into problems that have little to do with content but that are the result of interpersonal difficulties or intragroup process difficulties.

Groups concerned primarily with behavior change are focused more on self-directiveness of the group, permissiveness (especially where feelings are concerned), and listening to what is really said and less on content and interpretation. Again, involvement becomes important, as it is for all groups. The group atmosphere that contributes the most to therapeutic progress is characterized by increased member self-direction, shared leadership, honesty where feelings are concerned, group decisions, volunteering for tasks on the part of membership, a willingness to work for the group, hopefulness, informality, and humor. In general, the less authoritarian and the more humanitarian the leadership, the better the group for accomplishment of the therapeutic goals of the group.

The roles that individual members assume within the group may influence the total group function. It is interesting that not much is known about how change in the assumption of roles takes place, although it is known that the humanitarian influence of leadership appears to make a maturing role on the part of members more easily accepted. The role of a person within a group may be seen from two points of view—the group role and the individual need-meeting role. From the group view the person may be seen as any one of the following—initiator-contributor, information seeker, opinion seeker, information giver, elaborator, coordinator, orienter, evaluator critic, energizer, procedural technician, and recorder. From the individual view (meeting individual needs that may or may not be irrelevant to the group task) are the following roles—aggressor, blocker, recognition seeker, self-confessor, playboy clown, dominator, and self-seeking and special interest pleader. In these varying roles contributions toward or detractions from the therapeutic atmosphere are obvious. The problem becomes one of how to change the self-conception of the inward self and the conception of the self in relation to others that allows for growth and change in behavior. This would appear at the present moment in leadership that is humanely oriented, a permissive atmosphere that allows free exploration of feeling, the promotion of honest expression of feelings, and the honest facing of reality factors.

Groups, as do individuals, go through developmental stages, although group developmental stages have not been as clearly or definitely defined. There is a stage of orientation, a working stage, and a termination stage. The orientation phase is characterized by exploring, testing, defining, and decision-making. The working stage results in and may be characterized by periodic regression caused by poor orientation or threat from environmental or individual-need pressures. The regression may lead either to failure or to group decision-making that results in progress in behavior either by some individuals or by the total group. The smaller and the more stable the group, the more apt it is to go through coherent stages of development and to resolve its problems.

PRINCIPLES OF NURSING CARE

No definite, concrete directions as to how a nurse can most effectively function in the group setting of the hospital unit, the mental health clinic, or other social setting can yet be postulated with supreme conviction. Psychiatric nursing, however, in many instances can be thought of as primarily group nursing. By using skills in group interactions, nurses can create an atmosphere where patients learn to communicate in a healthier and more constructive fashion. Through this process, patients can realize their strengths and deal with their weaknesses. However, there is reason to believe that certain generalizations might at least be helpful guides for testing in action at the present time. The following principles are offered in this spirit.

It might also be wise to keep in mind that social therapy, to be effective, must have the participation of other groups in addition to nurses. Without administrative support, without the active assistance by aides and others involved in patient care, the nurse may well be faced with frustration. However, it might also be noted that in practically all of the successful experiments in social therapy, somewhere there has been a prime mover who instigated change and carried it through with the help of others.

Democratic group setting consistent with therapeutic goals. A group that functions under democratic processes rather than under authoritarian imposition is a group that holds therapeutic possibilities. Such a group recognizes individual worth and responsibility, yet it does not demand that the individual produce more than he is capable of doing. To the extent that the patient is able, this group does permit his participation in decisions affecting him and in carrying out those decisions.

Democracy is not mob rule. Authority exists in a democratic situation, but it resides in competency that is accepted by the group. Perhaps the greatest distinction between democratic and authoritarian approaches lies in the use of authority by each. In the authoritation approach, authority is used to impose decisions, to manipulate people, and to control situations in the interest of the authority figure. In the democratic approach, authority is used to promote the goals of the group. When mentally ill patients are in a democratic setting, the goals of such a group must necessarily be the improvement of patients' health status. Since this can hardly be achieved other than by patients, their participation in and commitment to this goal is imperative. Democratic processes foster such group orientation; authoritarian processes tend to negate it.

Therapeutic group characterized by permissiveness. A permissive group atmosphere is one in which patients are free to express and to explore their feelings. Such a group is feeling oriented rather than intellectually oriented. Patients are neither judged nor punished for expressed feelings, nor for what they do or have done. A premium is placed on facing emotional problems rather than on accomplishing things. This does not mean that patients are not brought face to face with the reaction of other patients to their behavior or expressions, but that the members of the group learn to focus on understanding themselves and others, rather than on judging and punishing each other.

A permissive atmosphere is one in which the patient is free to be himself. It includes respect for his limitations and for those abilities not limited by his illness. He is encouraged to assume all the responsibilities for himself that he can, and he is not required to assume responsibilities that he cannot handle.

Limitations within the group setting are clearly drawn and consistently enforced. These limitations are preferably set by the group within which the patient functions, including staff and patients, and all members of the group are responsible for the enforcement of limitations. Patients frequently show good insight into their own and other patients' behavior and can contribute much to defining and setting limitations. When group assets are used, however, the current level of behavior of the group must be the basis for approach. A unit of extremely regressed patients should be activated with limited goals, such as basic habit training for an immediate project. As patients improve, group goals can be raised.

Socialization and patient interaction with others supported and encouraged. The activity pattern of a ward unit should be organized to promote activities that encourage patient interaction with other patients and with staff. Activities that permit patients to function in isolated fashion without committing themselves in any personal or meaningful way to an activity are of doubtful value except as busy work. Tasks that can be carried out with others—that involve interpersonal contacts, joint decisions, joint planning, and joint activity—promote interaction. Such activities, particularly in a permissive setting, provide patients with an opportunity to explore their social skills and to improve them. The unit that allows or encourages patients to withdraw into themselves encourages regression.

If the staff will continually reach toward patients who tend to withdraw and allow them plenty of time to respond, personnel will forcibly realize that all too often the patient's ability to respond is vastly underestimated. Patients are aware of much that personnel do not recognize. They learn the pattern of behavior and the predominant social values of the setting in which they are placed and adapt themselves accordingly. If they are placed in a unit in which one of its primary goals is the interaction of the patients with others, the tendency to regress can often be reversed.

Therapeutic effect enhanced by close social relationship between staff and patients. The social distance between staff and patients in the traditional mental institution is wide. Most of the new social approaches to the treatment of patients have brought staff and patients more closely together, and they share meaningful tasks and participate in the life of the institution they share. In fact, there is some speculation that the factor that has produced results in patient improvement is related to this lessened social distance. Staff who become participants with patients, rather than observers or control agents, apparently positively affect the course of the illness of patients.

Actually, there exists a very close relationship between the interest and the involvement of staff and the participation of patients. There also exists a very close relationship between good therapeutic results and patient participation. It follows, therefore, that staff interest and personal involvement with patients has a genuine therapeutic effect.

Patients help themselves and each other. Given the opportunity, patients can help themselves get well. To a great extent, this has to do with the attitude of personnel who work with patients. Once this fact is accepted, it can then be carried into action. When the staff believes this, it becomes possible to offer patients such opportunities by respecting them as individuals and by permitting them to take an active part in their own therapy.

When patients are given an opportunity to help other patients, they are experiencing responsibility and satisfaction in a task that holds real meaning. There has been much discussion about the extent to which patients have helped each other get well. In some instances, recovered patients have testified that relationships with particular patients have been extremely helpful to them. In some of the more progressive hospitals, patients have definite assignments that include responsibility for the care of other patients. Such assignments range from responsibility for toileting a regressed patient to instructing groups of patients in a skill possessed by a particular patient. Such assignments and responsibilities for others have been demonstrated to be effective when the patient's ability to contribute has been carefully assessed and when the staff attitude toward the assigned task is positive.

Group approach more effective with patients who respond positively. When the nurse desires to approach a group with a suggestion or a question, it is usually more effective to direct the question or suggestion to a specific patient who can reasonably be expected to respond in a positive fashion. The pressure to conform, or not to disagree, that has infiltrated our society has also extended its influence into our hospitals, which reflect the society of which they are a part. Such an approach encourages others who are positively inclined to express themselves and brings some group pressure to support the desired outcome.

Social setting as realistic as patient limitations allow. The social organization of the therapeutic institution should not be at complete variance with the background from which patients come. If it is, the hospital can offer the patient little in better social adjustment and better social relationships on which to build in preparation for return to the community. This means that the institution should respect the rights of individuals, should be democratic in orientation, should allow for individual difference, and should value socially constructive behaviors.

In effect, it means that hospital organization, routines, and activities should support and encourage the kind of patient behavior that will be helpful to him when he returns to society.

Nurse's activities coordinated with all groups participating in patient care. When there is group participation in social therapy, the activities of all who have a part in the social situation must be coordinated in order to assure that the desired therapeutic goals are shared and implemented by all.

Groups within a therapeutic community exert influence on all persons within that community, both patients and staff. The nursing staff should be cognizant of such group processes and continuously observe and evaluate these processes so as to strengthen the therapeutic milieu. Since psychiatry is a multidisciplinary field there must be coordination and exploration of the roles of all the staff members, so as to enhance the effectiveness of the team. Team members can function smoothly, supporting each other in effecting positive patient intervention; or the team can be a highly destructive force within itself, thereby effecting negative therapeutic intervention.

REFERENCES

Aiken, L., and Aiken, J. L.: A systematic approach to the evaluation of interpersonal relationships, Am. J. Nurs. 73:863-867, 1973.

Alman, B.: Patients participate in nursing care conferences, Am. J. Nurs. 67:2331-2334, 1967.

American Nurses' Association: Standards for psychiatric mental health nursing practice, Kansas City, Mo., 1973, The Association.

Armstrong, S., and Rouslin, S.: Group psychotherapy in nursing practice, New York, 1963, The Macmillan Co.

Baumgartner, M.: Empathy. In Carlson, C. E., coordinator: behavioral concepts and nursing intervention, Philadelphia, 1970, J. B. Lippincott Co., pp. 29-31.

Bell, R. W.: Activity as a tool in group therapy, Perspect. Psychiatr. Care 8:84-91, 1970.

Berliner, A. K.: The two milieus in milieu therapy, Perspect. Psychiatr. Care 5:266-271, 1967.

Berne, E.: The structure and dynamics of organizations and groups, Philadelphia, 1963, J. B. Lippincott Co.

Bernstein, L., Brophy, M., McCarthy, M. J., and Roepe, R.: Teaching nurse-patient relationships; an experimental study, Nurs. Res. 3:80-84, 1954.

Caplan, G.: An approach to community mental health, New York, 1961, Grune & Stratton, Inc.

Duran, F. A., and Errion, G. D.: Perpetuation of chronicity in mental illness, Am. J. Nurs. 70:1707-1709, 1970.

Glasser, W.: Reality therapy, New York, 1965, Harper & Row, Publishers, pp. 5-41.

Goffman, E.: Asylums, New York, 1961, Doubleday & Co.

Goffman, E.: Stigma, Englewood Cliffs, N.J., 1965, Prentice-Hall, Inc.

Grob, S.: Psychiatric social clubs come of age! Proceedings of the Institute of Social Clubs for Former Psychiatric Patients, Hartford, 1968, The Connecticut Association for Mental Health.

Jones, M.: Beyond the therapeutic community, New Haven, Conn., 1968, Yale University Press.

Leininger, M.: The phenomenon of caring (part 5), American Nurses' Foundation, Nurs. Res. Rep. 12:2, 14, 1977.

Levin, P., and Berne, E.: Games nurses play, Am. J. Nurs. 72:483-487, 1972.

Luft, J.: Group processes: an introduction to group dynamics, Palo Alto, Calif., 1963, The National Press, p. 1.

Orlando, I. J.: The dynamic nurse-patient relationship, New York, 1961, G. P. Putnam's Sons.

Scheff, T. J.: Being mentally ill, Chicago, 1967, Aldine-Atherton, Inc.

Scheff, T. J., editor: Mental illness and social processes, New York, 1967, Harper & Row, Publishers.

Yalom, I. D.: The theory and practice of group psychotherapy, New York, 1970, Basic Books, Inc.

ADDITIONAL REFERENCES

Baker, F.: From community mental health to human service ideology, Am. J. Pub. Health 64:576-581, 1974.

Bentz, W. K., and Edgarton, J. W.: The consequences of labeling a person as mentally ill, Soc. Psychol. 6:29-33, 1971.

Bettelheim, B.: A home for the heart, New York, 1974, Alfred A. Knopf, Inc.

Bettelheim, B., and Sylvester, E.: Milieu therapy: indications and illustrations, Psychoanal. Rev. 36:54-68, 1949.

Chamberlain, A. S.: Visit to Gheel, Am. J. Nurs. 59:68-70, 1959.

Deloughery, G. W., Gebbie, K. M., and Newman, B. M.: Consultation and community organization in community mental health nursing, Baltimore, 1971, The Williams & Wilkins Co.

Eisenman, E. P.: Primary care in a mental health facility, Nurs. Outlook 24:640-645, 1976.

Marram, G. D.: The group approach in nursing practice, St. Louis, 1973, The C. V. Mosby Co.

Masserman, J., editor: Social psychiatry, vol. I, New York, 1974, Grune & Stratton, Inc.

Meldman, M. J., Neuman, B., Schaller, D., and Peterson, P.: Patients responses to nurse-psychotherapists, Am. J. Nurs. **71:**1150-1151, 1971.

Ozarin, L. D., and Spaner, F. E.: Mental health corporations: a new trend in providing services, Hosp. Community Psychiatry **25:**225-227, 1974.

Patterson, E. M.: Social system psychotherapy, Am. J. Psychother. **17:**396-409, 1973.

Rutledge, K. A.: The professional nurse as primary therapist: background perspective and opinion, J. Operational Psych. **5:**76-86, 1974.

Stubblebine, J. M., and Decker, J. B.: Are urban mental health centers worth it? Am. J. Psychother. **127:**909-912, 1971.

Underwood, P. R.: Communication through role playing, Am. J. Nurs. **71:**1184-1186, 1971.

CHAPTER 7

Crisis intervention, community psychiatry, and suicidal behavior

HISTORICAL DEVELOPMENT

The crisis approach to therapeutic intervention has been developed only within the past few decades and is based on a broad range of theories of human behavior, including those of Freud, Hartmann, Rado, Erikson, Lindemann, and Caplan. Its current acceptance as a recognized form of treatment cannot be directly related to any single theory of behavior; all have contributed to some degree. Our intent in presenting a historical overview is to create an awareness of the broad base of knowledge that is incorporated in its present practice. All theories of human behavior are not necessarily dependent on freudian concepts; however, the psychoanalytic theories of Freud are the major basis for further investigation of normal as well as abnormal human behavior.

Sigmund Freud was the first to demonstrate and apply the principle of causality as it relates to psychic determinism (Bellak and Small, 1965). Simply put, this principle states that every act of human behavior has its cause, or source, in the history and experience of the individual. It follows that causality is operative whether or not the individual is aware of the reason for his behavior. Psychic determinism is the theoretical foundation of psychotherapy and psychoanalysis.

An important outcome of Freud's deterministic position was his construction of a developmental or genetic psychology. Present behavior is understandable in terms of the life history or experience of the individual, and the crucial foundations for all future behavior are laid down in infancy and early childhood. Freud assumed that a reservoir of energy existing in the individual initiates all behavior. Events function as guiding influences, but they do not initiate behavior; they only serve to help mold it in certain directions (Ford and Urban, 1963).

Since the end of the nineteenth century, the concept of determinism has undergone many changes. Although the ego-analytic theorists have tended to go along with much of the freudian position, there are several respects in which they differ. As a group, they conclude that Freud had neglected the direct study of normal or healthy behavior (Ford and Urban, 1963).

Heinz Hartmann, an early ego analyst, postulated that the psychoanalytic theories of Freud could prove valid for normal as well as abnormal behavior. He emphasized that man's adaptation in early childhood as well as his ability to maintain his adaptation to his environment in later life must be considered. His concept of the ego as an organ of adaptation required further study of orientation to reality. He described man's searching for an environment as another form of adaptation, the fitting together of the individual and his society. Hartmann also believed that although the behavior of the individual is strongly influenced by his culture, there is a part of the personality that remains relatively free of this influence (Loewenstein, 1966).

Sandor Rado saw human behavior being based on the principles of motivation and adaptation. He viewed behavior in terms of its effect on the welfare of the individual, not just in terms of cause and effect. An organism achieves adaptation through interaction with its culture. The organism's patterns of interaction improve through adaptation, with the goal being the increase of possibilities for survival. Rado's adaptational psychotherapy emphasizes the immediate present without neglecting the influence of the developmental past. The primary concern is with failures in adaption *today*, what caused them, and what the individual must do to learn to overcome them. Interpretations always begin and end with the present; preoccupation with the past is discouraged. As quickly as insight is achieved, it is used to encourage the individual to enter his present, real-life situation repeatedly. Through practice the patient automatizes new patterns of healthy behavior. According to Rado, it is this automatization factor that is ultimately the curative process, not insight. He does not believe that it takes place passively in the doctor's office on a couch but actively in the reality of daily living (Salzman, 1962).

Erik Erikson further developed the theories of ego psychology, which complement those of Freud, Hartmann, and Rado, by focusing on the stages of development of the ego and on the theory of reality. His theory of development is characterized by an orderly sequence of development at particular stages, each depending on the other for successful completion. Erikson perceived eight stages of psychosocial development, spanning the entire life cycle of man and involving specific developmental tasks that must be solved in each phase. The solution that is achieved in each previous phase is applied in subsequent phases. Erikson's theory is important in that it offers an explanation of the individual's social development as a result of his encounters with his social environment. Another important element is his elaboration on the normal rather than the pathologic development of man's social interactions. Erikson integrated the biologic, cultural, and self-deterministic points of view in his eight stages of man's development and broadened the scope of traditional psychotherapy with his theoretic formulations of identity and identity crises. His theories have provided a basis for the work of others who further developed the concept of maturational crises and began serious consideration of situational crises and man's adaptation to his current environmental dilemma (Rappaport, 1959).

Lindemann's (1956) initial concern was in developing approaches that might contribute to the maintenance of good mental health and the prevention of emotional disorganization on a community level. In his study of bereavement reactions among the survivors of those killed in the Coconut Grove nightclub fire in Boston, he described both brief and abnormally prolonged grief reactions occurring in different individuals as a result of the loss of a significant person in their lives. Lindemann concluded that it could be profitable to develop a conceptual frame of reference constructed around the concept of an emotional crisis, as exemplified by the bereavement reactions. Certain events in the course of the life cycle of every individual can be described as hazardous situations—for example, bereavement, marriage, the birth of a child, and so forth. He speculated that in each of these situations emotional strain would be generated, stress would be experienced, and a series of adaptive mechanisms would occur that could lead either to mastery of the new situation or to failure with more or less lasting impairment of function. Lindemann's theoretical frame of reference led to the development of crisis intervention techniques, and in 1946 he and Caplan established a community-wide program of mental health in the Harvard area called the Wellesley Project.

According to Caplan (1961) the most important aspects of mental health are the state of the ego, the stage of its maturity, and the quality of its structure. Assessment of its state is based on three main areas: (1) the capacity of the person to withstand stress and anxiety and maintain ego equilibrium, (2) the degree of reality recognized and faced in solving problems, and (3) the repertoire of effective coping mechanisms available to the person in maintaining balance in his biopsychosocial field.

As a result of his work in Israel in 1948 and his later experiences in Massachusetts with Lindemann, Caplan evolved the concept of the importance of *crisis* periods in individual and group development.

Community psychiatry is now an established and recognized component of care. New concepts and new psychosocial problems arise continually. A difference is now perceived between long-term, psychoanalytic therapy of the individual and short-term, reality-oriented psychotherapy as practiced in community psychiatry.

According to Bellak (1964) community psychiatry evolved from multiple disciplines and is intrinsically bound to the development of psychoanalytic theory. The social and behavioral sciences that advanced during the first half of the century were predicated on psychodynamic hypotheses. At the same time, concepts of public health and epidemiology were advancing in community health programs.

The discovery and utilization of psychotropic drugs were important steps forward. They resulted in opportunities for open wards and rehabilitation of the hospitalized patient in his home milieu. It would be incorrect to assume that all of these factors merged spontaneously, creating a successful, structured cure for psychiatric illness. Rather, this was a slow process of trial and error, of widely different programs each striving to meet problems involving different interests, knowledge, and skills. Disciplines once separated in goals became aware of their interdependence in attaining mutually recognized goals. New, allied disciplines developed; roles changed and expanded. There was a diffusion of tasks, and lines between disciplines became more flexible.

The origin of day hospitals for the care of psychiatric patients grew out of a shortage of hospital beds, which forced premature discharges of patients to their homes, rather than as a treatment innovation. The first reported day hospital was associated with the First Psychiatric Hospital in Moscow in 1933. (Though this little known center probably had minimal effect on later developments in the western world [Dzhagarov, 1937] it is accurate to state that it was the first organized day hospital for individuals with severe mental illness.)

In the late 1930s, Bierer began the Marlborough Experiment in England. Patients lived outside the hospital as members of a therapeutic social club and were treated at day hospitals or part-time facilities. According to Bierer (1964), the primary goal of the program was to change the patient's concept of his role from that of a passive object of treatment to one of an active participant-collaborator. At the same time, the psychiatrist and staff had to reconceptualize the patient as a human being accessible to reason, emphasizing his strengths rather than concentrating on his psychopathology and conflicts. The reality of here and now was the focus of attention.

These innovations in attitude gave rise to the concept of the therapeutic community. The patient became a partner and collaborator with the staff and was granted equal rights, opportunities, and facilities. The medical staff and their assistants functioned as advisors. The patient group assumed responsibility for the behavior of its members, planned activities, planned their futures, and offered support to each other. Group and social methods that encouraged the constant interaction of the members were employed. With this frame of reference it was only natural that the general hospital should add to the various roles in which it serves the community that of becoming a focal point of preventive medicine and public health functions in psychiatry.

After the passage of the California Community Mental Health Act in 1958, the California Department of Mental Hygiene, in 1961, established the first state agency in the United States to undertake the training of specialists in community psychiatry. It was recognized that clinics were needed to accommodate those individuals in the community who were unfamiliar with established forms of psychiatric treatment. In January, 1962, the Benjamin Rush Center for Problems in Living, a division of the Los Angeles Psychiatric Service, a no-waiting, unrestricted intake, walk-in crisis intervention center, was opened. This center has several pertinent characteristics in its operation:

1. Treatment is usually offered the same day as the application, and always within 1 week.
2. There is a maximum of six visits, this limit in part being imposed by the theoretical consideration that a crisis is typically resolved within 4 to 6 weeks.
3. The major treatment emphasis is on specific problems of living, including life crises and/or psychiatric emergencies.
4. There has been an ongoing evaluation program since its opening.
5. Access is open without screening to persons regardless of diagnosis.

After more than 14 years of operation, the Benjamin Rush Center has accumulated considerable evidence that suggests that persons who come there are generally *not* the type who typically seek treatment in a traditional clinic. Their approach has been shown to bring forth persons who, while judged to be genuinely in need of psychiatric treatment, would not have sought traditional treatment because of reluctance to consider themselves sick, to assume the patient role, or to accept the stigma of psychiatric treatment. They seek short-term help but are unwilling or unable to make a long-term contractual agreement. The immediate-access feature of the Center undoubtedly allows persons to come into consultation who would have fallen by the wayside had there been a lengthy period of waiting.

THEORY AND METHODOLOGY

An understanding of the different meanings of the word "crisis" is necessary prior to the presentation of crisis methodology to avoid a multiplicity of confusion. The word "crisis" comes originally from the Greek word *krisis*, which means to separate or divide. In medicine, the word usually refers to that change in a disease process that indicates whether the result is to be recovery or death. In international relations a crisis often refers to an event or conflict, the outcome of which can determine war or peace. The Chinese characters that represent the word "crisis" mean either danger or opportunity. The outcome of a *psychologic crisis* can be either growth or deterioration—it is a decisive moment, a turning point.

Caplan (1961) states that crisis is characteristically self-limiting and lasts from 4 to 6 weeks. This constitutes a transitional period, representing both the danger of increased psychologic vulnerability and an opportunity for personality growth. In any situation the outcome may depend to a significant degree on the ready availability of appropriate help. Since time is at a premium, a therapeutic climate must be generated that commands the concentrated attention of both the therapist and the patient. A goal-oriented sense of commitment develops that is in sharp contrast to the more leisurely pace of traditional treatment modalities. The *minimum* therapeutic goal of crisis intervention is the psychologic resolution of the individual's immediate crisis and restoration to at least the level of functioning that existed prior to the crisis period. A *maximum* goal is improvement above the precrisis level.

Jacobson and associates (1968) state that crisis intervention can be divided into two major categories: generic or individual. The generic approach focuses on the characteristic course of the particular kind of crisis rather than on the psychodynamics of each individual in crisis. A treatment plan is directed toward an adaptive resolution of the crisis. Specific intervention measures are designed to be effective for all members of a given group rather than for the unique differences on one individual. Recognition of these behavioral patterns is an important aspect of preventive mental health.

The generic approaches to crisis intervention include "direct encouragement of adaptive behavior, general support, environmental manipulation, and anticipatory guidance. In brief, the generic approach emphasizes: specific events that occur to significant population groups, intervention oriented to crises related to these specific events, and intervention conducted by nonmental health professions" (Jacobson, Strickler, and Morley, 1968). This approach has been found to be an effective mode of intervention that can be learned and utilized by nonpsychiatric physicians, nurses, social workers, and the like.

The individual approach differs from the generic in its emphasis on assessment of the interpersonal and intrapsychic processes of the person in crisis. It is used in selected cases, usually those not responding to the generic approach. Intervention is planned to meet the unique needs of the individual in crisis and to reach a solution for the particular situation and circumstances that precipitated the crisis. This differs from the generic approach, which focuses on the characteristic course of a particular kind of crisis (Jacobson, Strickler, and Morley, 1968). Unlike extended psychotherapy, there is relatively little concern with the developmental part of the individual. Information from this source is seen as relevant only for the clues that may result in a better understanding of the present crisis situation.

Morley and his colleagues (1967) state there are certain specific steps involved in the technique of crisis intervention. Although each cannot be placed in a clearly defined category, typical intervention would pass through the following sequence of phases.

Assessment of the individual and his problem. This requires the therapist to focus on obtaining an accurate assessment of the precipitating event and the resulting crisis that brought the individual to seek professional help. One of the most important aspects of the assessment phase is to find out if the individual is suicidal or homicidal. The questions must be very direct and specific: "Are you planning to kill yourself . . . or someone else? How? When?" The therapist must find out and assess the lethality of the threat. Is the person merely thinking about it—or does he have a method picked out? Is it a lethal method—a loaded gun? Does he have a tall building or bridge picked out but will not reveal where? Can he tell when he plans to do it—for example, after the children leave for school? Usually, if the threat does not sound too immediate, the therapist can arrange for medication. However, if the method is carefully planned and the details specific, the individual should be sent for psychiatric evaluation and hospitalization in order to protect him or others in the community.

Planning for therapeutic intervention. After an accurate assessment is made of the crisis, intervention is planned. This is not designed to bring about major changes in the personality structure but to restore the person to at least his precrisis level of functioning. In this phase, determination is made of the length of time since the onset of the crisis. The precipitating event usually occurs from 1 to 2 weeks before the individual seeks help. It is important to determine how much the crisis has disrupted the individual's life and the effects of this disruption on others in his environment.

Intervention. The techniques of interventions depend greatly on the preexisting skills, creativity, originality, and flexibility of the therapist. Some of the following have been found to be useful.

1. Help the individual gain an intellectual understanding of his crisis situation. In many cases the individual can see *no* relationship between the hazardous situation that has occurred in his life and the extreme dis-

comfort he is feeling. A very direct approach must be used, describing to the individual the relationship between his feelings and the crisis and how it is affecting his life.

2. Help the individual bring out his current feelings that he has not been able to ventilate. Often the patient may have suppressed some of his true feelings, such as anger or hostility, toward someone he believes he should have nothing but love and respect for, such as a mother, father, or teacher. He may also deny feelings of grief or of guilt or not have completed the mourning and grief process after a bereavement. One immediate goal of intervention is to reduce tension by providing the opportunity for the individual to recognize his feelings and openly discuss them. It is sometimes vital to induce a mental catharsis to reduce immobilizing tension.

3. Explore his coping mechanisms. In this approach one assists the individual to examine alternative ways of coping with stress. If for some reason the coping behavior he has used in the past to successfully reduce tension and anxiety has not been tried, one can explore the possibility of its use in the current stressful situation.

4. Expand his social orbit. If his crisis has been precipitated by the loss of a significant individual in his life, it could be very effective if one introduces the possibility of new people to help fill the void. This can be very helpful if the supports and gratifications provided by the loss of a significant other can be achieved in a similar way from the establishing of new relationships.

Resolution of the crisis and anticipatory planning for the future. In this phase one reinforces those adaptive coping behaviors that the individual has used successfully to relieve his tension, anxiety/depression, and stress. As his coping abilities increase, positive changes occur and his ability to solve problems increases. These positive changes may be summarized for him to help him reexperience and reaffirm for himself the progress he has made. He can be assisted, as needed, in making realistic plans for the future. It is feasible to discuss the ways in which the present experience can help him cope in potential future crises.

SITUATIONAL AND MATURATIONAL CRISES

Whenever stressful events occur in an individual's life that threaten his biologic, psychologic, or social integrity, there is some degree of disequilibrium resulting and the concurrent possibility of a crisis. According to Rapoport (1962), when an instinctual need or a sense of integrity is threatened, the ego usually responds characteristically with anxiety; when loss or deprivation occur, the response is usually depression. On the other hand, if the threat or loss is viewed as a challenge, there is more likely to be a mobilization of energy toward purposeful problem-solving activities.

Something that may create only a feeling of mild concern in one person may create a high level of anxiety and tension in another. Studies have been made of behavior patterns that might be anticipated in response to common stressful situations. These studies have provided valuable clues to anticipatory planning for prevention as well as intervention in crisis situations. Some of these are combat neurosis (Glass, 1957), relocation through urban renewal (Brown, Burditt, and Lidell, 1965), rehabilitation of families after tornado disasters (Moore, 1958), hospitalized children and adolescents (Vernick, 1963), unwed mothers (Bernstein, 1960), and separation anxiety of hospitalized children (Bowlby, 1960). These studies suggest that there are certain patterned phases of reactions to unique stressful situations through which select groups of people can be expected to pass before equilibrium is restored. Preventive techniques of community psychiatry focus on anticipatory intervention; this is to prevent crises that could result from maladaptive responses as individuals attempt to return to equilibrium.

Situational crises refer to those events that may occur in the environment that may be stressful to the individual and thus may cause a crisis. Some of these events could be things like the birth of a baby. This requires a change in the living pattern. There may be feelings of inadequacy in caring for the infant or resentment because of a loss of freedom, either of which could be compounded by fatigue, since caring for a new baby is a 24-hour job. Even more stressful could be the birth of a premature baby or one handicapped either physically or mentally. There may be guilt feelings or a feeling of "What did I do wrong?" There may be shame and resentment: "How could I—who am so 'normal'—produce something so abnormal?"

A physical illness or accident can be, and usually is, a stressful event. There are many fears to contend with, such as "Will I live?" "Will I be all right?" "What about my future? my job? my family?" This is particularly true when it involves the loss of a body part, such as an arm, leg, eye, or breast. This is very threatening to body image and the self-concept.

Circumstances that are involved in divorce or separation can also be crisis-precipitating events. There is a feeling of loss or a sense of failure, and there may be guilt.

The death of a loved one is particularly stressful. There is a sense of loss and feelings of hopelessness and helplessness. Guilt feelings are common in those working through the grief process. But as with any loss the grief work, though painful, must be done. The family's reaction to the death of a member develops in stages varying in time. The death of a loved one must produce an active expression of feeling in the normal course of events. Omission of such a reaction is to be considered as much a variation from the normal as is an excess in time and intensity. Unmanifested grief will be found expressed in some way or another, and each new loss can cause grief for the current loss as well as reactivate the grieving process of previous episodes.

There are many other situations that can be stressful and thus produce a crisis. Some of these could be the loss of a job, loss of status, a promotion— almost anything that involves a loss or a change in life situations. This is why it is sometimes difficult to determine whether a crisis is caused by situational events or maturational events; sometimes there is an overlap, with one compounding the other.

Maturational crises have been described as normal processes of growth and development. They usually evolve over an extended period of time, such as the transition into adolescence, and they frequently require that the individual make many character changes. There may be an awareness of increased feelings of disequilibrium, but intellectual understanding of any correlation with normal developmental change may be inadequate.

Erikson (1950, 1959, 1963) believes that each maturational stage must be successfully negotiated, otherwise it creates problems later in life. Some of these stages are preschool, school age, preadolescence, adolescence, young adulthood (which involves studying for a specific career or seeking employment), late adulthood (with menopause and the male climacteric), and finally old age (with its problems of chronicity and retirement). We believe that "maturational crises" may be a misnomer. While it is true these stages produce stress, not every adolescent or every woman entering menopause, for example, develops a crisis.

According to Caplan (1964), man is constantly faced with a need to solve problems in order to maintain equilibrium. When he is confronted with an imbalance between the difficulty of a problem as he perceives it and his available coping skills, a crisis may be precipitated. If alternatives cannot be found or if solving the problem requires more time and energy than usual, disequilibrium occurs. Tension rises and discomfort is experienced, with feelings of anxiety, fear, guilt, shame, and helplessness.

One purpose of the crisis approach is to provide the services of a therapist skilled in problem-solving techniques. This does not mean that the therapist will have an answer to every problem. However, he will be expected to have a ready and knowledgeable competency in problem-solving, guiding and supporting the patient toward crisis resolution.

Problem-solving requires that a logical sequence of reasoning be applied to a situation in which an answer is required for a question and in which there is no immediate source of reliable information. This process may take place either consciously or unconsciously. Usually the need to find an answer or solution is felt more strongly where such a resolution is most difficult.

The problem-solving process follows a structured, logical order of steps, each depending on the preceding one. In the routine decision-making required in daily living, this process is rarely necessary. Most people are unaware that they may follow a defined, logical sequence of reasoning in making decisions, often only remarking that some solutions seem to have been reached more easily than others.

When professional help is sought because a person is in crisis, the therapist must use logic and background knowledge to define the problem and plan intervention. The model for problem-solving in the crisis approach will be readily familiar to nurses who have become skilled in making nursing judgments. It will be particularly familiar to mental health nurses.

It is important that both the therapist and the patient be able to define a situation clearly before taking any action to change it. Questions are asked such as "What do I need to know?" and "What must be done?" The more specifically the problem can be defined, the more likely it is that the "correct" answer will be sought. It is important to remember that the therapist's task is that of focusing on the immediate problem. There is not enough time and no need to go into the patient's past history in depth. The therapist could not care less what happened when the patient was 5 years old. Since they have *only* six weeks, the patient and the therapist have to work on solving the immediate problem.

In crisis the precipitating event usually occurs 10 to 14 days before the patient seeks help. Frequently it is something that happened the day before or the night before. It could be almost anything: threat of divorce, discovery of an extramarital affair, finding out that a son or daughter is on drugs, loss of a boyfriend or girlfriend, an unwanted pregnancy, and so forth. Between the perceived effects of a stressful situation and the resolution of the problem are three recognized balancing factors that may determine the state of equilibrium. Strengths or weaknesses in any one of these factors can be directly related to the onset of crisis or to its resolution. These are perception of the event, available situational supports, and coping mechanisms.

Perception of the event. If the event is perceived realistically, there will be recognition of the relationship between the event and feelings of stress. Problem-solving can be appropriately oriented toward reduction of tension, and successful solution of the stressful situation will be more probable.

If the perception of the event is distorted, there may be no recognition of a relationship between the event and feelings of stress. Thus attempts to solve the problem will be ineffective, and tension will not be reduced. In other words, what does the event mean to the individual? How is it going to affect his future? Can he look at it realistically, or does he distort its meaning?

Situational supports. By nature, man is social and dependent on others in his environment to supply him with reflected appraisals of his own intrinsic and extrinsic values. In establishing his life patterns, certain appraisals are more significant to him than others because they tend to reinforce the perception he has of himself. Dependency relationships may be more readily established with those whose appraisals tend to support the individual against feelings of insecurity and who reinforce feelings of ego integrity.

Loss, threatened loss, or feelings of inadequacy in a supportive relationship may leave the individual in a vulnerable position, so that when confronted with a stressful situation, the lack of situational support may lead to a state of disequilibrium and possible crisis.

Situational supports mean those persons who are available in the environment who can be depended on to help solve the problem. Who is his best friend? Whom does he trust? With whom does he live? Is there a family member he feels especially close to?

Coping mechanisms. Available coping mechanisms are what people usually do when they have a problem. They may sit down and try to think it out or talk it out with a friend. Some cry it out or try to get rid of their feelings of anger and hostility by swearing, kicking a chair or the cat, or slamming doors. Others may get into verbal battles with friends. Some may react by temporarily withdrawing from the situation in order to reassess the problem. These are just a few of the many coping methods people use to relieve their tension and anxiety when faced with a problem. Each of these has been used at some time in the developmental past of the individual, has been found effective to maintain emotional stability, and has become part of his life-style in meeting and dealing with the stresses of daily living.

SUICIDE

The development of suicide prevention centers is an important part of the broadly developing field of crisis intervention and community psychiatry. For one reason or another, suicide as a subject of serious study has been neglected. The basic assumption underlying all medical services, and those include many occupations, is that life is better than death. The goal of health services is to keep persons alive as long as possible. Those who negate the whole value system of the establishment by taking their own lives have posed serious value problems for the members of that establishment. Although it is not true in all cultures, in American culture suicide has been looked on as a sign of weakness or mental instability and has carried with it a stigma that is attached to all who survive a suicide attempt. Research has pointed out that the suicidal person is ambivalent toward life and death and that, as a consequence, prevention offers hitherto unsuspected opportunities. Suicidal thoughts and attempts have been labeled a cry for help. Suicide is a problem that affects and confronts all members of the community, especially those in the helping professions. They must learn how to hear the cry for help and respond to it appropriately.

Some of the statistics in regard to suicide and suicidal attempts are misleading. Reporting is not accurate. The yearly world death rate by suicide averages about thirteen persons in every 100,000. In the United States, one person dies by his own hand every 24 minutes. Suicide is the eleventh leading cause of death in the general population; it ranks second as a cause of death for adolescents and college students. This tragic loss of life is even greater than the known statistics indicate, since we must consider the unknown proportion of deaths classified as accidental poisonings, traffic accidents, and other untimely occurrences. Because of cultural and societal taboos, insurance coverage, and family protection, many deaths are assigned different causal factors. In addition, many authorities believe that the so-called accidental deaths from alcoholism and substance abuse are indeed hidden suicides.

Suicide does not limit itself to any particular age. Statistics show suicide as an ever-increasing problem of advanced age. For attempted suicide the pattern is different, since it is practiced more by young people. Traditionally, women attempt suicide more than men; however, recently young men are attempting suicide more frequently. Many of those who attempt suicide will try again, a number with lethal success. No single group, no race, or no class of people is free from self-inflicted death. Except for a very few cases most of the people who commit suicide want desperately to live—this is the irony!

Why does a man kill himself? Even a tragic upset does not alone explain why a person would take his own life. What makes this person different from others? Why do some give up? These questions have puzzled mankind for centuries, and within the last 100 years, certain scientifically tenable explanations have been found. Sociologic theories by Durkheim (1951) postulated three basic types of suicide, each a result of man's relationship to his society. Durkheim considered altruistic suicide as literally required by society. Customs and rules can demand suicide, as exemplified by the Japanese practice of hara-kiri and the Hindu widow who willingly cremates herself on her deceased husband's funeral pyre. In such cases, self-inflicted death is honorable. Durkheim saw most American suicides as egoistic. Egoistic suicide occurs in an individual who has too few ties with his community. In this case, there is no demand to live. He described anomic suicides as those suicides that occur when the established relationship between the individual and his society is suddenly shattered. Examples would include the shocking, immediate loss of a job, loss of a family member or close friend, or loss of wealth or possessions.

Freud fathered the psychologic explanations of suicide. To him, suicide was within the mind or the psyche of the person. Freud identified the aggressive destructive drive, thanatos, which is seen as the energy necessary to complete this act. A person ambivalently identifies with the object of his own love. In frustration, the aggressive side of ambivalence is directed in, against the internalized person. Psychoanalytically, suicide is seen as "murder in the 180th degree."

More recent theories, which have both sociologic and psychologic influence, are seeking to explain suicide. Hendin (1964) suggests suicide is a barometer of social tension. Suicide can be seen in terms of various levels of pressure on men; some of that pressure is causative to suicide. Thus, earlier traumatic experiences exerting underlying tensions, aggravated by unfortunate interpersonal experiences such as the end of a love affair, can precipitate an attempt at self-destruction. The toll of suicide cannot be communicated with statistics alone. It affects the lives of one out of ten people in the United States. The number of lives lost unnecessarily is incalculable. There is irrevocable damage to the survivors. All this has led to the demand that suicidal cries be heard. By 1966, more than 100 suicide prevention centers were functioning in the United States. At the same time, the federal government established The Center for Studies of Suicide Prevention in the National Institute of Mental Health. This agency supports research into suicide, its clues, causes, and prevention, and the agency prepares personnel to deal with suicide problems. The recent interest in the study prevention of suicide is long overdue.

The first concern with the prevention of suicide came from lay people rather than health personnel. The National Save-A-Life League was established in New York in 1906 by the Baptist minister, Henry Warren. In 1959, Father Kenneth Murphy organized Boston's Rescue, Incorporated. Although, as is so often true, private organizations blazed the way, with their efforts serving to demonstrate the need and the methods of meeting it, they were unable to meet the need itself.

One of the outstanding prototypes of the developing suicide centers, the Los Angeles Suicide Prevention Center, was established in 1958 by two clinical psychologists, Norman L. Faberow and Edwin S. Shneidman. The center with its ambitious goals was supported by federal funds. Three aspects of suicide prevention became its major goals. These were (1) saving of lives by identifying presuicidal persons and bringing them help, (2) using community resources to accomplish this goal, and (3) doing research into the total problem of suicide. As a result of their practice and research, these psychologists are now firmly convinced that suicide is preventable because persons who think about and commit suicide give indications in advance and are basically ambivalent about suicide itself.

Suicidal behavior. Almost anyone who seriously contemplates suicide leaves clues. Sometimes the clues are obvious hints, sometimes only subtle changes in behavior. The suicidal decision itself is not impulsive; it is often premeditated and at times meticulously prepared for. The suicidal act, in and of itself, may be impulsive in nature, but that decision has been given long consideration. It is not impossible, then, to spot potential suicide individuals.

The suicidal state of mind comes and goes. There is no single trait by which all individuals can be characterized. However, the person is disturbed and is often depressed. There is a feeling of hopelessness about the direction of his life and a feeling of helplessness concerning what to do about it. This attitude reflects itself in various verbal and behavioral clues. These clues are frequently the obvious self-pitying cries that threaten, "I'm going to kill myself" and "I can't stand it any longer." These threats should not be ignored since the individual usually means it; he just has not decided how or when. If conditions do not change for the person, the time and place will soon be set. All verbal indications of suicide should be taken seriously.

Behavioral hints of suicide attempts are usually quite obvious. A suicide attempt, no matter how feeble, is a serious indication of the suicidal intent. "He just wanted attention" is a jeering comment that often mocks a person following a suicide attempt. Without attention, however, the person may well succeed in his next attempt. Statistics suggest that four out of five persons who commit suicide have attempted to do so previously. Once a person has finally made the decision to kill himself, he begins to act differently. Patterns of acute withdrawal or relief of depression may occur. Withdrawal is severe, with decrease in eating and conversation, a change in sleeping habits, and a lack of sexual drive. It is as if the person were going on a long and distant trip. Conversely, severely depressed patients frequently look better. The decision-making process relieves the depression; hence, there is the necessary energy to carry out the planned act. At this point the safety precautions of those near the individual are often slackened, since it appears as if the person is getting better. Frequently, in both types of response the person gives away highly valued possessions.

That communication is one of the central and most important tools of suicide prevention should come as no surprise, but the fact that the telephone is one of the first lines of defense may come as a bit of surprise to some of the more traditional health professionals. In suicide prevention centers, prevention begins when the telephone rings. While listening is an important part of the process, information must also be obtained, and a judgment must be made as to whether the situation constitutes an immediate emergency. The person who answers the cry for help must assess the degree of the caller's stress, find out if the caller is a stable person responding to unusual situational pressure or an unstable person with a history of suicidal attempts, and determine whether he belongs to a group with the highest statistical risk. Among the more important information to be obtained is the caller's plan for committing suicide. The more specific and realistic the plan, the greater the danger. The staff member offers the caller a lifeline to the community resources that can help him. The crisis period is not the time for nondirective approaches.

The staff member cannot help to solve all the problems of the deeply troubled suicidal person. The imminent suicide attempt, however, can be averted, and the crisis can be managed. A person in this state actively seeking help, even though he might not verbally accept it, is displaying ambivalence, the wish to live and the wish to die. The goals of a suicide prevention service are limited. The primary goal is to stop the person from killing himself, not to remake a personality. When a person is floundering, a lifeline must be thrown to him. This is not the time to teach the drowning person how to swim. If the situation is critical, the staff member must come up with an answer to relieve the distress temporarily. Helping the person see life and his problem in a broader sense is important. In crisis, alternatives are difficult for the person to comprehend, since situations are seen rigidly—black or white, good or bad, yes or no, life or death. It is also important to arrange things for this person by setting up interviews that may provide further tension relief.

Perhaps the crisis intervention theorists, including those involved in suicide prevention, highlight most clearly the importance of individual nursing care plans and an understanding of the need for priorities in nursing care. The nurse needs a repertoire of behavioral responses and the ability to diagnose situations and people to respond appropriately. The only generalizations that seem to apply are the need for ego support for the individual in crisis and the mobilization and use of a wide range of resources.

Suicide prevention has also been of concern in the general hospital setting. Hospitalized patients who are depressed or confused present special problems concerning the identification of their suicide potential. Because hospitals are commonly thought of as places for prolonging, preserving, and enhancing life, the suicide of a hospitalized patient comes as a shock. Many persons feel the blow of such an action. Often there is suspicion or accusations of negligence and the threat of legal action. In terms of statistics the actual number is small, but in terms of responsibility the same number seems overwhelming.

Accident prevention and safety measure enforcement are imperative. How many confused and disoriented patients have gone out of windows, thinking they were doors? It is estimated that 200 hospitalized patients per year die in this manner. It is not uncommon to find suicidal attempts by overdosage. Some patients may save and hoard their pills as well as those of other patients. How many well-meaning but careless nurses have left medication at the patient's bedside, only to have it hoarded until the right time? Infrequently, but it still occurs, some patients remove the knife from the dinner tray, again in the preparation of a suicidal act. Most of these medical-surgical patients share common experiences, those of chronic illnesses, isolation, and a downhill course of events in their lives. There has often been a noticeable inability to adjust to the hospital. One fact remains clear; most of these patients gave clues and cries for help that went unheard or ignored!

For nurses everywhere, and especially for psychiatric nurses, the specter of patient suicide is ever present. When a patient communicates suicidal ideas, what is the nurse's responsibility, and what can be considered effective intervention?

Suicide is a cry for help. It is an act intended to stop an intolerable existence. Suicidal communication is a rescue operation. A person cries for help, and someone must be willing to hear that cry. Someone must also be capable of responding to that cry. Most well-intentioned and caring nurses do attempt to meet and respond to that cry. Often efforts are blocked in carrying out plans of approach. Unfortunately, at times cries are not heard, or they are neglected.

Appropriate intervention should lead to the dissolution of the need to threaten suicide. Of prime importance is the protection of the patient from his self-destructive behavior until he is able to protect himself. Again, we are dealing with the concept of ambivalence. Once time can be gained and a therapeutic relationship has begun, then the work can be focused on the underlying dynamics. The suicidal person must be helped to express his feelings of aggression and hostility outwardly and in a constructive manner, rather than turning them inward. Also, the person has to be helped to achieve a more realistic concept of himself.

A therapeutic nurse-patient relationship provides support and understanding based on a nonjudgmental approach to the manner in which the patient is acting out his problems. In assessing a nursing care plan of approach, one must consider long- and short-term goals. Long-term goals are integrating concepts to which the patient can eventually strive. As an example, long-term goals may include the broad concept of trust, the need to be accepted, the need for love, and the need for increasing independence and autonomy. Short-term goals are tools with which to move toward these integrating concepts. As an example, these goals may include being available to listen, being nonjudgmental in attitude, giving assurance that someone is interested and concerned, giving assurance by actions and by words that uncontrollable self-destructive behavior will be controlled by staff, seeking acceptable and constructive methods to deal with tension, not rewarding sick behavior, and providing continuity.

It must be stressed that these are only guidelines for basic assessment. Every person must be evaluated and assessed individually, based on his situation, his background, and, most importantly, his needs. The nursing care plan must be prepared by all the staff involved to ensure its accuracy and continuity; effort is needed to carry out the nursing plan. Time passes slowly when one awaits the results of long-term goals. A patient, or for that matter any person, does not build trust in another person or a group of people in a day or a week. It takes time, attention, and interest to jump the many hurdles in the challenge of developing a relationship.

The following case study is presented to illustrate the crisis model as a therapeutic modality as it is used in suicidal cases.

> Barbara was a 28-year-old, unmarried, attractive, and apparently intelligent young woman. She had moved to the city from a small midwest town approximately a year and a half ago. She had a responsible position in a nearby bank and stated that she did not particularly enjoy her work, since everyone was much older than she. She had only one close girlfriend, who lived in her apartment building; otherwise she was more or less a social isolate. When questioned about dating and boyfriends, she stated that she had been going steady with one young man, Phil, for the past 4 months.
>
> When questioned about her reasons for coming to the crisis center, she attempted to avoid answering the question by stating that she had been planning to enter therapy for some time because she had trouble making and keeping friends.
>
> Physically she appeared to be in rigid control of her emotions and feelings. She sat very straight in her chair with her hands clasped tightly in her lap. The therapist pointed out her rigidity to her and then asked her what she was really afraid of—what had happened that she felt she must have help today?
>
> Barbara was silent for a few moments and then blurted out, "I am afraid I am going to kill myself!" When asked why she felt this way she replied: "I tried before, in my home town, and under similar circumstances." She was asked, "What circumstances?" She replied that she had been dating a man, Jim, for 6 months and felt that he truly loved her; then he told her that he wasn't going to date her again because she was too possessive. When asked how she had attempted suicide before, she stated with a wry smile, "I almost was successful." Again she was asked "How?" She stated that she had taken an overdose of Seconal, stuffed towels under the doors and windows of her apart-

ment, turned on all the gas jets on the stove, and lay down in bed. She said that she was in the hospital for 3 weeks recuperating and was in a coma most of the time. The therapist asked if she had left a note or called anyone before she tried to kill herself. She replied, very emphatically, "*No, I wanted to die!*" When asked how she was found, she stated someone in the apartment building smelled gas and they started checking all of the apartments and discovered her barely alive.

The therapist focused on the "same circumstances" and asked Barbara to explain what she meant. She said that she and Phil were really becoming very close in their relationship and that she was afraid she was beginning to get possessive with him. Apparently, he had called to break a date, explaining that he had an unexpected business appointment, but she didn't believe him. She felt that he was getting ready to reject her because (1) he really didn't love her and (2) he was getting tired of driving up from the beach to date her.

The event that precipitated Barbara's crisis was believed to be her anticipation of rejection by Phil. Her past history of suicide, overdosing, is not high on the list of lethality; but her method (pills and gas), the fact that she did not attempt to let anyone know she was contemplating suicide (cry for help), and her impulsivity made her potentially a high risk for suicide. The immediate goal of intervention was to explore any method or plan she may have for suicide. The secondary goal was to get her to perceive the event realistically and provide situational support during the crisis period.

Because she was judged by the therapist to be high on suicidal lethality, this area was covered thoroughly during the first session. Barbara was questioned intently regarding any plans she had for suicide. She stated that she had purchased a revolver—to protect herself since she lived alone—and would use the gun: "This time I'll make it."

The therapist insisted on a written contract with Barbara. This included a commitment on her part that she would call her girlfriend and have her bring the gun in for the therapist to keep until it was felt that it would be safe for her to have it again. She was committed to call the therapist—day or night—if she felt depressed, anxious, or out of control. In the contract Barbara also agreed that she would not seek any other method of suicide while in therapy.

Barbara's girlfriend was called and she brought the gun (loaded) to the center. The therapist unloaded it, put Barbara's name and the date on it, and placed it in the safe. While waiting for the gun to arrive the therapist explored with Barbara her true feelings about Phil. She stated that she did love him and was hoping that they would eventually get married. When asked if Phil would come to the center to meet with the therapist she replied, "I don't know —but I'll ask him."

During the next sessions the therapist worked with Barbara and Phil. He was a very pleasant, ambitious young man. When questioned about his feelings about Barbara he stated that he too hoped that their relationship would lead to marriage. He did state that he felt that they should get to know each other better and that he *was* getting tired driving up from the beach to see her so often. This provoked laughter from all of them. The therapist asked Barbara if she would consider moving to the beach so they could see more of each other. She seemed startled and asked Phil what he thought; he was

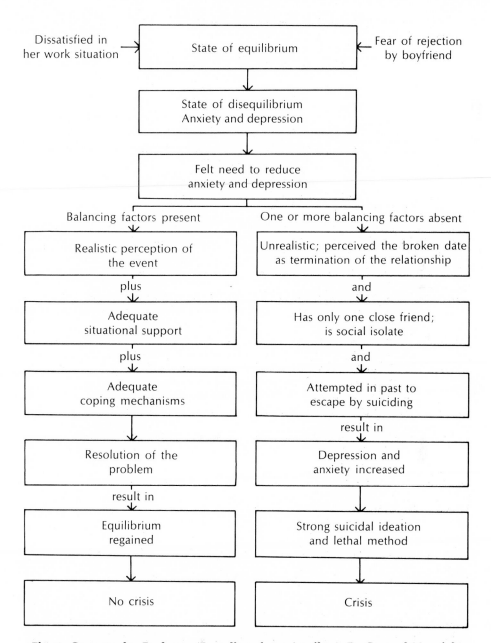

Fig. 1. Case study: Barbara. (Paradigm from Aguilera, D. C., and Messick, J. M.: Crisis intervention: theory and methodology, ed. 3, St. Louis, 1978, The C. V. Mosby Co.)

very enthusiastic and said he could probably get her an apartment in his building.

The rest of the sessions were spent with them making plans for Barbara's move to the beach. She had asked for and was granted a transfer from her present employment to a smaller branch bank at the beach. Phil had found her an apartment and they both appeared happy and relaxed. Time was spent in reviewing with Barbara the progress she had made and the need for her to have full, open communication not only with Phil but with all of her friends.

At the end of the last session the therapist gave Barbara her contract to tear up; she refused and said, "I want to keep it—to remember how stupid I was." When asked if she wanted the gun back, she laughed and said, "No way, I don't need it!" Termination was by mutual consent and Barbara was told that she could return to the center if she had any problems in the future.

This case study concerned a young woman with a high suicide potential. Assessment of the precipitating events indicated that Barbara was anticipating rejection from her boyfriend, Phil, and was unhappy in her work.

The focus of therapy was to minimize the suicidal potential, provide situational support, secure a contract, and help Barbara ventilate her feelings of inadequacy. Environmental manipulation was used by suggesting that she move to the beach to be closer to Phil. Collateral therapy was used when Phil agreed to attend the therapy sessions to help resolve the crisis.

REFERENCES

Aguilera, D. C., and Messick, J. M.: Crisis intervention: theory and methodology, ed. 3, St. Louis, 1978, The C. V. Mosby Co.

Bellak, L., editor: Handbook of community psychiatry and community mental health, New York, 1964, Grune & Stratton, Inc.

Bellak, L., and Small, L.: Emergency psychotherapy and brief psychotherapy, New York, 1965, Grune & Stratton, Inc.

Bernstein, R.: Are we still stereotyping the unmarried mother? Social Work 5:22-28, 1960.

Bierer, J.: The Marlborough experiment. In Bellak, L., editor: Handbook of community psychiatry and community mental health, New York, 1964, Grune & Stratton, Inc.

Bowlby, J.: Separation anxiety, Int. J. Psychoanal. 41:89-113, 1960.

Brown, H. F., Burditt, V. B., and Lidell, W. W.: The crisis of relocation. In Parad, H. J., editor: Crisis intervention, New York, 1965, Family Service Association of America, pp. 248-260.

Caplan, G.: An approach to community mental health, New York, 1961, Grune & Stratton, Inc.

Caplan, G.: Principles of preventive psychiatry, New York, 1964, Basic Books, Inc., Publishers.

Durkheim, E.: Suicide, New York, 1951, The Free Press. (First published in 1897.)

Dzhagarov, M. A.: Experience in organizing a day hospital for mental patients, Neuropathol. Psikhiatria 6:147, 1937.

Erikson, E. H.: Growth and crisis of the healthy personality. In Senn, M. J. E., editor: Symposium on the healthy personality, New York, 1950, Josiah Macy, Jr., Foundation.

Erikson, E. H.: Identity and the life cycle, Psychol. Issues 1(1):1959.

Erikson, E. H.: Childhood and society, ed. 2, New York, 1963, W. W. Norton & Co.

Faberow, N. L., and Shneidman, E. S.: The cry for help, New York, 1965, McGraw-Hill Book Co.

Fallon, B.: And certain thoughts go through my head, Am. J. Nurs. 72:1257-1259, 1972.

Ford, D. H., and Urban, H. B.: Systems of psychotherapy, New York, 1963, John Wiley & Sons, Inc.

Glass, A. T.: Observations upon the epidemiology of mental illness in troops during warfare, Symposium on Preventive and Social Psychiatry, Walter Reed Army Institute of Research, Washington, D.C., 1957, U.S. Government Printing Office.

Hendin, H.: Suicide and Scandinavia, New York, 1964, Grune & Stratton, Inc.

Jacobson, G., Strickler, M., and Morley, W.: Generic and individual approaches to crisis intervention, Am. J. Pub. Health 58:339-342, 1968.

Lindemann, E.: The meaning of crisis in individual and family, Teachers Coll. Rec. 57:310, 1956.

Loewenstein, R. M.: Psychology of the ego. In Alexander, F., Eisenstein, S., and Grotjahn, M., editors: Psychoanalytic pioneers, New York, 1966, Basic Books, Inc.

McCulloch, J. W., and Phillips, A. E.: Suicidal behavior, New York, 1972, Pergamon Press.

McLean, L. J.: Action and reaction in suicidal crisis, Nurs. Forum 8(1):29-41, 1969.

Moore, H. E.: Tornadoes over Texas; a study of Waco and San Angelo in disaster, Austin, 1958, University of Texas Press.

Morley, W. E., Messick, J. M., and Aguilera, D. C.: Crisis: paradigms of intervention, J. Psychiatr. Nurs. 5:537-538, 1967.

Rapoport, L.: The state of crisis: some theoretical considerations, Social Service Rec. 36:211-217, 1962.

Rappaport, D.: A historical survey of psychoanalytic ego psychology. In Klein, G. S., editor: Psychological issues, New York, 1959, International Universities Press.

Salzman, L.: Developments in psychoanalysis, New York, 1962, Grune & Stratton, Inc.

Shneidman, E. S., Faberow, N. L., and Litman, R. E.: The psychology of suicide, New York, 1970, Science House, Inc., pp. 125-245, 165-174, 259-273, 429-441, 449, 461.

Shneidman, E. S., and Mandelkorn, P.: How to prevent suicide, Public Affairs pamphlet no. 406, New York, 1967, Public Affairs Committee.

Umscheid, Sr. Theophane: With suicidal patients: caring for is caring about, Am. J. Nurs. 67:1230-1232, 1967.

Vernick, J.: The use of the life space interview on a medical ward, Social Casework 44:465-469, 1963.

Wallace, M. A.: The nurse and suicide prevention, Nurs. Outlook 15:55-57, 1967.

ADDITIONAL READINGS

Bahra, R. J.: The potential for suicide, Am. J. Nurs. 75(10):1782-1788, 1975.

Bayer, M.: Suicide: some children really mean it, RN 38(9):23, 1975.

Bayer, M.: Easing mental patient's return to their communities, Am. J. Nurs. 76(3):406-408, 1976.

Berry, C., and others: Community care for the mentally ill, Nurs. Times 72(21):804-805, 1976.

Bray, S. E.: When prevention fails: suicide, Part II, J. Pract. Nurs. 26(1):19-20, 1976.

Corsini, R. J., editor: Current psychotherapies, Itasca, Ill., 1973, F. E. Peacock Publishers, Inc.

Cunningham, R.: What do nurses do to help patients who attempt suicide? Can. Nurse 71(1):27-29, 1973.

Delbridge, P. M.: Identifying the suicidal person in the community, Can. Nurse 70(11):14-27, 1974.

Farewell, T.: Crisis intervention, Nurs. Mirror 143(10):60-61, 1976.

Fisher, S. A.: Suicide and crisis intervention, New York, 1973, Springer Publishing Co.

Friedeman, J. S.: Cry for help: suicide in the aged, J. Gerontol. Nurs. 2(3):28-32, 1976.

Merrifield, P. R., Guilford, J. P., Christensen, P. R., and Frick, J. W.: The role of intellectual factors in problem-solving, Psychol. Monogr. 76(10):12-16, 1962.

Sharpe, S.: Role of the community psychiatric nurse, Nurs. Mirror 141(16):60-62, 1975.

Shields, L.: Crisis intervention: implications for the nurse, J. Psychiatr. Nurs. 13(5):37-42, 1975.

Small, L.: The briefer psychotherapies, New York, 1971, Brunner/Mazel, Publishers.

Westercamp, T. M.: Suicide, Am. J. Nurs. 75(2):260-262, 1975.

PATIENTS WITH DYSFUNCTIONAL BEHAVIOR PATTERNS

CHAPTER 8

Patients with depressive and withdrawal patterns

DEPRESSION

Depression rivals anxiety as the most important and inclusive category in psychopathology. It is a neurotic symptom and is the salient feature of three psychoses: manic-depressive psychosis, involutional melancholia, and psychotic-depressive reaction. Even in other psychiatric conditions, depression is commonly a significant part of the symptomatology and a principal focus of therapeutic effort. Depression regularly accompanies serious physical illness and can be considered a normal response to the misfortunes of life. Nevertheless, much as pathologic anxiety can be contrasted with realistic fear, it is useful to contrast pathologic depression with normal disappointment, sadness, and grief.

Mild depression manifests itself largely by a loss of pleasurable interest in the usual affairs of life. Spontaneity is gone. Everything requires extra effort and provides less gratification than before. One does not feel physically ill but neither does one feel comfortable and well. Fatigue is excessive. Realistic worries and ordinary bodily discomforts are prominent in awareness, while encouraging memories, hopes, and plans are hard to keep in mind. A person with a mild depression does his work, meets his obligations, and appears normal to acquaintances. To himself and his intimate friends and family, however, something has changed.

In more severe depression the patient is frankly despondent or feels physically ill or both. He is usually gloomy, hopeless, helpless, and bereft of self-esteem. His thinking, speech, and movements may be slowed (psychomotor retardation) or he may be tense, hypervigilant, and restless (agitation). The agitated depressed patient is likely to complain endlessly about aches and pains, fatigue, feelings of unworthiness, or guilty fears. If the depression is of psychotic severity, the patient may actually believe things are as bad as he feels they are and he may have elaborate delusions, often hypochondriacal in nature.

Of the numerous physical symptoms, insomnia is the most prominent. Electroencephalographic (EEG) studies of depressed patients confirm that they tend to have a higher proportion of light or restless sleep and a shorter period of total sleep. In severe depressions, patients commonly awaken early after only enough sleep to take the edge off their exhaustion. These lonely vigils in the early morning hours are often the times of deepest despair.

Anorexia and weight loss are also characteristic of depression. Involuntary weight loss of 7 pounds or more in a month has been suggested as a diagnostic criterion for severe depression. Many other somatic complaints commonly occur in depression, particularly obscure pain, gastrointestinal symptoms, menstrual irregularities, and the whole range of psychophysiologic disorders. Sexual disinterest or incapacity—loss of libido—is described as a classic symptom. Briefly, the four major appetites are impaired: food, sleep, sex, and activity.

Dynamics of development. Although depression has been recognized as a clinical syndrome since ancient times, debate continues about whether it is a single well-defined entity of varying severity or a mixed category of qualitatively different disorders.

The difference between neurotic and psychotic depression is quantitative in the sense that both lie on a continuum with no precise distinction in the middle. From the viewpoint of planning nursing intervention, however, a mild depressive neurosis differs so greatly from a severe depressive psychosis that it is practical to think of the two as qualitatively different.

The concept of a resemblance between grieving and pathologic depression has been important as a starting point for contemporary psychodynamic theory and explanations of depression. In normal grieving, after the death of a parent, child, or spouse, there is dejection, diminished interest in the outside world, loss of capacity to love, inhibition of activity, a feeling of hopelessness, and intense preoccupation with different aspects of the lost person. This same picture characterizes pathologic depression except that the patient seems to be grieving over an inner loss, or absence, rather than the loss of an external love object. The individual ruminates not about a lost person but about himself—specifically, about those real or imagined aspects of himself that destroy his security or self-esteem. He may be very hostile toward himself, for example, belittling, accusing, and even reviling.

Modern psychodynamic formulations emphasize dependency as a primary issue in people prone to depression. Such individuals have exaggerated needs for nurturing, support, or approval. Some require special foods and bodily attentions from specific other people; others can get by if they have plentiful general conversation and companionship; for others, simple assurances that they are morally worthy or vocationally competent suffice, but they cannot get along *without* those assurances.

A very dependent person is always vulnerable to disappointment. Since he needs too much, he can never get enough. Because his needs are chronically unfulfilled, he has feelings of frustration and anger. Such a person is in a serious bind because expressing his anger will drive away or make hostile the very people on whom he is dependent. Therefore, he must hold in his anger, which seems to eat away at his insides, leading ultimately to feelings of helplessness and self-reproach. It is significant that the vicissitudes of anger and hostility remain part of every dynamic account of depression. It usually comes as a surprise to discover how angry the patient is, because superficially and consciously he blames no one but himself.

The anger becomes apparent when one attempts to reassure a depressed patient by asking him to be realistic or even optimistic about himself. Secondary gain in depression may be considerable. By being so miserable, the patient not only gains reassurance and sympathy from his friends but also makes them feel sad and guilty, thus gratifying his anger.

depressions are characterized by guilt, others by grief, some by anxiety, others by apathy; some mainly by physical symptoms, others purely by mental ones. In general, one can summarize the psychodynamic understanding of depression in this way. All of the mental symptoms of depression are correlates of a loss of self-esteem, no matter how it came about. The patient experiences hopelessness, guilt, or bodily discomfort in varying proportions. At one time or another, he reveals considerable anger, which he has directed largely toward himself. What *made* him angry is a loss, actual or symbolic. He is particularly vulnerable to loss because of excessive needs for nurturing or because his conscience is exceptionally vigilant, cruel, and unreasonable.

The nursing diagnosis of depression is easy when the patient understands that he is despondent and talks freely. The difficulty occurs when the patient's symptoms are predominately physical, or if he is withdrawn and uncommunicative.

When a depression manifests itself principally as physical symptoms—pain, insomnia, loss of appetite, and easy fatigability being the most common—the patient's symptoms may suggest a psychiatric illness. The most reliable clue is the apparent absence of organic disease. A recent depressing life event adds circumstantial evidence. Often such an event may be obvious to the family but not to the patient himself. The identification of a precipitating event or the presence of mental symptoms of depression is not conclusive evidence that physical disease is absent. A physical examination is essential before the presenting symptoms can be said to result from depression.

The recognition of depressive psychosis is important because hospitalization is usually necessary to effect prompt treatment and lessen the danger of suicide. In depressive psychosis, as contrasted with depressive neurosis, the mood disturbance is much more profound. It interferes with concentration and with memory. The patient often has guilty or hypochondriacal delusions. The insomnia is usually the early morning type, and weight loss is often considerable. The patient is unable to function normally, and family or friends are almost always certain that he is definitely sick, although they may not recognize that his sickness is depression.

The kind of depressive psychosis that involves the greatest risk of suicide is that in which agitation is a major symptom. Physical restlessness, handwringing, chain-smoking, or the expression of feelings that "You must do something" or that "I can't stand it anymore" are urgent pleas for close supervision, sedation, or perhaps a one-to-one suicidal watch in a quiet area on the unit.

An unresolved problem in a nursing diagnosis of depression is that of identifying the patient with masked depression, smiling depression, or depressive ～～～～ ～～～～ ～～～～ ～～～～ ～～～～ ～～～～ ～～～～ ～～～～ ～～～～ ～～～～ ～～～～ ions may appear in the guise of the usual somatic complaints or other psychiatric syndromes. In either case, the mood disturbance characteristic of depression is either absent or very hard to observe. The concept is valuable as a reminder that certain patients with pain or other obscure physical complaints have been dramatically relieved by electroconvulsive therapy (ECT) or other antidepressant therapy. It is also true that certain types of behavior—for example, unusual sexual activity or voluntary overwork—may be a substitute for or a defense against depression.

Types of behavior. Everyone worries and feels tension and anxiety, which tend to spread from one situation to another. Anxiety regarding one's competence in business may spread to anxiety concerning one's home. New doubts are added, and one may feel depressed, sad, and lonely. Activity and initiative slow up; mild agitation may result, or active and enforced gaiety may be used to cover up or dispel the feelings. Such responses in exaggeration become personality disorders.

Any of the deviations are usually precipitated by situations threatening enough to security to produce anxiety and tension over a long period. As indicated before, this is often related to the loss of a valued object, a term that can have varied meanings, including another person, a significant possession, a job, or one's own sense of competence.

A frequent precipitating factor in agitated depressions, for example, is the climacteric, or the menopause. The loss of sexual or socioeconomic status is a threat to self-esteem.

Agitated depression is a depressed emotional state accompanied by increased motor activity. Restlessness is characteristic, and activity is continual but limited in range. The patient paces back and forth wringing his hands, picking at his skin, and biting his nails. He is overwhelmed by a group of ideas or delusions of worthlessness, poverty, unreality, and sinfulness. He is completely preoccupied with this core of ideas centered about his sense of self-depreciation and self-reproach. He dreads the deserved punishment that awaits him and bitterly regrets the impending disaster he has brought on others. In the course of his illness he has neither the time nor the effort for sleep and food. Indecisiveness and uncooperativeness are common. The need for punishment is so deep that the danger of suicide is very real.

The following case study illustrates one type of agitated depression:

> J. M. was a man in his early fifties who was admitted to a psychiatric hospital on the insistence of his wife—because she felt he was "sick." Mr. M. was a tall, athletic-looking man with a tan, who stated to the nurse that he was a fireman. When asked why he looked so sad he stated that he knew he was going to be fired and that he deserved it. After further questioning and observation of his nonverbal clues—nail-biting and the inability to sit still for very long—the nurse was able to discover the apparent reason for his depression and guilt. Two years before, while fighting a fire, he had been on one side of a fence and his partner had thrown a hose, with a metal nozzle, over the fence to him. The nozzle touched the fence, which was electric, and his partner was instantly killed. After this happened he had said repeatedly, "I haven't felt the same since; it's my fault he is dead." The need for punishment, on his part, was tremendous. He felt worthless and was anticipating the doom of being fired.

Retarded depression is a depressed emotional state accompanied by a slowing down or retarding of thinking processes and motor activity. There is first a general slowing up that is accompanied by a feeling of sadness and dejection and a loss of initiative. Anxiety and tension persist throughout the episode, although their presence may be masked by later symptoms. A loss of weight occurs, and physical movements become slow and require much effort. The stream of thought becomes restricted and centers on ideas and delusions of personal unworthiness, self-depreciation, and convictions of failure in the past and the future. Thinking requires much effort, and only a limited range of ideas and simple thoughts can be handled. There is difficulty in concentrating on anything other than the hopeless and helpless ideas of self-rejection. Sitting in idleness, the head bowed and the face worn and haggard, the patient painfully endures his self-depreciation. He sleeps little and eats poorly. Practically the entire metabolic process is slowed down. The danger of suicide in this instance is greatest as the patient goes into and comes out of his depression. It is only at those times that the patient has sufficient energy available to plan and execute the suicidal act.

The *excitement pattern* is shown by elation or aggressive self-assertion that may reach delusional proportions. Delusions are usually fleeting and expansive, even grandiose, in nature. An energetic overactivity is displayed in which the patient rushes into reality and keeps himself preoccupied with his environment. The attention span is limited, and there is little ability to follow through or carry to completion any activity or thought. Focus of attention shifts so rapidly that a flight of ideas of varying degrees may occur. The patient may reach a goal idea by a devious roundabout pathway or may never reach it at all.

The flight of ideas may be shown by a quick reference to the objects or persons the patient sees or by quick jumps in ideas associated with the words used. Rhyming, punning, quips, and various witticisms may be seen. A general tendency to openly express primitive or purely biologic impulses is evidenced, and vulgarity and obscenity are common. The overactivity may include singing, shouting, and dancing. The patient often teases others and acts the clown. Through all this performance runs an impulsiveness that may include destructiveness (such as attacks on others). Irritability is usually marked, and the patient tolerates restrictions and restraints very poorly. Food, rest, and elimination are neglected, and the patient becomes dehydrated and loses weight. He is a ready prey to infections of any kind.

These three related syndromes are the most important of the aggressive reaction patterns. As has been pointed out, any combination of these patterns may occur, and they may include behavior not described here. There is a common tendency among these patients for both self-limiting episodic attacks and recurring attacks. The recovery rate from individual attacks is very high, but the high rate of recurrence reduces the hopeful outlook to some extent.

Nursing intervention. The problems presented by patients who are hostile or depressed are common throughout the range of nursing experience, and they form one of the cores of nursing practice. Such challenges are by no means restricted to psychiatric nursing. Nurses in all fields of clinical practice are faced with a variety of human behaviors that are fundamentally expressions of aggression and depression. The range of behaviors is as wide as the range of patients with whom the nurse comes in contact. Some behaviors may be the release of deep-seated trends within the personality, and some may be temporary reactions to health problems that threaten the self-image or self-control. The manifestations range from subtle to obvious. Every nurse knows the critical patient, the demanding patient, the self-deprecating patient, and the depressed patient. In all cases the patient is saying something, for all behavior has meaning and purpose. The patient's behavior also has meaning as far as his nursing care plan is concerned. Nursing intervention should be built as much on behavioral responses as on particular health problems. The meaning of the health problem to the patient is determined by its significance to the patient.

Nursing intervention should be based on the evident problems and assets of the patient. The nurse must decide where to intervene to relieve the depression. It is generally agreed that the nurse must be relatively active, since severe depressive symptoms make it impossible for the patient to take the responsibility for initial steps toward getting well. He is inclined to be discouraged and helpless. If psychotic, he may believe he deserves to be sick—or dead.

If the patient can accept reassurance and kind attention, these can be very helpful. In some types of depression, however, every gesture of affection or kind regard can "twist the knife" in the wound of the patient's guilty self-contempt. In such cases it may help to confront the patient sternly with his cruelty toward himself. The disapproving sternness gratifies his self-hate and at the same time helps him realize cognitively that he is not so bad as part of him claims he is.

Suicide risk must be evaluated in all cases of depression and in all illnesses associated with depression. Errors in the direction of understanding the danger of suicide usually occur when one has been hesitant to question the patient directly about his inclinations and intentions. In the course of treating a patient with a suicidal depression, special periods of danger occur after a setback —especially rejection by or the loss of a significant person; when agitation develops; when a patient with motor retardation becomes more active, and soon after going home after a period of hospitalization.

The nursing care of the identified psychiatric patient with depressive behavior directed outwardly as well as inwardly differs somewhat in the specific types of nursing problems likely to be presented. The pattern of illness, with its typical acute episodes that tend to be self-limited and also recurrent, suggests a plan for treatment that fits the episodic nature. Psychotherapy under the physician's direction takes advantage of the patient's better periods and concentrates on constructive interrelationships during the acute period to establish a good foundation for the later and more intensive psychic probing that will take place. The procedure is significant in its implications for nursing care.

The essence of a psychotherapeutic environment for depressed patients is that it be unchallenging and nonstimulating. A quietly pleasant ward in physical appearance and in psychologic atmosphere is necessary. Noise should be kept to a minimum, irritation avoided at all costs, and the administration of ward routine guided by the patient's needs. Allowance should be made for the slowness of depressed patients and the impulsive, distractable inefficiency of overactive patients. Since the underlying problem of hostility must be considered, the environment should restrict as far as possible the opportunities for its expression to be disastrous. The fact that stimulation can result from such varied things as bright colors, tension in others, a routine too closely calculated in regard to time, fatigue, noise, lack of outlet for energy, and numerous other factors should be taken into account when patient care is planned, both administratively and individually.

Facilities for the treatment of symptoms that are uncomfortable for the patient should be readily available. Overactivity feeds on overactivity and can set in motion a vicious cycle that leaves a patient exhausted and overstimulated by his own fatigue.

The advent of antidepressive drugs has reduced markedly the extent to which actual immediate patient control is a problem. These drugs are discussed in Chapter 13 and have introduced chemical control of depressive states of behavior. Hopefully, they have made patients more susceptible to the influence of interpersonal relationships.

Nurse-patient interpersonal relationships. The interpersonal relationship needs of a retarded personality are related to the patient's hostility and to the guilt it has aroused within him. The perception of himself as worthless and hopeless because of his hostility, his fear of expressing it, and punishment of himself for feeling it make the patient's nursing problems somewhat different in regard to overt behavior.

The goal in interpersonal relationships with this type of patient is to reassure the patient as to his worth as a person by making the acceptance of hostility easier for him and by reducing his deep-seated feelings of guilt. The reassurance of the worth of the patient as a person has dual implications. First, anything that may imply by word or behavior that the patient's opinion of himself is correct should be avoided. Second, positive action can be taken to help build the patient's self-esteem.

Since people tend to integrate and pay attention to the elements of experience that are pertinent to their own self-perception, the avoidance of any appearance of rejection calls for careful analysis of the behavior and attitudes of personnel. Certain characteristic situations hold specific dangers.

Life should be kept on a very simple level so that the patient is not confronted with demands he cannot meet, with resultant self-depreciation. The daily routine should be limited, and complex activities should be avoided. When the patient cannot care for himself, as in dressing or feeding, all necessary procedures should be done by personnel very matter-of-factly, without reminding the patient or others that it is necessary to do things for him. Routines should allow for the patient's slowness and protect him at the same time from any attention being called to that slowness. In other words, all routine and procedures should be reduced to the limits of the patient's level of thinking and behavior without in any way making his behavior conspicuous or an object of ridicule.

Hostility and self-depreciation may be expressed either openly or symbolically and should be quietly accepted. Failure to cooperate or making extra work for personnel may indicate hostility. The rejection or active avoidance of personnel may also express it. The right to feel this way belongs to the patient, and any criticism or rejection will increase his feeling of guilt, which is already one of his central problems. His behavior should therefore be analyzed for elements that might be an expression of hostility, and those specific forms of behavior should be accepted calmly with special care. The patient may also seek menial tasks as an expression of his need for self-punishment and should be permitted such tasks without comment.

The patient may verbalize his feelings of worthlessness and guilt, and care should be exercised in responding to such statements. Above all, they must not be treated lightly or thrust aside as temporary manifestations that are foolish or will disappear soon and be forgotten. They are profoundly important feelings to the patient and should be so accepted. If the nurse is certain that the feeling rather than the intellectual content is identified, the nurse may reflect the feeling, being careful to reflect no more than the patient has expressed. For example, if the patient comments, "My mother hated me, and she had reason to because I'm no good," the patient has expressed one feeling and hinted at another of which he is probably unaware. He feels self-deprecating, and he is probably, judging from his expression, attributing to his mother some of his own self-judgment. Hate from his mother, real or imagined, has some emotional response and may be quite significant in the patient's illness. However, the *feeling* expressed is self-depreciation, and it is real and important to the patient. To tell him that he is worth something is to reject him as he is, denying the importance of his feeling or implying that he should feel something else. To respond by saying, "You've felt disliked, haven't you?" accepts him, what he has said, and the feeling he has expressed. It neither condones or approves—it simply accepts. When in doubt, say nothing.

Another approach that can cause further depression is an emphasis on anything cheerful in the environment as a mistaken attempt to cheer the patient.

By contrast with such cheerfulness, the patient is apt to feel more deeply depressed. The contrast of opposites in this instance is likely to be detrimental.

In addition to not adding to the patient's feelings of self-depreciation, the nurse can take steps to help the patient support a positive feeling about himself. Of course, respect for the limitations his symptoms place on him has a positive aspect. It gives evidence that the patient is respected as the person he is here and now, which is probably the most effective reassurance that can be given under any circumstances. While avoiding too much verbalization about the matter, nurses can imply by overt and covert behavior that they believe the patient will get well. This can be done by quiet, personalized attention to the patient by seeking him out when routine does not demand it and by paying attention to the patient's expressed likes and dislikes whenever possible. Nurses can also help by not expecting the patient to appreciate what they do.

Most depressed patients have a period during the day, usually in the early evening, when their depression lifts slightly. This period of improvement should be exploited daily to reach the patient with personal interest. Simple activities may be shared at such periods, and every effort should be made to have them be as enjoyable as possible. Usually the early mornings present the most difficult period for the severely depressed patient.

The goal in interpersonal relationships with patients who are agitated and depressed is approximately the same as for overactive or retarded depressed patients. However, the problems encountered in reaching the goal combine some of the elements of both types. The problems arise because of overactivity and restlessness, preoccupation with ideas of sinfulness and guilt that produce the agitation, and insistence on reassurance that cannot be accepted more than momentarily. Such a combination results in a patient to whom cooperation and diversion are almost impossible during an acute phase. Acceptance may be given as indicated previously. Care should be taken to avoid by word, attitude, or implication any rejection or depreciation of the patient, and every opportunity should be used to build the patient's self-esteem.

The agitated patient, like the overactive patient, needs a rather neutral atmosphere as a buffer, although it must also be one that holds warmth and personal interest. Handling the demanded reassurances requires considerable patience and the ability to avoid impatient retorts under pressure. Impatient responses are apt to contribute to the patient's feelings of guilt.

The problem of communication centers about the patient's repeated convictions of poverty, sinfulness, and so on, which usually center around a specific group of ideas. Nurses should avoid being caught in this conversational trap and should keep their reassurance general rather than specific. No attempt should be made to reason the patient out of ideas that he is worse or more sinful than anyone else.

It is important to reach decisions quickly and firmly for agitated patients, since letting decisions be delayed by giving the patient an opportunity to make them tends to increase anxiety and tension. What is to be done must be indicated firmly and carried through at once. Explanations given must be short and specific. Resistance to routine and procedures indicates that diversion with the agitated patient is not as effective as diversion with the overactive patient; this occurs because the agitated patient is unable to attend to anything except his psychotic ideas. However, diversion should be tried.

Attention to personal appearance is often more effective with patients who show agitated depression than with patients who show retarded depression or a pattern of overactivity, and it is therefore an avenue of approach to be thoroughly exploited. It is also a means of reassuring the patient through personal attention. It is important to remember that hostility and guilt are the basic problems of the agitated depressed patient, and that expression of these feelings is to be accepted calmly and stimulation of these feelings is to be avoided.

The maintenance of adequate nutrition for patients with depressive patterns of behavior is essential and may be difficult. Frequent small feedings of easily digested foods are often necessary because metabolism is either speeded up or slowed down. Eating should be carefully supervised to ensure an adequate intake, and weight should be checked at least once weekly. Careful attention to personal likes and dislikes in regard to food and attractive servings are usually worth the effort. The overactive patient's needs for extra caloric intake should be met. Fluid intake is neglected by patients with these disorder patterns, and a regular schedule for giving fluids, reinforced with easily digested caloric content, should be instituted and followed through.

Elimination is a constant problem, and every effort should be made to avoid a resort to cathartics since their administration so often presents a psychologic problem. Adequate fluid intake, regular toilet schedule, and adequate diet roughage should be employed routinely.

The problem of insomnia is ever present, since the retarded and agitated depressed patient is too tense. Warm baths in preference to showers at bedtime, allowance of adequate time to settle down, and use of as many physical measures as possible are indicated. Warm milk at bedtime, the reduction of stimuli, a high pillow, back rubs, and a comfortable bed are all measures of importance. Careful observation as to the actual hours of sleep should be given in order that measures may be taken to avoid exhaustion.

Personal cleanliness is the responsibility of personnel for any patient in an acute stage. The period of bathing should be utilized to promote healthy personal relationships, but special attention should also be given to care of the skin, hair, and nails and to oral hygiene. Physical condition and physical well-being are closely related to emotional responses, and the patient should be kept as physically comfortable as possible in order to add no burden to his emotional problems. Personal appearance should be kept at the highest level possible because of its effect on the patient's self-opinion and on the response of others to him.

All depressive patients are careless in regard to personal appearance, personal cleanliness, and physical symptoms. Therefore careful observation in regard to symptoms of physical illness is necessary. In addition, slow healing is characteristic of these patients, so prompt and efficient attention to infections and their treatment is essential.

Self-injury short of suicide is fairly common in agitated depressed patients. Alert observation, distraction, and occupation of the patient in some constructive activity are usually the best preventive measures. The care of injuries presents quite a problem because of the patient's lack of ability to assist in treatment. Therefore prevention is the best measure.

The danger of suicide is marked in depressed patients and is present to some degree in overactive patients, since flashes of their underlying depression are often seen. The single best precaution against suicide is an alert and imaginative nurse who is aware of all the patient's potentialities, cognizant of the possible suicide methods open to the patient, and acutely sensitive as to how the patient actually feels. If such assurance is lacking, various measures may be used in a precautionary manner. A special close observation of the patient may be ordered, with responsibility specifically delegated to one person at all times. A depressed patient is always a suicidal danger, and the nurse should be conscious of the fact that the patient's life may depend on the ability to observe him and to understand how he feels. When caution to prevent suicide is being exercised, there is always the danger that concern for such prevention dominates thinking, feeling, and acting on the part of the personnel to the extent that other aspects of care become subordinated. Actually, suicide prevention is probably enhanced when other aspects of care, such as acceptance and attention to patients for purposes other than suicide prevention, are carried out faithfully.

Relationships with other patients. The retarded depressed patient will isolate himself if possible, but he should be encouraged to be with other patients even though he does not participate actively in a verbal sense or share too much in physical activities. The presence of others like himself is somewhat reassuring since it does not make him seem so alone and so different.

Associations only with patients like himself would not result in any specific stimulation; therefore, he should be exposed to more active patients. He should be allowed to advance to more shared activities at his own rate of speed, since socialization is not the urgent necessity that it is for a patient with a withdrawal pattern. Depressions tend to self-limitation, and the period for more aggressive therapy is during their absence.

Agitated depressions also tend to be self-limited, and for these patients it is fortunate. They invariably irritate other patients and tend to be a source of group discontent. They may function to unite the group against them, which is not particularly good for the patient although it may be good for members of the group. The example of personnel attitude may help patients tolerate the agitated one. However, isolation from the group is more frequently indicated than in other types of illness. The prognosis for this particular behavior pattern is good; therefore, the acute phase may be handled in terms of the patient's ultimate recovery.

The convalescent period is one of return of responsibility to the patient for his own behavior and destiny. More patients actually succeed in committing suicide during the convalescent period than during the acute period, especially the retarded depressed patient. The nurse must therefore be extremely alert and not lulled into a false security by the patient's seeming normality. The nurse must always be accessible to the patient and encourage his free discussion of any topic in order to have an opportunity to assess his true emotional state. The nurse must also be very tactful about this.

It is quite customary to see the patient go through a mild swing in the direction opposite from his illness, and the nurse should expect and be prepared for this. The overactive patient often has a mildly depressed period, and the depressed patient often has a mildly elated period. Signs of ominous significance during the convalescent stage are insomnia, loss of appetite or weight, and irritability. Another signal of significance is a sudden comfortable relaxation in the midst of obvious tension. Such an occurrence usually indicates that the patient has made a decision, and a decision made under such conditions may be unwise even to the point of determination of a definite method of suicide.

Approaches to normal should be quietly encouraged. If the patient wishes to talk about his experience, well and good. The nurse should encourage it. However, a patient should not be embarrassed by talking about his acute period unless he indicates he wishes it. Even then, no judgment should ever be passed.

If the patient presents the opportunity, encouragement should be given him to utilize his better adjustment through continued psychotherapy. The patient should also be encouraged to recognize signs in his own behavior that may indicate a relapse and need for a return to treatment.

WITHDRAWN BEHAVIOR

The behavior pattern characterized by the individual in withdrawal has as its central theme the refusal to invest emotional energy or to attach any enduring emotional interest to persons or objects outside the self. Depending on past experience and the incorporated standards of behavior of significant other people, withdrawal may vary in degree and in its method of expression. Withdrawn behavior is not a simple, clear-cut diagnostic category. It is essential to understand that many forms of behavior exemplify the withdrawal pattern; the failure to externalize emotional attachment is the significant starting point of difficulties. The compensation developed to overcome the threat to security, growing out of the resultant loneliness, may take various forms with different individuals. The compensatory mechanisms will, however, carry through consistently the withholding of emotional investment in the environment.

The failure to respond to external situations or to invest anything in the environment leads to inconsistencies in behavior that range from mild to rather complete personality disorganization. Most behavior, viewed from the outside, holds at least some degree of reasonableness in the eye of the viewer. In the withdrawn person, thought, emotion, and action responses may differ from each other and may appear to be inappropriate to the situation. The failure to respond behaviorally to the checks and balances of reality results in actions and expressions that are difficult for the uninitiated, and many times the initiated, to understand.

The symptoms shown by a patient who becomes mentally ill are an indication of what is happening to his self-organization and its integration with others. Persons with a normal introverted personality do exist, and many get along well without *serious* difficulties. It is not abnormal or sick to have a quiet, reticent personality, just as it is not abnormal to be extroverted and verbal. The difference lies in the manner in which the individual is able to feel about himself and in his ability to function at his full physical, intellectual, and emotional capacity. This reemphasizes the concept of the continuum of mental health and mental illness. All human behavior fits in this continuum. The world would be dull and boring if all behavior were normal (whatever that is) and if there were no human variations. It is these variations that have led to some of the superior struggles and gifts of man. The existence of compensatory devices has long been acknowledged in the fields of science, sports, art, and music, thus giving leverage to personality.

Corrective experience with significant people may integrate into the introverted personality a core of warmth that may support it well. Environmental stress may not be sufficient to precipitate a breakdown. In addition, experience is not often consistent enough to produce a "pure" introvert. Most persons are a mixture of introversion and extroversion. If the introversion, however, is markedly predominant and if experience *does* produce a disorganization of the self, the disorganization will probably be in the direction of withdrawal from reality to the realm of intellectual fantasy.

The patient's pattern of behavior is usually an indication of the illness that is to follow. There will have been past difficulty in socialization with others; many times this appears in combination with a quiet, studious, well-behaved exterior. Some persons tend to daydream frequently, and if they are outstanding in any area, it is usually in the intellectual field.

Physically, such patients do not show a consistent pattern of any type of defect, although some of them do not seem generally well equipped to meet life adequately on a physical basis. The implications of this fact are uncertain since what positive findings have been shown, such as irregularities in carbohydrate metabolism and poor vasomotor control, are not consistent, nor can the findings be shown positively to be either cause or effect. Considerable work has been done in the last two generations exploring the possible underlying causes of the withdrawal pattern of behavior. Genetic inadequacy, biochemical disturbances, family influences, cultural influences, and psychologic factors have been areas of study, but not one of the intensive studies has produced conclusive evidence. Current thinking still leans toward psychologic causation, with early life experience, family life, and cultural factors considered especially significant. More evidence than we have now is needed before any conclusions are definite.

Recently, there was considerable hope aroused when it was thought that the administration of certain experimental drugs, such as lysergic acid diethylamide (LSD) and mescaline, produced typical responses that resembled the psychotic symptoms of the withdrawn patient. This pointed toward a biochemical causation. However, further research tied the results achieved by the administration of such medications to the familiar toxic psychoses rather than the withdrawal pattern of behavior. Lysergic acid diethylamide, an ergot derivative, and psilocybin have been used experimentally in therapy, although there is a strong controversy over the use of the so-called consciousness-expanding drugs.

The following symptoms of withdrawn patients are the result of regression: (1) autistic thinking, characteristic of infancy, when self and environment are not clearly distinguished and meaning is highly personal in character, (2) no check on behavior that would ordinarily be inhibited by the influence of reality, and (3) inability to distinguish between a symbol and the thing symbolized. *How* regression will be expressed will depend on the past experience of the individual. The reason we do not see the actual behavior of an infant is that the patient carries back with him in his regression the tools of adult living, such as language, which are then misused on an infantile level. In addition, certain integrated parts of the personality from higher levels may persist.

The gross interference with the function of personality is shown in motor behavior, in intellectual activity, and in emotional responses. Behavior may show a complete indifference to surroundings, and the patient will be content to sit alone and daydream. Symbolic, ritualistic dancing or posturing may express primitive or sexual wishes. Behavior may show an active resistance to any form of suggestion or influence from the environment. There may be periods of overactivity that may or may not be wholly impulsive and that seem purposeless to the observer. Common to all of these patients is the rejection of reality and its loss of influence on conduct. Social criteria do not apply.

Emotional responses may be inadequate, inappropriate, and apathetic, or the patient may show extreme tension that is discharged in sudden bursts of overactivity. The patient may show these reactions in combination or in sequence or may show one type of reaction consistently. These emotional responses can be understood if we remember that the patient is feeling at an autistic level, where experience has its own personal meaning, unchecked by reality, and that both the self-system and the dissociated self are being expressed openly and often independently.

Some patients simply show a lack of interest, are totally devoid of ambition, and drift whither circumstances send them. They show little response to social criteria, and their emotional lives are superficial since they form no real or enduring attachments to anything or anyone. Their passive course does not carry through to behavior bizarre enough to attract undue attention. The village ne'er-do-wells, the town drunkards, hobos, prostitutes, and the bowery bums number many such persons among their ranks. A general belief is held that these patients do not respond well to treatment, but this is difficult to state categorically, since only a small percentage of them ever comes under treatment.

There may occur a sudden, violent upheaval characterized by silliness, grimacing, posturing, delusions, and hallucinations of fantastic or grotesque nature. Behavior may be markedly impulsive and emotional response totally inappropriate. The strong emotional response usually dies out fairly quickly.

Another form occurs in which conduct peculiarity is marked. The patient swings from periods of stupor to excitement. Impulsive but stereotyped behavior, hallucinations, and a strong negativistic reaction to all suggestion from the environment occur. The patient approaches the area of magic here and identifies with cosmic forces, which are the battleground of good and evil. During periods of stupor the patient maintains a rigidly assumed position and shows the famous waxy flexibility that is *almost* diagnostic. The patient will hold rigidly, and for hours on end, a position in which he is placed. The excited period tends to be explosive, and sudden attacks on the environment or self are fairly common.

A coloring of projection may be added to the form of illness in that any of these patients may develop suspiciousness and fear of the intent of the environment. Traits from one of the three types of withdrawal briefly described may appear in either of the other two types, but a particular behavior pattern will usually predominate.

Withdrawal, as a pattern of behavior, is encountered in all clinical areas and in many types of patients. Withdrawn behavior is not characteristic only of psychiatric patients. Withdrawal may occur as an individual's response to crisis situations in health, as part of the person's response pattern to almost any type of situation, as a temporary incident, or as an exacerbation of an underlying trait during stress. Withdrawal may be expressed in a wide variety of behaviors, all serving the purpose of evading the demands of the immediate situation and limiting contact with and responses to others. The reaction may range from mild and temporary to severe with indications of permanence. A person reacts to threats in terms of personal perceptions and existing repertoires of behavioral responses. The nursing care plans of such patients should take cognizance of the basic health problems. Factors to be taken into consideration are the adequacy of the patient's previous adjustment, the meaning of the health problem to the patient, the extent to which the nurse must bear responsibility for the establishment of trust, and the probable, if predictable, course of events.

The following case study illustrates the behavior of a withdrawn patient.

> Mrs. B. had been on a hospital unit for 3 weeks. She was withdrawn and uncommunicative. She refused all interaction with the staff and her fellow patients. Staff members accepted her withdrawn behavior and were content to see that she was clean, comfortable, and well fed. Mrs. B. was taken to all of the group activities but would only sit passively in a chair, doing nothing. Mrs. B. was not permitted to isolate herself in her room and since she did not like being in the dayroom with the other patients, a chair was placed outside her door so that she could observe the activities of others.
>
> One afternoon, as a psychiatric attendant passed her in the hall, Mrs. B. got out of her chair, picked it up, and hit him with it. She didn't say a word while being led to her room, but she exhibited clues of intense hostility by

her resistance to the staff. Shortly thereafter she began to talk to the staff about her anger and apologized for hitting the attendant.

Nursing intervention. The bizarre and seemingly illogical behavior of psychiatric patients who have rejected reality seems often so incomprehensible to the average nurse that she is bewildered as to what her function in the care of such patients may be. Analysis of the patient's behavior will indicate certain needs that are paramount in combating his illness. The focus must be placed on the patient as a person, rather than on the symptoms he shows. One of the most challenging nursing problems that exists is to help back to healthy social participation the patient who has emphatically turned his back on interpersonal relationships and the society in which he lives. This is not an easy task.

The recovery of a patient with a severe withdrawal pattern of behavior must be based on reeducation of his perception of himself in relation to others. He must be able to see himself as he is, lose his negative attitude toward himself, and rebuild a new perception in its place. Normal society has failed to accomplish this; therefore, a new type of existence, oriented to make such reeducation possible, is indicated.

Security is one of the patient's first and greatest needs; his opinion of himself must be supported consistently. Such an opinion and a realistic self-image that supports contacts with others represent resources that the patient needs to be able to move toward the reintegration into society that he must achieve. The physical environment can do this in several ways. The consistent attitude of personnel that the patient is a person with human dignity helps. It is primarily through this attitude that the establishment of trust in others must occur. The routines should make reasonable expectations of behavior, with the stimulus to which the patient will be exposed offering the opportunity for response. Demands made on the patient for response should offer him some degree of success and should call for increasingly complex behavior.

There is a growing realization that the more treatment of behavior disorders that can be carried out in the community and the more the hospital approaches the reality situation from which the patient comes, the better. The belief in this fact applies to general as well as to psychiatric facilities. The patient may show deficiencies in some social abilities, and some decisions may be made for him, especially in emergencies, but he should never be allowed to become completely comfortable with total irresponsibility for himself.

Nurse-patient interpersonal relationships. Certain problems in the establishment of interpersonal relationships with these patients are characteristic of withdrawal patterns of behavior. Healthy interpersonal relationships cannot be established at once, and, in fact, *any* establishment is the immediate problem. However, from the beginning an attempt can be made to build rapport on a foundation that will lend itself to healthy growth by the patient.

The first and most important problem is to reach the patient emotionally and to establish a bond with him. In view of the patient's rejection of people, the initiative must rest with personnel. It must be a consistent, steady attempt to draw the patient into some response, without, at the same time, demanding a specific response. The patient *must* be left free to respond as he wishes. This means one-sided conversations, one-sided interest in the patient's appearance, and one-sided interest in everything the patient does. Such a program must be carried through for a long period, always sincerely and always without retaliation for the patient's failure to respond. When a response does come, mature techniques of social skill should not be expected, and the patient's fumbling and often inept social responses should be accepted with the same grace and tolerance with which indifference was accepted. At the same time, the response must be recognized for what it is, a step in the right direction. Sudden verbal lashings, incoherent language, grimacing, and absurd and silly behavior should be expected. It is wise to remember that the labels given such behavior in the immediately preceding sentence reflect our judgments, which must not be referred to the patient. Could we understand the meaning of his behavior as it appears to him, the patient might well be justified in reversing the judgment and applying it to us.

The problem of verbal communication is not an easy one. The patient uses language in a highly personal way and has his own individual meaning for words, phrases, and sentences. Experience unchecked by reality may be quite distorted, and fantasy may reign unchecked. Therefore, if the patient shows such symptoms, it is wise to keep communication directed toward him in simple language. Also, communication occurs on more than verbal and intellectual levels; emotional communication may be even more important in this instance. The constant awareness and seeking out of the patient at every opportunity communicates the nurse's interest. Sitting quietly beside a patient saying nothing for brief but consistent periods conveys its message. It is wise not to get trapped in the patient's intellectual fantasies, not to argue about them, and not to attempt to reason them away. Acceptance of the patient without criticism and without ignorning him while ignoring his behavior does not necessarily sanction his behavior. However, the withdrawn person must be sought—he will not seek others.

In relationships with patients, all efforts must be centered around the attempt to build the patient's badly shattered opinion of himself. Encouragement and praise may be used, but only when they are justified and can be accepted by the patient. The most important thing another person can do for us is to be interested in us. That in itself, if it is consistent, helps. The sensitive ego must be nourished carefully. Until it has been rebuilt, it cannot tolerate the little rebuffs and the give-and-take of ordinary relationships.

Certain protective needs of patients with withdrawal patterns grow out of their particular syndrome. Since their intellectual processes tend to digress from routine and expected patterns, the degree of predictability in regard to their behavior is reduced. Hence, behavior that seems purposeless and impulsive to the outside observer can and frequently does occur. Patients need alert and imaginative observation to protect them from the possible consequences of impulsive and unself-disciplined acts. Sudden attacks on others, often without any evident personal animosity, can occur, as well as sudden jumps or wall-diving that may result in personal injury or death.

One of the patient's needs is to be protected from idleness and unbridled indulgence in fantasy. An effort to keep the patient actively participating in life within the hospital routine and at some task that requires a contact with reality must always be made.

Relationships with other patients. Withdrawn patients pose some real problems in relationships with other members in the hospital unit. A predominance of passively withdrawn patients can hold group interaction to a depressive minimum, and a predominance of actively withdrawn patients can completely disrupt a group. As a minority within a group, they tend individually to be isolates. Although they perhaps are not verbally interacting with other patients, nonetheless they are definitely part of the group emotionally; their presence has its effect on other members, and other members affect the withdrawn patient. Participation occurs on levels other than verbal.

In group relations, the withdrawn patient is always in danger of attack from the more aggressive patient. The aggressive patient may need a safe outlet for his aggression and may realize that the withdrawn patient can be this safe outlet, or he may resent the withdrawn patient's seeming lack of pressure of activity that plagues him. If the group comes to the patient's defense, well and good; this supportive action then conveys an acceptance of the patient, which he needs whether he can acknowledge it or not. In such an instance the aggressive patient needs help. If, however, it falls on the nurse to rescue the withdrawn patient, this must be done tactfully through diversion of the aggressive patient. To openly champion the quieter person may isolate him further from the group.

When a patient is being guided to participate in socialized activities, encouragement and support are useful. The patient may be placed with another patient much like himself to start with, and then the two are later fitted into a slightly larger group containing perhaps more active members. The membership of the group should remain fairly constant unless the group reaction is unfortunate and some members must be replaced to create a better working group. In regard to activity within the group, the particular form of occupation chosen for or by the patient may be something he can do alone. Shared activities may be introduced later, with the element of competition held to a minimum, until the patient seems comfortable in the group.

Nurses should at all times avoid placing their relationship with the patient on a footing that isolates him from the group of patients. Competition for their favors will occur, and behavior that results in rejection of the patient by others deprives him of one of the real values of hospitalization.

During the convalescent period the withdrawn person usually needs further support for his ego and reassurance in regard to his return to society. One of the best ways to develop an objective attitude toward his mental illness is through nurses' matter-of-fact, objective acceptance of it. The patient should be encouraged to talk through his feelings about going home. Socialized activities should be encouraged, and the patient should be given opportunities to develop social skills until he feels relatively sure of himself if possible. Bridge, dancing, and other activities that can be enjoyably shared should be practiced until they can be done well, on the simple principle that most persons enjoy doing what they can do well, and the withdrawn patient's greatest need is for things he can do well with others.

Attention should be focused on the value of day-by-day experience and the acquisition of good health habits, including a balanced program of work and play. Realistic ideas concerning future plans should be supported; unrealistic ideas should be faced matter-of-factly. Requested information should be given freely on the level of the patient's understanding, and advice should be abjured.

The patient should be given gradual and increased responsibility for himself and his decisions so that he begins to outgrow his dependence before he leaves the hospital. In addition, this is an excellent period for learning from the patient, for most patients have some skill, knowledge, or understanding they can impart.

DELUSIONS

A delusion is a false belief, usually unique to the individual, which is not susceptible to modification or correction by logical persuasion or by compelling contrary evidence. At times, as in folie à deux, a delusion may be shared with another person who is dominated by the delusional patient, typically the spouse.

A delusional system is an elaborate complex based on the delusional premise, that is, a person who falsely believes he is being persecuted develops a delusional system that consists of the reasons for his being singled out, the identity of his persecutors, the means they use, and the "evidence" to support his convictions.

The explanation of delusions in their purest form, as in the paranoid state, is not clearly established. Two main theoretical views are prevalent. One is that a specific biochemical or physiologic dysfunction underlies the disease process and that the delusion results from faulty perceptions or interpretation caused by this dysfunction. The alternative view is that delusion formation is a psychologic defense mechanism that enables the patient to cope with painful or threatening impulses, needs, or conflicts even at the cost of loosening his contact with reality. According to this view the patient is using the same mechanisms of denial and projection that everyone uses at times, but to an exaggerated and pathologic degree.

Some of the most common forms of delusions are the following.

1. *Paranoid delusions.* Ideas of persecution: of being followed, watched, slandered, having one's mind controlled or influenced, being harmed physically, or having plots against one's life. The weapons of the persecutors are not readily amenable to confirmation or repudiation—that is, electronic devices or telepathy.

2. *Depressive delusions.* Ideas of guilt, poverty, incurable disease, having no feeling, being dead, or the world having ceased to exist.

3. *Grandiose delusions.* Ideas of having great wealth, influence, or power or of being an outstanding, famous, or notorious person or a historic or religious figure.

4. *Erotic delusions.* Ideas, most commonly paranoid, of infidelity, sexual molestation, or change of sex; but sometimes grandiose, such as being loved by someone, often a movie star, who is unable to make his or her feelings known.

5. *Diffuse delusions.* Confused and poorly defined beliefs that oneself or one's surroundings are strange, unreal, or different. They may vary in content and in the earnestness with which they are held.

The possibility that a patient might act on his delusional belief must always be considered. Some patients may dissociate their ideation and behavior, so that a patient who believes himself to be omnipotent may nevertheless submit meekly to direction. On the other hand, a patient who believes himself to be threatened may take violent action in self-defense.

In working with a patient who has delusions, an attitude of noncommittal respect and willingness to listen to the patient's ideas without prejudgment is desirable. Expressions of incredulity or amusement or a patronizing pretense of agreement must be avoided. An empathic recognition of the patient's affective response to his beliefs should be maintained. No attempt should be made to argue with the patient or persuade him of the falsity of his ideas, since any such attempt interferes with rapport and may cause the patient to incorporate the nurse into his delusional system.

No special treatment is required for delusions; they usually disappear as the underlying mental illness abates. Rarely, they may continue in circumscribed form in an otherwise well-recovered patient; in these instances, the patient has at least partial insight and does not permit the delusions to affect his behavior.

HALLUCINATIONS

Hallucinations are spontaneous, unwilled sense perceptions, experienced as arising outside the self, for which there is no external basis. Awareness of the unreality of the perception (insight) may or may not be present. Volition and consciousness are essential considerations in distinguishing hallucinations from certain other mental phenomena. Volition, as used here, refers to mental activity that is voluntary and willed as opposed to that which is involuntary, spontaneous, and uncontrolled. In the former, there is a sense of the mental experience occurring inwardly; in the latter, a sense of "out-thereness" about the experience. Dreams are sometimes cited as examples of hallucinations in normal experience, but they probably should not be so considered since they occur during sleep, when consciousness is largely absent. Daydreams are ▇▇sness nor volition is absolute, a sharp distinction between hallucinations and these other mental phenomena is frequently impossible.

Any sensory modality may be involved in hallucinations, that is, hearing, vision, taste, smell, and touch. These may occur singly or in combination. Hallucinations vary in clarity, vividness, intensity, and associated affect according to the varying circumstances in which they occur. The significance of hallucinations depends on many factors. They are not necessarily indicative of a mental disorder.

Fleeting visual hallucinations may be part of the clinical picture associated with prolonged extreme physical exertion or starvation. Factors such as sleep deprivation and electrolyte imbalance probably play a role.

Hallucinatory experiences in persons subjected to prolonged isolation, such as shipwrecked sailors and polar explorers, have long been recognized. In recent years, many investigators have reported the occurrence of hallucinations in volunteers subjected to isolation and sensory deprivation.

Hallucinations may be part of a delirious state after surgery in persons who exhibited no sign of mental illness preoperatively. The cause of such delirious states is obscure; the anesthetic agent used, infection, and electrolyte imbalances are among the possibilities. The possibility of a functional reactive psychosis should also be kept in mind.

Hallucinatory states following cardiac surgery are common and may be particularly complex both because of the intense emotional stresses involved and because various types of physiologic shocks are unavoidable.

Hallucinations, usually visual, are common among primitive people during trance states. They are benign in nature and disappear with the termination of the trance. Similar hallucinations occur in various delirious states, for example as a symptom of drug-taking with such drugs as LSD, mescaline, and peyote.

In some cases it is quite apparent that patients are hallucinating. They appear to be listening to or seeing something not present, or they may voluntarily tell you about their hallucinations. On the other hand, many patients will deny or withhold their hallucinatory experiences. The nurse should note repetitive eye movements, movements of the lips, and any other behavior that suggests that the patient may be responding to hallucinations.

Patients whose contact with reality is obviously disturbed may be asked directly if they hear voices or see strange things. Less direct inquiry may be called for with other patients. Frequently, they will say something that, if pursued, will bring out the presence of hallucinations. Questions such as the following may be useful: "Do you ever hear your own thoughts out loud?" "Have you ever had what seemed like a dream when you were awake?"

It is important also to ask patients if they smell unusual odors, have peculiar tastes in their mouths, or feel things on their skin that they cannot see.

REFERENCES

Aguilera, D. C.: Review of psychiatric nursing, St. Louis, 1977, The C. V. Mosby Co.

Arieti, S.: Manic depressive psychoses. In Arieti, S., editor: American handbook of psychiatry, vol. 1, New York, 1959, Basic Books, Inc.

Arthur, A. Z.: Theories and explanations of delusions, Am. J. Psychiatry 121:105-115, 1964.

Burgess, A., and Lazare, A.: Psychiatric nursing in the hospital and the community, ed. 2, New York, 1976, Prentice-Hall, Inc.

Cammer, L.: Up from depression, New York, 1969, Simon & Schuster, Inc.

Cole, J. O.: Depression, Am. J. Psychiatry 131:204, 1974.

Crary, W. G., and Crary, G. C.: Depression, Am. J. Nurs. 73:472-475, 1973.

Field, W. E., and Ruelke, W.: Hallucinations and how to deal with them, Am. J. Nurs. 73:638-640, 1973.

Giffin, K.: Interpersonal trust in the helping professions, Am. J. Nurs. 69:1491-1492, 1969.

Keup, W., editor: Hallucinations, New York, 1970, Plenum Press.

Kolb, L. C.: Modern clinical psychiatry, ed. 8, Philadelphia, 1973, W. B. Saunders Co.

Kyes, J., and Hofling, C.: Basic psychiatric concepts in nursing, ed. 3, Philadelphia, 1974, J. B. Lippincott Co.

Lenarz, D. M.: Caring is the essence of practice, Am. J. Nurs. 71:704-707, 1971.

Mellow, J.: Nursing therapy, Am. J. Nurs. 68:2365-2369, 1968.

Moser, D. H.: Communicating with a schizophrenic patient, Perspect. Psychiatr. Care 8:36-45, 1970.

Solomon, P., and Mendelson, J.: Hallucinations in sensory deprivation. In West, L. J., editor: Hallucinations, New York, 1972, Grune & Stratton, Inc., p. 137.

Solomon, P., and Patch, V.: Handbook of psychiatry, Los Altos, Calif., 1974, Lange Medical Publications.

Sullivan, H. S.: Conceptions of modern psychiatry, Washington, D.C., 1947, William Alanson White Psychiatric Foundation.

Thaler, O. F.: Grief and depression, Nurs. Forum 5(2):8-22, 1966.

Tudor, G. E.: A sociopsychiatric nursing approach to intervention in a problem of mutual withdrawal on a mental hospital ward, Perspect. Psychiatr. Care 8:11-35, 1970.

Ujhely, G. B.: Grief and depression—implications for preventive and therapeutic nursing care, Nurs. Forum 5(2):23-35, 1966.

Winokur, G.: Depression in the menopause, Am. J. Psychiatry 130:92-93, 1973.

ADDITIONAL READINGS

Arieti, S.: Affective disorders: manic-depressive psychosis and psychotic depression. In Arieti, S., editor: American handbook of psychiatry, vol. 3, New York, 1974, Basic Books, Inc., pp. 449-490.

Ayd, F.: Recognizing the depressed patient, New York, 1961, Grune & Stratton, Inc., pp. 118-125.

Beck, A. T.: Depressive neurosis. In Arieti, S., editor: American handbook of psychiatry, vol. 3, New York, 1974, Basic Books, Inc., pp. 61-90.

Maoz, B.: Female attitudes to menopause, Soc. Psychiatry 5(1):35-40, 1970.

Modell, A. H.: Hallucinations in schizophrenia patients and their relation to psychic structure. In West, L. J., editor: Hallucinations, New York, 1962, Grune & Stratton, Inc.

Schwab, J. H., Brown, J. M., Holzer, C. E., and Sokolof, M.: Current concepts of depression: the sociocultural, Int. J. Soc. Psychiatry 14(3):226-234, 1968.

Secunda, S. K.: The depressive disorders: special report: 1973, Department of Health, Education and Welfare Publication No. (HSM) 73-9157, Washington, D.C., 1973, U.S. Government Printing Office.

Silverman, C.: The epidemiology of depression, Baltimore, 1968, Johns Hopkins Press.

Solzhenitsyn, A.: Cancer ward, New York, 1969, Farrar, Strauss and Giroux, Inc.

Tudo, G. E.: A sociopsychiatric nursing approach to intervention in a problem of mutual withdrawal on a mental hospital ward, Psychiatry 15:193-217, 1952.

Ward, A. H.: My silent patient, Perspect. Psychiatr. Care 7(2):87-91, 1969.

West, L. J., editor: Hallucinations, New York, 1962, Grune & Stratton, Inc.

Williams, H. L., Morris, G. O., and Lubin, A.: Illusions, hallucinations and sleep loss. In West, L. J., editor: Hallucinations, New York, 1962, Grune & Stratton, Inc.

Wilmer, H.: Social psychiatry in action, Springfield, Ill., 1958, Charles C Thomas, Publisher.

CHAPTER 9

Patients with aggressive and projective patterns

AGGRESSIVE PATTERNS

At one time much of the aggressive instinct was referred to as the death instinct. It includes all of the destructive and hostile forces in the human psyche. The derivatives include the impulse to self-assertion, ambition, competition, the desire to win, and the drive to succeed. There are often fusions between sexual and aggressive drives—for example, competition for the object of one's love and active measures of self-protection such as fighting to protect one's home and loved ones. Overt sadistic and masochistic activities are pathologic fusions of the two sets of instincts, with the aggression directed toward others in sadism and toward oneself in masochism. There is a release of sexual tension in both activities.

Dynamics of development. As a child develops, the pathways of discharge of aggression change; for example, between early childhood and latency, words take the place of muscular action. It is in this phase that swear words are relished by the child, serving as a defense against aggression taking the form of muscular action; it is also here that the child is taught to count to ten before acting. Aggression in psychotic children may occur for many reasons, one of them being a healthful discharge of aggressive impulses. Other aggressive acts may be for the purpose of defending the ego, for example, when defenses are weakening, as a defense against anxiety, as a reaction of the superego against id impulses, and also as an expression of a sort of powerless rage.

Bender (1969) states that hostile or destructive aggression in children is the result of developmental pathology in the context of a disturbing situation that has disorganized the normal drives of the developing child. She further states that murderous, hostile aggression is not a normal pattern for children.

Freud (1957) thought that aggressive behavior rests on different physiologic aspects of the body.

According to Anna Freud (1972), the child's pleasure in constructive activity is libidinal, whereas his pleasure in destruction is aggressive; they exist together and each is the derivative of a primary id tendency. Furthermore, the observation of early aggression in young children shows that attack derives expressly from the aggressive drive. Children are extremely aggressive toward each other; they bite, kick, pull hair, and hit but initially the victim of the attack dissolves into tears instead of defending himself. Only later does the youngster learn self-defense. One might conclude that aggression in service of defense is learned and mediated by the ego.

Mahler and colleagues (1973) describe a period of growth and development in the child in which the euphoric aspects require assistance from others, namely the mother figure; if these aspects are submerged, the aggressive drive becomes uppermost and is projected onto others. As a result, the world may be divided into good and bad and consequently the child divides himself into good and bad. Mahler also thinks that these mechanisms may provide the beginnings of paranoid features; behaviorally, the child clings and is moody and coercive.

The frustration-aggression hypothesis of Dollard and associates (1939) purports that frustration increases with rank and territory of man. Berkowitz (1962) views aggression as not automatically accompanying frustration or threat; instead, he sees it as relative to the degree and amount of frustration, the power of the individual to react against the aggressive act, and one's values against aggression.

In the past, aggressive acts might have led to a duel, for example, which was socially acceptable at the time. Dueling served as a sanctioned outlet for individuals or groups in conflict. After the duel, amicable relations were expected to resume.

In modern times, competitive sports are ritualized forms of aggressive behavior. In the highly ritualized sport of tennis, one may symbolically "wipe out" one's opponent by winning the game; afterward both parties approach each other, smile, shake hands at the net, and thank each other for a good game.

Although some groups are more aggressive than others, all cultures experience aggression to some degree. Man has survived by developing his biologic endowments for communal living. But communal living is always a potentially violent existence, and especially so in the modern world, with its general fragmentation of social systems in times when there is no major external threat to create a sense of internal solidarity with one's countrymen.

Violent aggression as a manifestation of social unrest or protest is a transcultural phenomenon that appears to be most common in ex-colonial societies with competing racial, ethnic, and religious groups such as Cyprus, Ireland, Indonesia, Nigeria, and Pakistan. Carstairs (1969) lays great emphasis on overcrowding as an indirect cause of violence and anticipates serious consequences if recent population trends are allowed to continue. He traces the alienation and despair of the dispossessed who are the product of overcrowding and their victimization by mentally unstable but charismatic demagogues. When the latter stimulate extravagant aspirations that cannot be met, group violence is bound to occur. Similarly, in overcrowded universities where students have lost contact with teachers and the aims of the curricula—examples would include Berkeley, Columbia, Kent State, and universities in Paris, Rome, and Tokyo—mild protest movements become violent when confronted with countermeasures aimed at preserving public order. In his inquiry into the psychology of violence, Toch (1969) offers realistic suggestions for prevention. Nonviolent behavior presupposes an opportunity structure available to all and a corresponding improvement in the quality of interpersonal relationships. He also stressed the importance of child-rearing and recommends the participation of the violence-prone individual himself in research activities as a potent educative influence.

Gorney (1971) proposes that in societies where we see the most intense interpersonal relationships, we also see the highest level of cultural achievement and intrapsychic conflict. He poses the thought that aggression and mental disorder might be diminished by reducing the intensity of interpersonal relationships.

Aggression is usually easily perceived, and the concept of constructive aggression is well known. The child who uses magical thinking to release aggression may also experience guilt when he wishes that his brother would die and the brother does in fact die. A guilt reaction to unexpressed aggression is probably normal for the adolescent. In the 10 to 15 year old, depression is usually linked to unexpressed aggression. Sadism and murder are extreme forms of outward aggression; masochism and suicide are examples of extreme inward aggression. A classic example of hatred raises the question of the origins of aggression, for example, Hitler's annihilation of the Jews. A study by Silver and co-workers (1969) covering three generations of families of abused children supports the view that violence breeds violence and that a child who experiences violence has the potential of becoming a violent member of society as he grows older.

Release of aggression. Release of aggression as in play, hunting, work, and other physical activities may be greatly altered when patients are hospitalized, at times of other stresses, and when usual outlets for aggression are not available. For example, a blind man may verbally attack an agency, reject it, or make excessive demands on it. Nurses are familiar with the many biting remarks that some patients make about the hospitals serving them and about other professionals caring for them. The intimacy, sustained close contact, and heightened interaction that nurses experience with patients provide fertile ground for arousal of hostility and tension as well as the more positive affects of rapport (Coser, 1956). The rivalry—for example, the traditional dislike of the French for the Germans and vice versa—between nations also serves as a channel for release of aggressive feelings. The competitiveness between nations symbolized by the Olympic Games can now be experienced vicariously throughout the world via the medium of television.

Inappropriate aggression. Suspicion is the imagination of the existence of some fault, defect, guilt, or falsity when there may be slight or no evidence for its existence. Suspicion precedes hostility. The suspicious person tends to question motives of others over minute matters, mull over the consequences, and later confront individuals with long, involved analyses of their motives. Hostility refers to an unfriendly, antagonistic manner, to resentment, grudges, and resentful acts. All humans experience hostility. It is common for everyone to feel aggressive when frustration is encountered and handle it by adjusting, adapting, changing one's perceptions, or leaving. Hostility usually emerges after much rumination over an imagined slight. Buss (1961) makes the point that a hostile remark such as "I hate you" voiced by a person who is alone is not aggressive until there is someone to hear it. Hostility is one way that patients who feel threatened react to the threat. If the threat can be removed, the hostility is not needed.

The following terms describe behavior of hostile patients: picky, resentful, argumentative, antagonistic, uncooperative, aggressive, irritable, sarcastic, rude, critical, resistant, demanding, complaining, derogating, threatening, and rejecting. Inflicting physical injury, making barbed remarks, and joking at someone else's expense are all examples of hostility.

Nursing intervention. Aggressiveness in patients may create anxiety in the nurse. The patient who is sarcastic, irritable, and resentful and who complains about the hospital, the doctors, and other staff members puts the nurse in a defensive position without actually knowing whether the patient's complaints are justifiable. The nurse should try to discover whether there is a basis for his sarcasm. If there is none, perhaps the patient is releasing aggression because his normal manner of handling it is unavailable. The nurse can help by listening, offering alternative solutions to problems, and helping the patient to feel secure enough so that his aggressive behavior is no longer necessary.

Signs of mounting tension can be noted by the nurse, who can prevent the patient from hurting others, destroying objects, and injuring himself. Increased motor activity, angry facial expressions, stereotyped movements, and tremulousness may be some of the clues. The nurse should remove the patient from others, take him to his room, remain with him, touch him, and talk with him. A one-to-one relationship with someone he trusts provides continuity of care.

Aggressive patients need contact with persons who can accept them as they are and who function as neutral but warm human buffers who accept them as people and against whom they can test themselves without retaliation or judgment. Patients must be able to express their hostility and ambivalence in a calm accepting atmosphere in which their guilt is not reinforced. The limitations placed on them by their symptoms must not be used against them.

The overactive patient presents certain problems in interpersonal relationships. He is too active physically and therefore has a high nuisance value, he resents authority, he tends to be domineering, he is sarcastic and fond of ridicule, he enjoys embarrassing others, he is impulsive, he has a limited attention span, his sense of humor is often crude, his wit and verbal punning are often too funny, he demands attention and will not be ignored, he is profane and vulgar, and he is very sensitive.

Above all, the overactive patient needs a person with good self-control who can see and understand objectively what is happening. He needs a person who can be calm and collected under all or most circumstances and whose judgment can surmount the annoyances of the patient's behavior. The answer lies in the ability to accept a person without necessarily sanctioning his behavior. This can be done in the following manner. The patient should first of all be protected from overstimulation. His resentment of the necessary restrictions of a psychiatric hospital should be respected by limiting him tactfully and by allowing him to verbalize his annoyance. Critical comments should be met matter-of-factly, and no attempt should be made to talk him out of it; his verbal attacks on personnel should not be met with self-defense or explanation. One of the favorite traps in an overactive patient's attack on his environment is to force personnel into a defense of themselves, their behavior, or their weaknesses. Such attacks must again be met with tolerance, even when they sting, as they so often do. Fairness in treatment and attitude toward the patient must be maintained. Profanity and vulgarity should also be faced without prudishness. In summary, the aggressiveness, the resentment of authority, the criticalness, the vulgarity, and the attempt to belittle and challenge personnel are best met by a calm, matter-of-fact manner, and further hurt to the patient should be avoided by not increasing his feeling of guilt in relation to any such manifestations of behavior.

The achievement of such serenity is not an easy task and as a rule comes as the result of deliberate cultivation. A sudden verbal thrust at a weakness is not a pleasant experience, and, since, the nurse is a human being, the necessity for self-defense and retaliation is part of the nurse's personality as well as of the patient's. The criterion to apply to each situation is the question: What have I done *for* the patient? It may lead to control if the nurse is emotionally mature enough to apply it objectively.

The problem of communication with overactive patients should take into consideration the patient's poor attention span, his distractibility, his tendency to be funny, his need to express hostility, and his sensitivity. Complicated ideas and long, involved explanations and discussions are contraindicated. Short, simple answers and comments, direct and to the point, are more effective. Rhetorical questions are often used by such patients, and silence is then best employed, since the patient usually neither wants nor expects an answer and is annoyed when given one. Direct commands are not well accepted, particularly if given in a sharp tone. The patient is easily distracted, and this symptom should be exploited to avoid difficult situations whenever possible.

In this connection, it is well to remember that studies have shown that patients have a tendency to be somewhat more tolerant of psychotic behavior than personnel, and what may appear to be a difficult situation for a nurse may not seem so to other patients. This is especially true of conversations and behavior related to crudeness. When the patient's conversation is very witty or funny, it is wise to guard carefully against the tendency to encourage the patient and overstimulate him. In addition, the nurse must learn the distinction between laughing at and laughing with patients. Patients are acutely aware of the difference and sensitive to its implications. Free verbalization of hostility as shown by sarcasm and ridicule should be tolerated by personnel, since the patient needs an opportunity to share his negative emotional feelings to learn to evaluate them. Care should be taken in comments so as not to imply rejection. Comparison of the patient with other patients or comparison of his behavior with previous days should be avoided. The statement "I like you because you are better behaved today" is a subtle threat to withdraw approval if the patient does not continue the better behavior. Encouragement and praise should be given with tact and an awareness of the possible implications of what is said. Verbal punishment and threats are taboo. Overactive patients present so many problems so often that the temptation to give an impatient response is great. Such temptation should be resisted.

As can be recognized from the description of such patients, there are limitations that must be placed on interpersonal relationships and physical activities. Limitations are necessary, but the manner of their enforcement may present difficulties. No one person—patient, nurse, or other—is ever allowed free and complete expression of his immediate wishes and wants. Limitations in a psychiatric or any hospital, however, are or should be determined by the patient's needs. For this type of behavior, limitations are imposed because of several important considerations. The patient should not be allowed to injure himself or others, so limitations in his behavior are determined by this criterion. An expression of his hostility and ambivalent feelings is necessary, so he is allowed to go as far in this conduct as is safe for himself and those around him. Exhaustion is an experience he should be spared; therefore, limitations are placed on how overactive he may be in terms of this factor. Limitations should be agreed on and *consistently* enforced so that the patient has the security derived from knowing what to expect. Verbal explanations in regard to limitations are of not too much value and so should be very brief. Patients will learn best by experience.

It is interesting to note the close relationship between the physical status and clinical condition of patients with aggressive patterns of behavior. A loss of appetite and weight goes along with an increase in severity of symptoms, and an increase in weight and hours of sleep often presages clinical improvement. For this reason, if for no other, serious efforts to improve the general physical status of the patient should be included in the general plan of treatment, and their importance should not be minimized.

The protective needs of patients with aggressive behavior patterns are quite high. Exhaustion, injury to others and to self, and suicide are common enough occurrences to warrant constant alertness directed toward their prevention.

Exhaustion can be produced by overactivity, agitation, or tension. The physical condition of such patients should be carefully observed, and indications for intercession should be acted on. The nurse should not be confused as to the reserves of patient energy by the degree of output. Measures to avoid exhaustion are the limitation of activity by physical or chemical means, the careful avoidance of stimulation and irritation, and the maintenance of fluid and caloric intake and elimination. Accurate observation and reporting are essential.

Injury to others may occur through the impulsive gestures of overactive and aggressive patients. Close observation and thorough knowledge of the patient's behavior patterns are aids in preventing such injuries. Recognition of mounting tension as indicated by voice changes, muscular signs of tensions, and increasing irritation are indications to take action to avoid possibly injury to others. In addition, objects that can be used for assault should be restricted.

Relationships with other patients. The overactive, aggressive patient is far from being a total loss in a group. Unless there are too many like him, which can be extremely disruptive, he can be an asset. His values are derived from the fact that he can initiate activity, although he may not carry it through, and that he can stimulate responses from withdrawn and retarded patients that a person in an authoritarian position may not be able to do. The danger to him lies in the fact that his domineering aggressiveness may draw group reaction against him, and his sensitivity may render him quite susceptible to hurt. Also, his aggressiveness may secure for him an undue amount of time and attention from personnel, which may result in a group united against him. If these precautions are kept in mind, his entrance in groups may be promoted, and assistance may be given him when he is in difficulty by distracting him from his course of action and by substituting another activity that will bring peace for the moment. For him, this substitution is all that is necessary since he is more or less at the mercy of environmental stimulation. The association with quiet patients may also tone him down somewhat since they are not particularly stimulating. If, however, their very quietness irritates him, contact with such patients should be minimized as far as possible.

The following case study illustrates one method of nursing intervention with an aggressive, hostile patient.

> Mr. N. was well known on the hospital unit for his verbal and physical aggressiveness. He was over 6 feet tall and was very muscular, which alone intimidated most of the staff. There was only one staff member—a young, slightly built attendant named John—with whom he appeared to be fairly comfortable. His teasing with John was funnier than it was bitter and sarcastic. One day during group therapy Mr. N. was obviously becoming very irritated with another patient; his voice became louder, his remarks more caustic, and his movements more restless. John observed his behavior through the door and decided Mr. N. was eventually going to lose control. He asked the therapist if Mr. N. could be excused from the session; this was granted, and John took Mr. N. for a long walk on the grounds. Mr. N. was able to verbally express his aggression, and this combined with walking and talking with John enabled him to calm down.

PROJECTIVE PATTERNS

The projective disorders characteristically occur in middle-aged persons. This finding is consistent with a better retained personality organization, since the patient has managed to crystallize some adjustive techniques that have served to carry him well into adulthood.

A tendency to develop a suspicious attitude and projective techniques of adjustment is found in persons who childhood produced hatred, chronic insecurity, suspiciousness, pride, inability to develop social skills, and a rigid, self-centered personality organization. Such a tendency is usually produced by a combination of factors in early experience. The child first develops a sensitivity to situations that made him feel inadequate and inferior, usually because this is his parents' perception of him. This feeling of inadequacy is reinforced by patterns of suspiciousness that are characteristic of the significant adults in his life. Also, rather extravagant demands are made on the child, and the standards of performance and conformity to which he is expected to adhere are unfortunately high. This overcompensatory insistence on status and prestige and on higher standards than others in the immediate environment, which reflects the parents' insecurity, produces several results in the child. It renders him sensitive to the opinions of others, and it strengthens narcissistic tendencies. It also arouses deep hostility that the child is afraid to express and must learn to hide.

The result is a person with a hostility-laden outlook, chronic insecurity, sensitivity, pride, and suspiciousness, all of which make it extremely difficult for the growing personality to develop social skills in interpersonal relationships. A proud person finds it hard to talk problems over with others since it necessitates the admission to another that all is not well. The accompanying suspiciousness further checks any effort to establish satisfactory relationships with others. Brooding or introspection becomes a fixed method for dealing with personal problems. Because of his inability to establish relationships with others, the individual finds it harder and harder to understand or appreciate any viewpoint except his own. As a result, reality-testing becomes a lost art. Personality organization becomes increasingly rigid as outside influence finds it more difficult to make an impression. Yet a sensitivity to outside opinions is retained, without the ability to evaluate them objectively.

Within the matrix of such a personality, which is unable to tolerate suspense, prolonged anxiety, or sustained tension, the projection of self-inadequacies and self-criticism to others follows readily. By this means, the basic hatred within the patient and his unacceptable impulses and wishes are denied as part of himself and projected to others around him, even if he has to invent someone as the object of projection. Personal faults and failures are attributed to others and disclaimed for the self. The process not only produces comfort by ridding the self of unacceptable facets, but it also makes one feel comfortably superior by comparison. It serves the purpose of avoiding loss of prestige or affection.

The ability to check this tendency by validating conclusions objectively against what has actually happened is defeated by the personality structure. When tension and anxiety are built up and sustained, events are misinterpreted, and significance is attached to the environmental happenings that are in accord with the self-criticism and pride of the individual. Gradually the environmental forces are believed to be aligned in a plot or plan to harm the suspicious person. This offers at least an explanation for what is going on and gives some relief from doubt and suspense. Delusions of persecution have developed. Since the individual has been unable to develop techniques for retesting and analyzing situations in which he is personally involved and has arrived at the conclusion that he is persecuted, this conclusion is extremely difficult to change. Feedback from real situations is misinterpreted. Further inferences are made on the basis of the assumption of persecution, and those parts of experience that support it or can be misinterpreted to support it are selected for attention. The delusional system becomes more or less systematized. Past events are recalled to support the assumption and distorted to confirm the delusions.

The rigidity and self-centeredness of the individual, along with his sensitivity and the almost inevitable gap between his demands on himself and his capacities, render him vulnerable to the use of projective patterns to defend himself in his own self-esteem. The projective pattern bolsters the ego since it both makes one important enough to be persecuted and gives a solid alibi for failure. If the anxiety and threat to security produced by the emotional response to the persecutory delusional system continue, delusions of grandeur may be the next resort. They may simply be a direct reaction to the self-criticism expressed in the original delusional system or they may result as an outgrowth of fantasied achievement with which the patient consoles himself.

Types of behavior. The degree to which projective methods of adjustment are used varies widely, and the behavior that results is a reflection of that degree. All of us behave to some extent on the assumption that other persons are as we are—that they share the same values, feelings, attitudes, and dislikes. The less experienced the individual, the more likely he is to act on this assumption in situations in which it is unwarranted. In addition, projection is more likely to operate in areas that involve socially forbidden and unacceptable actions. We quite frequently ascribe to the behavior of others motives of selfishness, evil intentions, and malice aforethought, although we are eager and anxious to disclaim any such motives on our own part. This is quite similar to the tendency of children to avoid punishment by denying bad behavior and placing responsibility on others or, if caught outright, to try to implicate others. When confronted suddenly with criticism or blame, the majority of adults will find some quick alibi that places blame on circumstances or persons other than themselves.

When a vulnerable, suspicious personality is exposed to prolonged tension and anxiety, it becomes necessary to protect self-esteem. The mechanism of projection is used as a bolster. The domination of the patient's behavior by delusional ideas is the point at which he usually shows a frank mental illness. One of the first symptoms to appear is rigidity of thought and loss of flexibility.

The patient becomes unable to form correct judgments concerning events that occur. As the delusional ideas come to dominate the patient's behavior, the failure in judgment becomes apparent. The suspiciousness and brooding sensitivity become more marked. Ideas of reference follow in which the patient relates all happenings in his surroundings to himself and feels that everything that goes on has some special significance for him. Events are misinterpreted. Suddenly, things clear up. The patient realizes that a conspiracy against him is afoot. At first such false beliefs, or delusions, are fairly well organized, but they spread. The longer these delusions exist, the more is woven into them, and the less logic there is to them. The Federal Bureau of Investigation is out to prove that he is a Communist; the world and its environs are united against him. Ideas of influence then appear; that is, the patient feels his behavior is influenced by outside forces. Radar messages are transmitted to him that force him to commit acts against his will. Electric wires are attached to his brain, and derogatory messages are sent to him constantly. The patient's wife or husband, anxious to engage in an undisturbed extramarital affair, has had the innocent patient committed to the hospital and has planted nurses and attendants in the institution to make obscene remarks and to drive the patient crazy. If perchance the patient is driven to take defensive or vengeful action toward his tormentors, counteraggression is automatically called forth; this reinforces the patient's delusions.

Hallucinations may occur in the more serious manifestations. The patient hears voices accusing him of homosexual behavior or making threats against him. Grandiose delusions may make their appearance, and the patient believes he is Christ, Napoleon, or someone else of stature.

The emotional reaction to the psychotic behavior and ideas may range from completely adequate and appropriate to completely inadequate and inappropriate. The patient may feel a natural resentment against the forces aligned against him, may be mildly annoyed, or may discuss his delusional content with complete indifference. The adequacy of the emotional response is often fairly well correlated with the degree of logic of systematization of the delusions.

Nursing intervention. The individual who isolates himself from sharing experiences with others is not a happy person, nor is he easy to reeducate. Persons for whom he reaches or who reach toward him are frustrated and thwarted by the reactions he calls forth, reactions that make friendship and warmth difficult under ordinary circumstances. The patient can admit no fault in himself and no virtue in others, a trait that is uncomfortably irritating until it is recognized that a fault in himself or a virtue in others threatens him seriously. His tendency to misinterpret situations and read into them derogatory motivations threatens the persons about him; hence, nursing intervention is often more easily planned than carried out.

The use of the pattern of projective behavior is ubiquitous. Everyone uses the mechanism of projection at one time or another, and its use becomes more important as a factor in behavior as it tends to become a major method of adaptation. Its purpose is ultimately defensive. Temporary projection is not serious, but permanent projection is serious. Such trends become one of the factors that influence nursing care in all clinical settings.

One of the basic ingredients of the psychotherapeutic environment must be a lack of counteraggression or retaliation against the patient for his ideas, because at this point the vicious circle can be broken. The patient's symptoms defeat his attempts to reach security and reasonable self-esteem because they call forth counteraggression, which confirms the defensive need for the symptoms. The environment must reduce sharply the difference between the standards expected of the patient and his abilities. It must offend his sense of importance no more than is absolutely necessary. Activities must be available that offer some satisfaction, and the ward routine should have some intellectual challenge while being systematic enough to contribute to security. The environment should also offer the patient full opportunity to explore relationships and to explore such relationships within the limits of safety.

Nurse-patient interpersonal relationships. The ultimate goal of interpersonal relationships with the patient is a contribution to his security in relationships with others, a building of his sense of importance and prestige within the framework of reality, and a sensible reduction of the demands he makes on himself. The patient's symptoms become obstacles in the path to this goal. This is the factor that has made it impossible for society to meet the patient's needs. The obstacles are superior attitude, sarcasm and ridicule, extreme pride and sensitivity, overemphasis on status and prestige, inability to see any other viewpoint, self-centeredness, misinterpretation of the behavior of others, and inflexibility.

A superior attitude is invariably accompanied by the implication that all others are thereby inferior. Conceit, justified or otherwise, does not make for popularity because it makes other persons uncomfortable, places them on the defensive, and encourages attack and retaliation. It is important for nurses to be aware of this response since they will most certainly feel it, and in the interest of the patient, they must recognize and control it. The superior attitude meets a deep-seated emotional need of the patient—it builds his self-esteem. To retaliate, to "teach the patient his place," makes certain that the patient will continue his behavior. Nurses must accept the patient's attitude and recognize its purpose. If the patient were superior, he would not need the attitude.

Nurses can constructively contribute to his sense of importance by giving praise for real ability and accomplishments. In the meantime, the patient should be permitted to express his feelings, and the nurse, without agreeing with these feelings, must still accept the patient as a person and maintain involvement with him. The pressure on the patient to accept reality should not be reduced, but at the same time he should not be punished for his behavior.

Sarcasm and ridicule are used by the patient as a support for his superior attitude and his sense of importance. The purpose behind such behavior is to reduce the status of others and to make the patient appear better by comparison. Sarcasm and ridicule should be met with a matter-of-fact manner, and explanation, justification, and self-denfense should be foregone. This again is not easy, since few persons are so completely secure that they are comfortable under direct attack. However, since the patient needs the attitude and the behavior that spring from his basic self-doubt, it is important that the response to him contain acceptance as a person and the challenge to face reality.

The extreme pride and sensitivity of the patient make imaginative tact and courtesy necessary. Slights and offenses tend to be taken when none is intended. The particular points on which the patient is most sensitive should be learned and respected. Thoughtless comments and answers can cause a great deal of difficulty.

The patient's overemphasis on status and prestige may lead to certain problems in interpersonal relationships that can be difficult to handle. The patient may hold himself completely aloof from others and consider himself apart from and above everyone else, including personnel. He may identify with personnel in an attempt to set up a pseudointimate relationship that places him above other patients in status. Such behavior should be quietly accepted, but if group retaliation against the patient is to be avoided, the patient should be tactfully guided into channels that involve participation in activities with other patients. The nurse should remember that at the moment he is not an individual capable of tolerance for the weaknesses of others and therefore should not be turned loose on others who are acutely sensitive to open attack on their faults. On the other hand, the benefits of status and prestige should be conferred wherever possible for constructive accomplishments.

The tendency for the patient to misinterpret behavior in terms of his emotional needs should be recognized, and such misinterpretation should be assessed for its worth. If, for example, the patient is praised for three accomplishments and reprimanded for one mistake, the reprimand will receive more selective attention and be responded to more strongly than the praise. Such elements leading to self-doubt should be avoided if possible. When the patient does misinterpret, reason is not a particularly effective method of dealing with the symptom. Misinterpretation of events and conversation is a symptom; the cause rather than the symptom should be the source of response. Only when negative emotions and behavior are calmly accepted by others does the patient have an opportunity to see them objectively himself.

The self-centeredness, inflexibility, and inability to see any other viewpoint must be recognized for their implications in nursing intervention. Reason is useless until the patient has attained sufficient security to lose the need to be so rigid. Lengthy explanations and attempts to justify someone else's viewpoint are blocked and are therefore irritating to the patient. An approach that emphasizes altruistic motives, doing things for others, and having tolerance for others is doomed to defeat and makes the patient uncomfortable. In addition, such an approach demands something the patient cannot give and therefore increases his self-doubt.

The matter of how to respond to the psychotic ideas expressed by the patient is of paramount importance. That the entire personnel of the Federal Bureau of Investigation and the Secret Service are persecuting an innocent individual is rather absurd when checked against reality. The first step is to listen in full to the patient's expression without either agreeing or disagreeing. Frequently many of the patient's questions are rhetorical, and if personnel do not interrupt the flow of conversation to answer questions, the patient goes on. Actually, the patient is much less interested in what other people think than in what he thinks and feels. Direct contradiction of the patient's ideas should be avoided, and they should not be brushed aside as nonsense, nor should any indication be given that the patient's statements are accepted as true. As a rule the patient has been shushed, called absurd, and reasoned with beyond endurance. The nurse must listen to him first and at length and note carefully what is said and record it. During an acute phase, the nurse should do no more than let the patient talk and avoid doing any talking about the patient's ideas.

Hostility expressed in vengeful attack on the environment or persons in that environment should be controlled without punishing the patient for his behavior.

Because of his suspiciousness and his delusions of persecution, the patient frequently presents problems in the maintenance of nutrition. If he fears being poisoned, a careful study should be made of ways to get him to eat, up to and including indulgence of his rituals to make sure that his food is free from poison. Tube feeding should be avoided if at all possible because it is an invitation to the patient to misinterpret the procedure as counteraggression. If the patient's illness is chronic, attention to the details of personal appearance and cleanliness may be the responsibility of personnel.

The protection of the projective patient centers around the symptoms he has developed to protect his ego. Since he sees himself as a person largely sinned against, he is always a potential danger to others because he may take action against what appears to him to be a vindictively hostile world. The patient should have adequate observation, and the possibility of attack on others should be guarded against. Two particular situations warrant special attention. If the patient retains a strong and appropriate emotional response to his psychotic ideas, retaliation on his part is more likely to occur. If, however, he recites his long list of persecutions without seeming to be disturbed by them, the danger is less. Projection against specific persons in the immediate environment is also an indication for alertness to possible danger. If the patient weaves the physician, the nurse, the attendant, or another patient into his delusional system, the persecutor is handy for retaliatory action. In such an instance, the personnel member should be warned, or if a patient is involved, protection should be afforded him.

Early stages of the illness may be accompanied by depression, which is an indication of the danger of suicide. The patient may also react to his psychotic ideas with depression because he feels overwhelmed by an environment with which he cannot cope. In either instance, precautions against suicide should be taken.

If one remembers that the patient believes that all is right with him and all is wrong with the rest of the world, it is easy to understand that his hospitalization is a cruel and unnecessary step against him. Personnel should be alerted to the fact that such patients present an elopement threat. There is so much psychologic trauma involved in an elopement and forcible return to the hospital that it is well worth the effort to prevent escapes. If one does occur and the patient is returned to the hospital, his feelings in regard to the matter should be spared at all costs.

Relationships with other patients. The patient who leans heavily on the mechanism of projection tends to be isolated emotionally from the group. If he is at all active, he is likely to be a mild trouble center because of his seeming sense of importance, his suspicion of the motives of others, and his intolerance for the faults of others. However, relationships with hospital personnel can be an extremely constructive experience for the patient and may lay the groundwork for the later establishment of closer relationships in the hospital group and in society.

The patient should be encouraged to work or to play with other patients, starting with a limited number. Large groups either overwhelm him or afford him a screen behind which he can hide. Intellectual activities and detail work are usually his forte and should be permitted. Any activity that can be shared should be encouraged, since skill in social relationships is a real need for this individual. He likes the importance of responsibility and may be allowed to help with slower and more withdrawn patients. In such situations the contribution to his own self-esteem may curb his expression of contempt for others. The appeal for such efforts should be directed to the patient's personal gain rather than to the benefits that will be derived by others. The projective patient cannot afford the luxury of altruism.

It may be necessary to protect other patients from this patient, but it is also necessary to realize that there are times when he himself may need protection. He can usually defend himself verbally against any onslaught, but the very act of defending himself indicates that his pride and sensitivity have been hurt. At such times he needs diversion from group activities and support. He should also be prevented from completely isolating himself and remaining aloof.

As the patient's behavior improves, it is not unusual for him to go through a long period during which he retains his psychotic ideas but does not let them govern his behavior so completely or express them so freely. During this period, direct contradiction of the ideas he holds or admits having held is still not wise. Other explanations may be given for the patient to think about, but there should be no demands on his acceptance of such explanations. If the patient insists on an answer as to whether personnel believe his persecutory or grandiose ideas, a frank "no" may be given with the proviso that the patient is made aware that he has as much right to think "yes" as personnel have to think "no."

As the time approaches for a return to society, the patient's self-responsibility should be returned him, and any evidence of recrudescence of the illness should be carefully watched for.

Social skills should be emphasized and encouraged during this period. The underlying sensitivity will probably always be a part of the patient; therefore, development of social skills without making the patient uncomfortable will require unusual tact. This patient rarely experiences the sense of relief that a convalescing overactive or depressed patient does on escaping from the acute phase of his illness. He is very likely to be somewhat ashamed of his episode and to rationalize to justify it. Matter-of-factness toward mental illness on the part of personnel at this stage is very important to him. He may give the nurse little direct opportunity to demonstrate it in discussions with him, but he will be very alert as to how it is discussed with others within his hearing and as to how the nurse behaves toward mentally ill patients generally.

The patient in his convalescence needs as much support as can be given for realistic future plans. If he goes from the hospital retaining a wide discrepancy between what he expects of himself and what he is capable of accomplishing, he is vulnerable to a relapse. For that reason discussion of his future plans, which will give him an opportunity to see how they sound and to develop some objectivity toward them, should be encouraged. Advice should not be given, and no decisions should be suggested. The patient must be permitted to retain responsibility for himself.

The following case study illustrates the behavior of a patient with projective patterns.

> While hospitalized on a psychiatric unit Mrs. S. was visited regularly by her husband. Mr. S. was a very concerned, gentle, patient man who tried desperately to meet all of Mrs. S.'s needs. He was very attentive, brought her small gifts, commented on how well she was looking, stated frequently how much he and the children missed her, and so forth.
>
> Mrs. S. rejected all of his attentions and told him (and any staff member that would listen to her) that he was not concerned about her, didn't love her, and so forth. The *only* reasons for his visits was to see one of the staff nurses—with whom he was having an affair. Nothing Mr. S. or the staff could say could shake her adamant conviction that her husband was having an affair.

REFERENCES

Aguilera, D. C.: Review of psychiatric nursing, St. Louis, 1977, The C. V. Mosby Co.

Bender, L.: Hostile aggression in children. In Garattini, S., and others, editors: Aggressive behavior, New York, 1969, John Wiley & Sons, Inc.

Berkowitz, L.: Aggression: a social psychological analysis, New York, 1962, McGraw-Hill Book Co.

Buss, A. H.: The psychology of aggression, New York, 1961, John Wiley & Sons, Inc.

Cameron, N.: Paranoid conditions and paranoia. In Arieti, S., editor: American handbook of psychiatry, vol. 1, New York, 1959, Basic Books, Inc.

Carstairs, G. M.: Overcrowding and human aggression. In Graham, H. D., and Gurr, T. R., editors: Violence in America, New York, 1969, Bantam Books.

Carter, F. M.: Psychosocial nursing, New York, 1976, The Macmillan Co.

Coser, L. A.: The functions of social conflict, New York, 1956, The Free Press of Glencoe.

Dollard, J., Dobb, L. W., Miller, N. E., Mowrer, O. H., and Sears, R. R.: Frustration and aggression, New Haven, Conn., 1939, Yale University Press.

Freud, A.: Comments on aggression, Int. J. Psychoanal. **53:**163-169, 1972.

Freud, S.: On narcissism: an introduction. In Standard edition of the complete psychological works of Sigmund Freud, vol. XIV, London, 1957, Hogarth Press, pp. 73-102.

Gorney, R.: Interpersonal intensity, competition and synergy: determinants of achievement, aggression, and mental illness, Am. J. Psychiatry **128:**4:436-445, 1971.

Kolb, L. C.: Modern clinical psychiatry, ed. 8, Philadelphia, 1973, W. B. Saunders Co.

Mahler, M. S., Berman, A., and Pine, F.: Danger signals in the separation-individuation process, unpublished paper, 1973.

Silver, L. B., Dublin, C. C., and Laurie, R.: Does violence breed violence? Am. J. Psychiatry **126**(3):404-407, 1969.

Solomon, P., and Patch, V.: Handbook of psychiatry, ed. 3, Los Altos, Calif., 1974, Lange Medical Publications.

Stankiewicz, B.: Guides to nursing intervention in the projective patterns of suspicious patient, Perspect. Psychiatr. Care **2:**39-45, 1964.

Sullivan, H. S.: Conceptions of modern psychiatry, Washington, D.C., 1947, William Alanson White Psychiatric Foundation.

Toch, H.: Violent men: an inquiry into the psychology of violence, Chicago, 1969, Aldine-Atherton, Inc.

ADDITIONAL READINGS

De Felippo, A. M.: Preventing assaultive behavior in a psychiatric unit, Superv. Nurse 7(6):62-65, 1976.

Matheson, W., and others: Coping with the aggressive patient: an alternative to punishment, Can. Nurse 72(7):18-19, 1976.

Scoggins, J. B.: Communicate, dammit, RN 39(3):38-41, 1976.

CHAPTER 10

Patients with antisocial patterns

Antisocial personality is currently considered the official term for what was first called moral insanity, then constitutional psychopathic inferiority or psychopathic personality, and then sociopathic personality disturbance with the subcategories antisocial reaction, dyssocial reaction, sexual deviation and substance abuse.

The person with an antisocial personality gets into repeated conflict with society. He has no loyalty or concern for others, ignores social codes or values, and acts only in response to his own desires and impulses. Punishment does not touch him, and experience teaches him little. He cannot resist temptation since he cannot tolerate frustration, and he blames others skillfully when he is caught.

Since many people flout the rules of society to satisfy their own desires at one time or another, a diagnosis of antisocial personality depends on both quantitative and qualitative data and on an assessment of a patient's total lifestyle. One must consider *how much* disregard for the ethical standards of society the patient has shown, *how long* he has shown this disregard, and *how basically* unsocialized and unsocializable he is.

The antisocial personality is usually first manifested in childhood or early adolescence by such behavioral problems as truancy, theft, running away, incorrigibility, associating with bad companions, impulsiveness, lying, and a poor record of achievement in school or employment. Enuresis is often part of the history, for some unknown reason.

It is generally considered that the patient with an antisocial personality is unable to postpone immediate pleasure or gratification of an impulse, lacks the capacity for maintaining a close relationship with another person, and feels no guilt or anxiety over his antisocial acts. Such persons dissipate anxiety by immediate and impulsive actions with essentially no delay between stimulus and response.

The symptoms and signs persist into adult life as poor marital adjustment, bad work history, repeated arrests, impulsiveness, pathologic lying, sexual promiscuity, vagrancy, and social isolation. In women, the history usually includes prostitution, venereal disease, and illegitimacy.

The antisocial person is not a stupid individual who has been unable to learn the rules of society; he may be very bright or even brilliant. Most of these individuals have great social charm, usually developed over a lifetime of practice in the art of cunning, conning, and guile—all directed toward immediate gratification of desires. The con men and the manipulators are apt to be found in this category, along with those who use other people for their own ends with little regard for consequences.

Cleckley (1976) has formulated a set of criteria for the antisocial syndrome, some of which are summarized as follows:

1. Average or superior intelligence
2. Absence of irrationality and other commonly accepted symptoms of psychosis
3. No sense of responsibility
4. Disregard for truth
5. No sense of shame
6. Antisocial behavior without apparent regret
7. Inability to learn from experience
8. General poverty of affect
9. Lack of genuine insight
10. Little response to special consideration or kindness
11. No history of *sincere* suicide attempts

Dynamics of development. Since much antisocial behavior violates social norms, it is not surprising that many investigators have focused on the primary agent of socialization, the family, in their search for the explanation of such behavior. Many antisocial individuals have apparently experienced the trauma of losing a parent. Greer (1964) found that 60% of his sample of diagnosed sociopaths had lost at least one parent during childhood. Similarly, McCord and McCord (1964) concluded that lack of affection and severe parental rejection were the primary causes of antisocial behavior. Other studies have related antisocial behavior to the parents' inconsistencies in disciplining the child and in teaching him his responsibilities to others (Becker, 1963). Also, the fathers of sociopaths are likely to display antisocial behavior.

Much of the behavior of patients whose difficulty seems to be disregard for social standards with little personal discomfort seems explicable in terms of a deep lack of emotional capacity that is not always obvious to the casual observer. The individual who does not feel so deeply as others or is unable to feel with others misses most of the significance of human experience. Experience has not the same meaning for such a person, nor can he appreciate what is important to others. An outlook on life that does not include the usual depth of the experiences of love, hate, and shame, for example, makes the integration of experience difficult and incredibly hampers the growth toward a mature personality. After all, the first steps toward growth come through strong emotional response to reward and punishment. Without the emotional component, approval and disapproval are not strong enough to mold the growing individual into accepted patterns of behavior. Characteristically, patients with this defect usually show a long history of maladjustment that grows increasingly evident as they age and more mature criteria are used as a standard for comparison with their behavior. Also in keeping with this basic assumption—that the central defect in the personality structure is a severe limitation of emotional capacity—is the fact that such patients are rarely modified by experience or treatment. The need for approval as a means of security is an important motivating factor in mental health, but antisocial individuals are not susceptible to motivation of this sort.

Extremely severe emotional trauma early in life, especially in a sensitive child, might possibly lead to a rejection of the emotional aspect of existence, although a repression so deep and so complete of what ordinarily constitutes a major portion of experience would require very severe trauma.

Another possibility is the effect of parents who mechanize human relationships, who are capable of living only with the intellect. The absence of warmth in parents, especially if the child is isolated from other contacts before school age, may result in personality growth being forever stunted by the effect of growing up in an emotional refrigerator. The traits of such parents are exaggerated in the child. It would be necessary for both parents to participate in such a pattern or for the pattern to be determined by one parent who completely dominated the child.

The hypothesis that patients with antisocial patterns of behavior are victims of some lack at birth has been frequently advanced. This theory has never been adequately proved or disproved.

The psychodynamic understanding of this condition is much the same as for the passive-aggressive personality. The pattern arises from grossly faulty mothering, ambivalent parental relationships, and unresolved oedipal conflicts. Behaviorists stress the lack of opportunity to learn the values of society from socially acceptable models. They emphasize that antisocial behavior can be consciously or unconsciously taught to a developing child. The father who lies and cheats to his son's certain knowledge is teaching him that the rules of society are for other people—that it is all right to lie, cheat, and steal and that one does not need to feel guilty about it.

Psychotherapy has had little success in the treatment of these individuals. Classically, the approach is to confront the patient and convince him that his problems are not with the outside world but within himself. Having thus in a sense converted his problem to a neurosis, the usual psychotherapy for the neurosis is instituted.

Since many people with antisocial personalities spend time in prison where facilities for individual psychotherapy are limited, it is not surprising that milieu treatment and group therapy have enjoyed some vogue with these patients. Any psychologic approach that offers no rewards for antisocial behavior and definite rewards for social behavior would seem a valid approach based on learning principles. When a social situation is provided from which the patient cannot easily escape, as with milieu or group therapy in prison, the consequences of his antisocial behavior are forced on him; that is, since he cannot run away impulsively as he would ordinarily do, he is forced to come to grips with some aspects of society. Only limited success has been reported with these types of therapy, but they perhaps represent the best hope for future therapeutic approaches to this treatment-resistant group of patients.

Some antisocial persons, despite lack of ability to learn from experience, seem to "burn out" in their thirties and become respectable citizens.

The following case study depicts the classic antisocial individual, the intervention, and results of the intervention:

Michael, age 36, a tall, handsome, and extremely well-dressed man, appeared at a crisis center. He was asked to come into the office, have a seat, and to tell what had motivated him to seek help at the center. Michael sat down, unbuttoned his suit jacket (revealing an automatic gun in a holster on his belt), and smiled pleasantly. He was asked by the nurse-therapist if he was a police officer; he replied "no," which increased the therapist's anxiety considerably! He was asked why he was wearing the gun. He replied, "I never go anywhere without it." He smiled and added, "It's a jungle out there."

When asked why he came to the center, his expression sobered and he replied, "I *think* I've got a problem." He was asked to elaborate. He stated that he was out of jail on bail, that he was a "three-time loser," and that he did not want to spend the rest of his life in jail. He also stated that he had two forged passports under two assumed names and that he planned to go to Canada or to Australia. When he was told that it was not the therapist's role to make his decision for him—merely to explore the alternatives of his possible action with him—he asked if what would be discussed would remain *completely* confidential. He was assured that a patient and therapist have a fiduciary relationship, like attorney and client, and that the only conditions under which a therapist would, by law, be requested to release information about sessions would be if he said he was going to murder someone and named the person, time, and place. He was also told that a therapeutic relationship, to be effective, involved complete honesty and trust between the therapist and the patient.

He sat back in his chair, looked directly at the therapist, and remained silent—as if testing the therapist. Neither said anything for approximately 3 minutes. Michael then smiled faintly and said, "O.K., I'll tell you what is *really* bothering me." (It was obvious that he was expecting negative reactions from the therapist regarding the gun, being out on bail, being a "three-time loser" or a "hardened criminal," and possessing forged passports and contemplating forfeiting the bail and leaving the country illegally.) He then related his "lousy" childhood. His mother had left his father when he was 3 years old and he had lived with various relatives sporadically, when he was not in juvenile hall or in a correctional institution. He stated he had only one friend, one person who had stuck by him "through thick and thin," a distant cousin named Chuck.

Chuck had recently married and his wife was expecting a child. Chuck had started a business that was beginning to be very successful. When Michael was picked up for armed robbery—"It was a stupid thing; I didn't need the money, I was doing it for kicks"—his bail was set at $30,000 because of his past police record. Chuck made arrangements with a bail bondsman by signing over all of his equity and property in his business and home to get Michael out on bail.

Michael said this was his dilemma: he did not want to go back to jail but he also didn't want Chuck to lose his business. He stated that he had never before felt any compunction about jumping bail or committing any of his numerous crimes . . . and they were numerous! He couldn't understand why he was feeling "so rotten . . . couldn't make a decision . . . why he had ever come to the center . . . why he felt he needed help—he had managed without it for 36 years . . ." and so forth.

The therapist let him ventilate his feelings fully—it was apparent that he could not understand his own behavior at this time. He was asked whether he just might be beginning to mature, to begin to think of others rather than just himself, to *care* if Chuck lost his business because of him. He replied that he really didn't know, he just felt rotten. Michael was asked if he would commit himself to coming for therapy for 6 weeks. He replied hesitantly, "I think so, but I don't know; I may leave the country tomorrow." He was asked to come back the next week, if he didn't leave the country—and if he did leave the country, to send an unsigned postcard from wherever he was. He laughed and seemed to relax, and said, "I'll see you next week at the same time." He and the therapist shook hands when he left—trust and honesty had been established.

Michael kept his appointments—always on time. He and the therapist worked on his new feelings and what they could mean. At the fourth session Michael was asked if he thought he was benefiting from therapy and he replied with a very strong "Yes." The therapist told him about a maximum security prison in the state that had excellent therapists and the regimen of milieu and group therapy sessions for those who truly wanted to change and stay out of prison. The therapist asked, "If I could get the judge to consent, would you be interested? It would also mean a reduced sentence if you sincerely complied with the therapeutic regimen." Michael looked at the therapist intently and said: "Do you really think I can be helped?" The reply was, "Yes, you have already begun to change." He looked very thoughtful and replied, "You would *really* try to get me in there, wouldn't you?" Again the answer was, "Yes, Michael." He stood up and paced the floor, looking at the therapist occasionally. He stopped and leaned over the desk and said, "Thank you for caring; try to get me in—if you can." The therapist stood up, smiled, and said, "I'll do everything I can; keep in touch daily, and I'll give you a progress report."

The judge was contacted and a meeting was arranged. He listened to Michael's story and progress and answered, "If you can give him a chance, so can I; have him call me—the sooner the better." Michael did very well while in prison and corresponded frequently with the judge and the therapist. He was released, apparently cured; he left the state, is working and doing well, is married, and has a child.

Types of behavior. The types of behavior shown by antisocial patients are not easily described. There is not complete agreement on who is included in the grouping, and the types of classification within the species vary with the clinician's personal experience and attitude toward patients as well as numerous other factors. The descriptions that follow are not intended to be wholly inclusive or exclusive. A patient need not show all of them to be an antisocial individual, nor would the existence of symptoms other than those mentioned exclude him from consideration as antisocial.

Patients in this category usually possess superficial charm and high intelligence. They sound quite interesting and interested, can discuss numerous subjects, nearly always say the right thing and say it well. That they do not mean what they say is not apparent on first or casual acquaintance. Met only on a verbal level, they seem to be thoroughly competent. If they could live life as well as they talk it, all would be in order. These persons, however, are completely unreliable. They lack a sense of responsibility in both trivial and serious matters and further confuse observers with spasmodic periods of conforming behavior. Closer observation usually reveals that these periods of conformity cost the conformer little in terms of energy and nothing in terms of personal sacrifice.

A pattern of frequent failure is characteristic. Although the patient gives evidence of having the potential to succeed in his chosen field, he rarely stays with it and frequently quits for seemingly trivial reasons. He lacks perseverance. He may look good for a little while, but given time, he shows his inadequacy.

Insincerity and untruthfulness are hallmarks of this group of patients, yet they sound as though they mean every word they say. It is only when they fail to carry through into behavior that the insincerity and lack of honesty become apparent. They may protest a deep affection for a spouse, spend the night with someone else, come back the next day with the same protestation of deep affection, and see no incongruity in their words and their actions. Further, they will be annoyed and indignant if criticized.

A complete egocentricity is also characteristic of the antisocial individual. What emotional capacity he has is centered on himself, and he seems incapable of any real emotional investment in others. Deep and lasting affection for another is utterly foreign to his nature. His readiness of expression is often confused with strength of feeling. In all situations he suffers from lack of enduring emotional responses. Remorse and shame are beyond him; although he can and does convincingly apologize, he repeats his offense at the first opportunity. He learns little from experience and seems never to think of the consequences of his behavior. His antisocial acts often seem to have little reason behind them, and he shows no remorse for the pain he causes others. He usually shows impatience at the idea that he should be punished or constrained from following his wishes. His judgment is poor; he steals when he is sure to be caught, spends his money on pleasure when he needs it to pay his bills, and repeats the same mistakes again and again. Kindness, special consideration, and trust are taken for granted and arouse no response of appreciation. His sex life is impersonal and poorly integrated. As would be suspected, he is often sexually promiscuous, but the act itself is without any deep personal significance for him. He cannot evaluate himself or his behavior realistically and rationalizes easily by way of explanation. He is irresponsible and completely undisturbed about it. He has no life plan and cannot follow one consistently. In other words, only the present is significant; the past matters little, and the future does not count.

The specific expressions of the disorder are to be found in sexual promiscuity and perversions, lying, stealing, recklessness, and substance abuse. They are seen in a whole range of minor and major infractions of the law, such as forgeries, arson, assault, and robbery. The constant use of other people for personal and casual satisfaction is also a specific expression of the disorder.

In summary, behavior characterized by the following traits, shown in social aggression rather than psychotic symptoms, is considered antisocial. The traits include inability to profit from experience, poor judgment, living for the present, emotional deficiency with cold-blooded self-centeredness and little or no capacity for remorse, quick and facile emotional responses without depth or duration, amorality, lack of a sense of responsibility, explosiveness under pressure, and a tendency to repeat mistakes. Many of these characteristics are not obvious on first acquaintance; only when the patient is better known do his difficulties become obvious.

Problems in intervention. The inadequate knowledge concerning antisocial personalities may be one of the reasons for the generally held nihilistic attitude toward therapy. In recent years a more hopeful attitude has been expressed from several quarters, but such voices are few. This attitude is understandable in view of the fact that so little is known concerning causative factors in the development of an antisocial personality. Few of these patients are ever completely cured. When our knowledge expands, as it has recently in so many other areas of personality disorders, a marked advance in the therapy of patients with aggressive personality disorders may occur.

The antisocial person's uncooperativeness toward treatment and his peculiar legal status make it exceedingly difficult to get him under treatment and to keep him there. By legal definition, such patients are not psychotic, which makes them ineligible for psychiatric hospitalization except in private institutions where the cost of care is prohibitive. The great majority of psychiatric patients are in governmental hospitals of one type or another, where they cannot remain unless their problems are complicated by a psychotic episode. Under such circumstances relatively little effort has been expended on the problem of understanding them, since more extensive and urgent problems of other types of disorders confront the psychiatric health team in their working environment.

Because of their inability to abide by rules and regulations that conflict with their impulses and immediate wishes, antisocial individuals frequently come into conflict with the law, which results in jail sentences. Many of these patients show real ability at evading paying the consequences of their behavior. Although they *do* serve jail sentences, there are many more occasions in which additional or longer penalties would have seemed indicated.

Even though the personal history may indicate quite clearly that society needs protection from these individuals and will continue to need protection during his lifetime, the patient can be sentenced only for the period his particular offense merits and then must be released to transgress again. This is not to imply that all antisocial individuals are criminals or that all criminals are antisocial individuals. However, many of them do come in conflict with the law and pose a severe problem in rehabilitation.

If all treatment fails, there is no way to adequately protect the person from himself and society from him. Therapy is frustrated by his inability to integrate new experience and to alter his personality development through corrective experience. He does not profit by mistakes, and thus his poor judgment has little opportunity to improve. The traits that characterize his developmental defect operate to prevent his improvement.

Nursing intervention. What is said here concerning nursing intervention of antisocial patients is a series of tentative suggestions that may prove false in any specific instance. These suggestions hould be checked carefully against experience and revised as deemed necessary.

Relatively few antisocial individuals will be found in psychiatric hospitals. Because their incidence in the general population is not small, it is important to recognize them for what they are and to be able to identify them. They make poor friends and poor wives and husbands, and the payment for becoming emotionally involved with them comes high in personal unhappiness.

With our present knowledge, all we can say concerning the type of environment necessary for an antisocial personality is that it should provide a considerable degree of control over the patient. In line with developing knowledge, however, it seems safe to add that the environment should also be one in which the atmosphere is oriented toward understanding the fact that the patient's behavior is symptomatic of a personality defect and in which careful observation and study of the patient is possible.

It is not known whether the cultural milieu of a psychiatric hospital, which abounds with frankly psychotic patients, is the best place for attempted treatment of antisocial personalities. It may be that a different type of institution needs to be developed.

Nurse-patient interpersonal relationships. The major problem in interpersonal relationships with antisocial personalities is to avoid being taken in by their smooth and often charming exteriors. With their verbal fluency and seemingly intact intelligence, they often appear to be extremely well-adjusted people who have wandered into the hospital by mistake. They are quite believable and play on the sympathies of personnel. The danger of being taken in lies in the fact that they use other people for their own purposes, ruthlessly and without remorse. When a member of the staff is suddenly confronted with the patient's defects, the natural reaction is to apply normal standards of conduct for judgment and to be quite angry. If the staff expects the patient to lie, to steal, to stir up trouble, and to project his defects to personnel, it is much easier to accept the patient's behavior quietly and not put any additional pressure on him. Such a patient tends to be explosive under pressure. In other words, the approach to be used with the antisocial personality is to remain constantly on guard to be able to quietly accept his amoral or antisocial behavior when it does appear. On the surface he seems so charmingly normal that it is hard to curb the tendency to retaliate when he does not wear well. The patient needs acceptance as he is, and it is not good for him to have his capacities overestimated.

The protective needs of the antisocial individual are usually more in the nature of protecting others from him. He should be protected from the results of indulging in impulsive expression of primitive tendencies. Most of the difficulty for such patients is in the area of adjusting to social control applied to themselves or others.

The antisocial individual is often casually cruel to others, and sensitive patients may need to be protected from contact with him. He is often the source of forbidden materials for such patients, and this trait should be carefully watched for and guarded against. He is the person who finds razor blades for the depressed patient and matches for the confused and bewildered patient who is unsafe with them.

Relationships with other patients. As a rule, the antisocial individual makes a good initial impression on the group, but this impression does not last long. He often causes arguments without being involved himself, he helps other patients break rules and laughs at their resulting difficulties, and he makes fun of the psychotic ideas of patients. He is an extremely disruptive group member and needs careful attention to keep him constructively occupied. His defective social judgment becomes most apparent in his group relationships. He often shows a tendency in a hospital situation to identify himself with personnel and should not be encouraged in the practice if the effect is detrimental to other patients. If it is not, however, this trait can be used to keep the patient occupied.

Firmness in keeping the patient on routine will still be necessary, and every encouragement to accept continued treatment should be given him. Above all, careful and objective observation of the patient and detailed charting are important. More research in this particular area is vitally needed.

SEXUAL DEVIATE BEHAVIOR

A sexual deviation, perversion, or paraphilia is defined as a pattern of sexual behavior in which the predominant source of sexual gratification is by means other than normal heterosexual intercourse. Sexually deviant acts are usually impulsive and compulsive in character. Individuals who practice them may seem outwardly as normal as anyone else; in fact, a man's wife, for example, may be ignorant of his sexually deviant tendencies for years. The legal status of sexually deviant acts is often culturally influenced—for example, homosexuality between consenting adults is no longer a crime in England but it is in most of the United States. From a legal standpoint, homosexuality in the female is more acceptable than in the male. However, tolerance of homosexuality in general seems to be growing rapidly.

Types of behavior

Homosexuality. Homosexuality is defined as desire for sexual contact with persons of one's own sex. However, a history of isolated homosexual experiences, usually in adolescence, does not constitute homosexuality. Homosexual behavior between women is termed lesbianism. Men or women who enjoy sexual contact with both sexes are termed bisexual. It is generally considered that most bisexuals are primarily homosexual, although they can bring themselves to perform heterosexually, and even enjoy it somewhat.

Homosexuality is the most common of the sexual deviations. Its prevalence is not precisely known and varies in different societies. Homosexuals congregate largely in urban areas. Most homosexual pickups are made at certain locally known sections of town—such as gay bars, or Turkish baths—or by cruising the streets. Homosexual prostitution is not unusual. Some individuals live open, exclusively homosexual lives, whereas others are more discreet and live—and pass—in a predominately heterosexual world. In recent years homosexuals have begun to portray themselves as an oppressed minority and are beginning to fight for their rights openly.

Some homosexuals attempt to emulate heterosexual relationships and may even be "married"; after a passionate start these relationships might break up or continue for many years.

The following case study illustrates some of the problems homosexuals encounter.

Jane, a fairly attractive, 29-year-old executive secretary for a state government official, came to a crisis center seeking help. She stated emphatically that she did *not* want a female therapist: "a woman would not understand or be able to accept my problem." She was informed that the only therapist available was female, and that if she wanted to wait for a male therapist they would put her on a waiting list for the first available one. She reluctantly agreed to see the female therapist but stated, "It won't work."

When Jane came into the office, the nurse-therapist introduced herself, shook hands, and asked Jane to be seated and discuss what was bothering her. Jane sat rigidly in the chair with a defiant look on her face and said, "I doubt if *you* can help me." The therapist smiled and replied, "I can't—if you don't tell me what your problem is!" Jane very reluctantly began talking, watching the therapist's face constantly for any clues of disgust or repugnance.

Jane stated that she was a lesbian and had been "all of my life, I guess," and that no one knew. Everyone at work thought she was straight; her days were spent in passing and her evenings in the gay world. She stated that she and her lover, Nikki, had been living together for 6 years and that they had a beautiful relationship and encountered very little difficulty in getting along with each other. Jane stated, "I work and earn the money and Nikki takes care of the house."

The therapist asked again, "Then what is the problem, Jane?" She circumvented answering by explaining her childhood and how she always knew she was "different." Jane grew up in a small midwestern town, was an excellent student, and was the youngest child, having two older brothers. She described her early home life as great. Her father, a physician, was delighted to have a daughter—at last—and her brothers and mother spoiled her rotten, at first. When she was 3 years old, her father died of a heart attack. After the estate was settled the family discovered that the father had been speculating in the stock market and had left no money and many unpaid debts. Her mother was very bitter because she had assumed there would be more than enough money for them to continue to live quite comfortably. Her mother found a job, for a small salary, as a receptionist in a physician's office and her brothers took part-time jobs to help out. Jane stated, "I really don't remember too much— only that no one was happy, and I felt like I was a nuisance."

Apparently, the family remained more or less the same during Jane's formative years, with her mother becoming more bitter and dominating each day. Jane's only happiness came when she was in school. Her teachers thought she was an ideal student: quiet, studious, and well behaved.

When Jane graduated from high school with top honors she went to a large city near her home town to attend a secretarial school. Again she was the ideal student and was able to get an excellent job when she graduated. She stated that she was really too busy to date and that she wasn't asked out that often— "I was too quiet and reserved."

One evening the office manager, Miss B., asked her to work late so they could complete a large order that had to go out that evening. Jane agreed and they worked until 7:30 P.M. Miss B. invited Jane to her apartment for a drink and dinner and Jane agreed. After dinner and several drinks, Miss B. began to make sexual advances toward Jane. Jane said, "Maybe I was a little drunk— but it seemed so natural and she was so sweet and patient with me—I knew that I really loved her." Their relationship continued for 2 years until Jane felt someone might find out, so she quit her job and moved to the west coast.

She had no difficulty in getting her present position but stated that she was very cautious about her evening activities, because she knew she would be fired if it were discovered she was a lesbian.

Again the therapist tried to get Jane to focus on the current problem. Jane had apparently not detected any overt or covert signs of disapproval from the therapist because she was a lesbian. She appeared to relax and stated that her first lover, Miss B., had found out where she was working and had called and stated that she was coming out so they could be together again. Jane was in a panic because (1) she did not want Nikki to know about Miss B., (2) she really didn't want to see Miss B. again, and (3) she was afraid that if she didn't see her, Miss B. might call her boss and reveal all and she would lose her job.

The therapist asked Jane when Miss B. was expected and she blurted out, "This afternoon at 3:30 P.M.; I have to meet her at the airport." Jane was then asked if she wanted the therapist to be with her when she explained her new situation to Miss B. Jane looked incredulous and said, "Would you really?" The answer was "Yes, bring her here from the airport and you can tell her in my office, with me here." Jane started to cry with relief; the therapist gave her some tissues and told her jokingly to repair her makeup—or Miss B. *might* think she was crying because she was so happy to see her! She stopped crying and both had a good laugh.

Jane and Miss B. appeared at the center and were seen by the therapist together. Jane explained about Nikki and about her job to Miss B. Miss B. listened and said, "I understand—Nikki sounds great. I won't try to move in with you, but don't you think I could stay in a hotel and get a week's vacation? I've always wanted to visit here, and the plane fare was expensive!" Jane laughed and said, "I'll see that you get a good tour guide."

The next day the therapist received a gorgeous bouquet of flowers; the card read, "Thanks, all 'straights' aren't 'square,' Love, Jane and Nikki."

While this case study does not illustrate *all* of the problems of homosexuality, hopefully it does give some insight into the multiplicity of problems that confront patients when deviations from the expected norm are present.

Exhibitionism. Exhibitionism is a common deviation defined as deliberate and compulsive exposure of the genitals in public, almost always by a male, as a means of achieving sexual gratification. Exhibitionistic play is common in preadolescence and is not a perversion. In the pervert, exposure leads to sexual excitement that culminates in orgasm, either spontaneously or, more commonly, by masturbation. Exhibitionistic behavior is often a compulsive and repetitive act, committed usually around strangers and in busy streets or theaters, with much guilt after the act. Exhibitionists usually have inadequate personalities and sadistic and masochistic tendencies. They also tend to return to the scene of the incident and are therefore often apprehended.

Voyeurism. Voyeurism is obtaining sexual gratification through observing sexual organs and sexual activities of others, usually women. It is common in preadolescence purely as seeking sexual excitement. In adults, voyeuristic traits may be normal, as in foreplay prior to intercourse. The deviant, however, obtains his major satisfaction by compulsively and repetitively observing others, often at great risk. His methods vary from Peeping Tom activities to prearranged observations of elaborate sexual performances.

Transvestism. Transvestism is obtaining sexual arousal and gratification by wearing clothes appropriate to the opposite sex. It must be distinguished from transsexuality. The male transvestite may have a complete wardrobe of feminine attire that he wears in secret. Orgasm usually occurs by masturbating in contact with this clothing.

Fetishism. Fetishism is defined as obtaining sexual arousal and gratification from inanimate objects (for example, shoes or lingerie) or from parts of the body (such as the feet or hair) of persons of the opposite sex. It is predominately a male form of sexual deviation. Fetishism is an exaggeration of the normal sexual overevaluation of certain articles associated with the love object. The female fetishist sometimes engages in compulsive kleptomania, which may have unconscious sexual significance. In males, excessive attention to certain parts of the female body—such as breasts, buttocks, or legs—is called *partialism*.

Sadism and masochism. Sadism consists of obtaining sexual arousal or gratification by inflicting pain or humiliation on the partner; masochism is sexual pleasure derived from suffering pain or humiliation. The two are always present together—although one or the other is apt to be dominant—and are referred to as sadomasochism. The terms are derived from the Marquis de Sade, a French writer, and Leopold von Sacher-Masoch, an Austrian novelist who wrote on this subject.

Transsexuality. Transsexuality is the conscious, compelling desire to change one's sex. A male transexual is a person who thinks, feels, and acts like a female but is biologically male. In contrast, the hermaphrodite has biologic abnormalities of both sexes, but usually the sex-role orientation is appropriate to the predominant external sexual characteristics.

In recent years, male transsexuals have become increasingly successful in inducing legitimate surgeons to perform plastic surgery on them, with castration and the provision of a vagina-like organ. Female transsexuals resort to mastectomy and prosthesis.

Causes of sexual deviations. The causes of sexual deviations are unknown. The psychoanalytic view, which is plausible, stresses the defense against castration anxiety in deeply buried oedipal conflicts. The specific deviation seems to be determined by the pathologic experiences of childhood, reinforced by parental rejection, hostility, or ambivalence.

Treatment. As one would suppose, since the sexual deviate perceives his symptomatic behavior primarily as a source of gratification and only secondarily as a means of his getting into trouble, in uncomplicated cases it is not common for him to ask for treatment. The most hopeful situation would be one in which the sexual deviate, for strong, positive motives of his own—for example, to save a marriage that is valued and meaningful—seeks treatment on his own initiative.

The psychiatric treatment of sexual deviation is by intensive psychotherapy or psychoanalysis. No physical or chemical mode of treatment appears to be of any value in affecting the underlying disturbance. If the patient's total personality happens to be of such a nature that his judgment and discretion are impaired, therapy should begin in a hospital setting; in most instances therapy can be undertaken on an outpatient basis. The initial objective of therapy is that of enabling the patient to understand his deviate sexual activities as being dictated by anxiety more than by choice.

REFERENCES

Aguilera, D. C.: Review of psychiatric nursing, St. Louis, 1977, The C. V. Mosby Co.

Becker, H. S. Outsiders: studies in the sociology of deviance, New York, 1963, The Free Press.

Cadoret, R., and King, L.: Psychiatry in primary care, St. Louis, 1974, The C. V. Mosby Co.

Cleckley, H. M.: Psychopathic states. In Arieti, S., editor: American handbook of psychiatry, vol. 1, New York, 1959, Basic Books, Inc., pp. 567-588.

Cleckley, H. M.: The mask of sanity, ed. 5, St. Louis, 1976, The C. V. Mosby Co.

Davison, G. C., and Neale, J. M.: Abnormal psychology, New York, 1974, John Wiley & Sons, Inc.

Greer, S.: Study of parental loss in neurotics and sociopaths, Arch. Gen. Psychiatry 11:177-180, 1964.

Kolb, L. C.: Modern clinical psychiatry, ed. 8, Philadelphia, 1973, W. B. Saunders Co., pp. 494-502.

Kyes, J., and Hofling, C.: Basic psychiatric concepts in nursing, ed. 3, Philadelphia, 1974, J. B. Lippincott Co.

Lindner, R.: Rebel without a cause, New York, 1944, Grune & Stratton, Inc.

McCord, W., and McCord, J.: The psychopath: an essay on the criminal mind, New York, 1964, Van Nostrand Reinhold Co.

Solomon, P., and Patch, V. D.: Handbook of psychiatry, Los Altos, Calif., 1974, Lange Medical Publications.

ADDITIONAL READINGS

Aichorn, A.: Wayward youth, New York, 1955, Viking Press.

Alexander, F., and Stauf, H.: The criminal, the judge, and the public, translated by Gregory Zilborg, New York, 1931, The Macmillan Co.

American Psychiatric Association: A psychiatric glossary, Washington, D.C., 1969, American Psychiatric Association.

Bettelheim, B.: Truants from life: the rehabilitation of emotionally disturbed children, New York, 1955, The Free Press.

Blos, P.: The concept of acting out in relation to the adolescent process. In Rexford, E. N., editor: A developmental approach to acting out, New York, 1966, International Universities Press, Inc., p. 136.

Bowlby, J.: Attachment and loss: attachment, vol. I, New York, 1969, Basic Books, Inc.

Bowlby, J.: Attachment and loss: separation, anxiety and anger, vol. II, New York, 1973, Basic Books, Inc.

Freud, S.: Criminality from a sense of guilt. In Collected papers, vol. IV, London, 1949, Hogarth Press, p. 343.

Gianascol, A. J.: Psychiatry and the juvenile court: patterns of collaboration and the use of compulsive psychotherapy. In Szurek, S. A., and others, editors: The antisocial child: his family and his community, Palo Alto, Calif., 1969, Science and Behavior Books, pp. 149-159.

Johnson, A. M., and Szurek, S. A.: The genesis of antisocial acting out in children and adults. In Szurek, S. A., and others, editors: The antisocial child: his family and his community, Palo Alto, Calif., 1969, Science and Behavior Books, pp. 13-28.

Rappeport, J. R.: Antisocial behavior. In Arieti, S., editor: American handbook of psychiatry, vol. III, New York, 1974, Basic Books, Inc., pp. 255-269.

Report of the Panel on Youth of the President's Science Advisory Committee: Youth: transition to adulthood, Washington, D.C., 1973, U.S. Government Printing Office.

Schimel, J. L.: Problems of delinquency and their treatment. In Arieti, S., editor: American handbook of psychiatry, vol. II, New York, 1974, Basic Books, Inc., pp. 264-274.

CHAPTER 11

Patients with psychophysiologic patterns

Psychophysiologic, also termed *psychosomatic*, disorders are organic dysfunctions in which emotional disturbances presumably play an important etiologic or contributory role. The autonomic nervous system is most frequently involved. The organic symptoms are actually produced or aggravated by emotional disorders and are not symbolic substitutes for them, as in the neuroses. Ultimately, pathologic changes may result. *Neurotic conversion* symptoms are produced by the transformation of an anxiety state into a bodily dysfunction, usually with partial or complete relief of the anxiety. The voluntary motor and sensory systems are frequently involved, and the particular organ or body part in the symptom is often a symbolic expression of the emotional conflict. *Psychogenic-functional* disorders refer to clinical manifestations of psychic origin of any sort. A functional disorder is one in which there is no morphologic change and for which no known organic cause exists. There is widespread agreement that, in general practice as well as most specialties in medicine, over 50% of the cases and probably 75% of physical complaints are functional in origin.

In the study of psychophysiologic disease, the concept of a specific, single causation has gradually given way to the modern view that a variety of factors are usually operative. Early researchers did not distinguish between hysterical conversion reactions and psychophysiologic reactions. The leading figures in the field of psychophysiologic medicine have been Cannon (1929), Selye (1956), Dunbar (1954), Alexander (1950), and Mirsky (1957). Cannon presented excellent physiologic evidence of his fight-or-flight hypothesis, expounding the role of epinephrine secretion. Selye's concept of diseases of adaptation em-

235

phasized the role of the adrenal-pituitary axis in its reaction to stress as being responsible for various disease states. Dunbar's specific personality profile—hypertensive character, ulcer personality—described statistical correlations between diseases and personality types, for example, coronary thrombosis and striving, goal-oriented, confident, and aggressive individuals.

Franz Alexander introduced the concept of the common underlying psychodynamic conflict, conflict specificity, where overt personalities differed but there was a specific relationship between certain emotional constellations and certain physiologic responses, for example, the wish to receive love-dependency conflict and peptic ulcer, or the fear of maternal separation and asthma. Conflicts thus could change in the same patient over the years. In this manner, one could explain two psychophysiologic disorders in one patient—for example, rheumatoid arthritis and peptic ulcer, bronchial asthma and coronary artery disease.

In addition to emotional trauma, personality profiles, and emotional conflict, constitutional factors have also been implicated. Mirsky's studies of individual variability of peptic acid secretion are noteworthy contributions in this area. Current beliefs emphasize multifactorial, etiologic components that interact and produce changes through complex neurophysiologic and neurochemical pathways.

Dynamics of development. A constellation of early influences usually combines to produce a high degree of sensitivity to the normal function of the body and a deeper concern than is customary with physical health. Actually, in our particular culture a certain attention toward care and concern for the body is necessarily inculcated in all of us. Since everyone learns early to note body changes, such as pain, and to report them, a tendency develops to consider physiologic inadequacy as a threat to security. A rather high degree of concern over physical status is normal to western culture. In fact, only sin and sex can compete with constipation, weight, and physical illness as topics of conversation. However, when solicitude over health or physical symptoms without an organic basis persists indefinitely in the face of contrary evidence and becomes a dominant factor in the pattern of living, then the point of normality has been transgressed.

Parental models are usually an important factor in the development of such a behavior pattern, since children often adopt uncritically whole patterns of behavior from adults important to them without realizing or understanding what is happening. Fortunately for most of us, parents come in pairs, and one parent may counteract the destructive influence of the other. If the parents share the same pattern, the likelihood of the child's adopting that pattern is increased. Even if the child later, as a result of experiences outside the family, begins to drop a pattern so acquired, there remains the strong tendency to reactivate it in periods of stress and personal insecurity.

If the parents tend to be chronically anxious persons who respect and bestow attention on fatigue, this is the pattern the child is likely to follow. If attention and increased affection are focused on physical complaints and the parents use this type of behavior on the child, this is the pattern the child is likely to follow. If a great deal of attention is bestowed on awareness of body function, this is the pattern the child is likely to follow. The disproportionate use of fatigue and physical complaints by the parents or by the parent who has the greater influence on the child can predispose the growing personality to a similar defect in development.

Another form of parental behavior that tends to strengthen and overemphasize body concern is oversolicitude. The oversolicitude may be adopted as the child's own attitude toward himself, and, depending on which particular type of body concern brings the greatest satisfaction, the groundwork may be laid for a fatigue syndrome, a morbid preoccupation with health, or a definite physical disturbance.

Illness or injury during the early years or at times of stress may be the precipitating factor in overconcern with the body. This is particularly true if some degree of chronic insecurity is built into the personality structure. An individual, perhaps not too happy with himself and others, suddenly finds himself the center of attention, showered with sympathy, and reassured of his importance to others. It is a nice comfortable feeling, and the urge to experience it again can be very strong. When insecurity, anxiety, and tension mount again, the pattern of gaining reassurance and security through physical illness may be resorted to unconsciously. Repetition can build the habit firmly into the personality.

Extremely traumatic experiences, especially during early childhood, accompanied by severe anxiety can be instrumental in establishing the use of physiologic and pseudodisease processes as methods of adjustment. Strong emotions are accompanied by definite visceral changes that can be felt. It is not at all unusual for severe emotional disturbances to be obscure in origin to the person affected. The art of repression can be employed, and the individual reacts to the body sensations accompanying the emotional upheaval rather than to the cause. In fact the visceral changes may be perceived as the cause. The original precipitating factor in the emotional upset is pushed into the unconscious and cannot be brought to awareness. The anxiety produced is displaced onto the body processes in a sort of body protest. This happens most often in humiliating or dangerous situations. Such an experience or a succession of experiences may lead to overconcern with body function.

Add to any of these experiences a large element of credulity, and an interesting phenomenon in behavior may occur. An individual brought up in a superstitious and uninformed atmosphere is likely to show unusual hypersuggestibility and naivete. Placed under severe stress or strain, he may show an unusual physical symptom that results in inactivation of some part of the body. This may be, for example, the unscientific stocking-and-glove anesthesia in which the anesthesia corresponds to the patient's idea of the function of the part of the body and not to the actual nerve distribution. Other selective losses of function may occur, such as blindness, deafness, or inability to eat. The part of the body involved is usually psychologically related to the anxiety-producing conflicts, and the function of the illness, the control of anxiety, is often clearly hinted at by the patient's emotional calmness toward his symptom. This form of difficulty may also be deomonstrated in episodic behavior disorders when an isolated behavior fragment temporarily appears to take over the personality. In such cases, multiple personalities and amnesias may be seen. The pattern just described is a naive one and is more commonly found in uninformed persons. Its incidence has been somewhat reduced by wide publicity.

All of these patterns serve common purposes. They either express anxiety or defend against it. In addition, they gain attention and interest and give the afflicted one a socially acceptable topic of conversation. Most of these patterns can, however, exhaust this effect since the persons around the patient eventually become annoyed, and rejection of the patient may finally occur. By this time the behavior pattern is so overlearned that it is difficult to change. The rejection increases the patient's tension and anxiety and leads to an accentuation of his behavior.

An element of compensation may enter the picture since the patient derives actual satisfaction from his behavior and the reception it gets. This can become a substitute satisfaction for the more usual ones the patient cannot achieve. One important factor in the pattern of body overconcern is that it supplies a rationalization for failures and inadequacies and has the advantage of being a socially acceptable one. Not so much is expected from the individual, and there is a ready excuse for his failure to meet even moderate demands that are placed on him.

The same pattern can also be used aggressively to punish others. A paralyzed bedridden person can be a tyrant who rules the household with an iron rod. A husband who ventures a criticism of the management of the household finances can be brought in line by his wife's severe headache that forces her to bed. He caused the headache, he misses his golf game, he cooks the supper, and he is kept busy carrying icecaps and reassurance to the bedside.

All of these techniques are part of an escape or evasion of the demands of one's self and of reality. They control anxiety and bring peace, but at a price; the price is the denial of a full, rich life.

MAJOR PSYCHOPHYSIOLOGIC DISORDERS

Peptic ulcer. Peptic ulcer has been described as a disease in which the "hungry" stomach eats itself. The longed-for food is equated with love or mother's milk. The typical ulcer patient has been epitomized as the tough, hard-driving executive who will not acknowledge his passive dependent yearnings and thus falls into unconscious conflict and resultant illness. Although this characterization is applicable to many peptic ulcer patients, it certainly does not describe a large number of others.

It is difficult for some individuals to acknowledge their dependency needs. Appropriate dependency needs are just as natural as the need for independence. Dependency is desirable in the patient being treated, in the student being educated, in the learner being trained; interdependency is essential in team sports, orchestras, government, war, sex, and marriage. The denial of dependency in men is often associated with an unconscious fear of homosexuality and the submissiveness connected with it. In women, the denial of dependency may be part of the rejection of the feminine role. Thus pseudomasculinity in men and masculinity in women have been considered by some to be characteristic of the "ulcer picture."

Ulcerative colitis. Tension and emotional stress are known to cause bowel disturbances in many individuals. In ulcerative colitis, the onset or relapse is often clearly and repeatedly associated with emotional duress.

The overactive colon is thought by some to be a means of expressing unconscious defiling hostility. Associated reactions may include enormous guilt and severe infantile dependency. Many patients with ulcerative colitis are considered to be fixated at the anal-expulsive stage of development. The anal personality in these patients may also demonstrate the genetically earlier anal-retentive aspects of character, for example, parsimony, compulsiveness, meticulousness, scrupulous promptness, excessive cleanliness, and zealous honesty. They are often unable to express aggressive or hostile feelings in a direct manner, but they make their relatives suffer secondarily as a result of their illness.

In the management of ulcerative colitis, it is important to consider that the patient's ego may be as friable as his bowel mucosa. Treatment should be gentle and considerate, with no attempts at deep-going or interpretative psychotherapy. These patients need strong emotional support. If a major way of dealing with the environment—diarrhea—is taken away from some of these patients, they must be given some alternative or the resultant depression may lead to suicide.

Bronchial asthma. Psychic factors are believed to play a large role in either causing or aggravating bronchial asthma. The wheeze of asthma has been likened to the cry for the mother, and it is true that asthmatics often give a history of a poor mother-child relationship. Attacks are said to be precipitated by threats of loss or separation from the mother or mother substitute. The asthma personality has been described as preoral or respiratory, where the fixation on the mother antedates all other relationships and is of such vital and immediate nature that even brief separation, if threatened as permanent, is reacted to as though potentially fatal.

Hypertension. When the popular "raising your blood pressure" occurs without apparent emotional provocation or organic explanation, hypertensive disease is considered to have an underlying psychotic basis. Overly controlled, suppressed rage can act like a pressure cooker with the lid screwed on tight. The distinction between essential and malignant hypertension is still uncertain despite great advances in the pathophysiologic understanding of hypertension. It is not known whether emotional factors are the initial causes of hypertension. Medical care should be supplemented by opportunities for emotional ventilation and better self-understanding. Psychotherapy can be relatively effective in the treatment of hypertension.

Arthritis. It has been said that the arthritis patient is able to get his hostility out only as far as his fists, where chronic tension and muscular contractions cause impaired circulation and articular changes. The rheumatoid personality has been described as extroverted, athletic, hyperactive, jovial, and overambitious.

Organic factors to be considered are repeated trauma, perhaps partly resulting from unconscious volition; metabolic disturbances such as gout, collagen disease, and autoimmune disorders; infections such as gonorrhea; and associated systemic disease.

In addition to medical treatment, one should provide ample opportunities for verbal expression of suppressed resentments and bitterness. Harsh words may be healthier than clenched fists. Muscular activities of various sorts should be encouraged. A well-earned fatigue may be preferable to taut muscles and pent-up feelings.

Migraine. In the patient with migraine the hostility is so deeply repressed that it cannot even be thought of. The typical migraine patient is a hardworking intellectual, with high standards for himself and others and uncompromising with the world. Migraine should be differentiated from other types of recurrent severe headache, including anxiety tension headaches and headaches of a vascular nature, neuralgia, and toxic and infectious states. Migraine patients often do well in prolonged intensive psychotherapy that permits them to bring unconscious resentments to the surface.

Obesity. For years there has been controversy as to whether nature or nurture is responsible for obesity. The condition of being obese and the process of overeating must be considered separately in order to understand the underlying drives and needs. Being obese may serve as a means of escape from sexuality, social interaction, maturity, responsibility, reality, or life itself. The layers of fat may be insulating in multiple fashion. Overeating in response to a need for love, security, and pleasure occurs in infantile, dependent, passive individuals with poor ego strength who are unable to obtain their gratification and sustenance in more mature ways. Elements of hostility and aggression may be involved.

Anorexia nervosa. Anorexia nervosa is a serious disease with a substantial mortality rate. It is seen frequently in adolescent girls but also in women in their twenties and thirties. Occasionally there is a history of obesity, and the onset of anorexia nervosa may be associated with—but not caused by— extreme and overconscientious dieting. Secondary amenorrhea is a constant feature. These patients are immature and narcissistic; often they are obsessive or hysterical in personality makeup, and many of them are preclinically psychotic. They center their lives around a totally irrational approach to food. No known organic cause exists.

Treatment consists largely of psychotherapy. Patients are often seen several times a week, usually for many months or years. Hospitalization, tube feeding, and electroconvulsive therapy should be considered when necessary.

Types of behavior. The range of behavior shown by persons with this particular group of disorders has already been indicated to some extent. The fatigue syndrome is one so closely related to normal that it is only under stringent criteria that it can be classified otherwise. Fatigue can be produced by overexertion or by lack of rest and is a common experience. The degree of resistance also varies from time to time in individuals, and the fluctuation is often a measure of interest in the task to be done. When fatigue consistently appears too readily, when it is out of proportion to the exertion involved, when it impairs social effectiveness over a prolonged period, or when an individual's life becomes organized around it, the behavior is deviating from normal. The usual presenting complaint is a feeling of exhaustion, of being utterly wornout. The slightest exertion produces weakness, and it is necessary to plan routines and activities that are restricted to a mild output of energy. Secondary symptoms usually occur, including headaches, heightened sensitivity to any sensory stimulation, discouragement, irritability, and difficulty in remembering or concentrating. This is a picture that we can identify in ourselves at one time or another.

The personality disorders centered around physiologic functions and complaints related to them are extremely varied in manifestation and may involve almost any part of the anatomy. The gastrointestinal tract probably leads all others in incidence of involvement. This is reasonable since early habit training involves a great deal of emphasis on the processes of eating and elimination. Strong cultural attitudes, taboos, and rituals continue to be associated with the use of both ends of the alimentary tract throughout life. In addition, the function of the gastrointestinal tract is easily observed, is open to some degree of control, and is an acceptable topic of social conversation. The actual range of complaints that leads the patient to a physician may involve any part or all of the system and may include heartburn, indigestion, nervous stomach, pains related to the eating period, diarrhea, constipation, and inability to eat. The actual task of distinguishing between the use of such complaints as a method of behavior adjustment and actual gastrointestinal disease is not always easy. Other systems frequently involved are the cardiovascular, the respiratory, the genitourinary, and the neuromuscular. The symptoms of almost any disease of these systems can be the original complaint of the patient, and the pattern of complaints may not fit any particular illness. In each instance, careful evaluation of the actual physical status of the patient is necessary to rule out a psychophysiologic disease. The most common symptoms related to the cardiovascular system are rapid pulse, palpitation, breathlessness, pain, dizziness or faintness, and throbbing blood vessels. Many of these can be symptoms of actual cardiovascular disease, but they can also be the visceral expression of strong emotional responses. The genitourinary tract is used more often by women in a neurotic adjustment, probably because of the menstrual cycle, the more dramatic climacteric, and the incidence of serious gynecologic diseases among women.

The particular organ or system around which the patient organizes his life is largely a matter of personal experience. Any symptom or combinations of symptoms found in a medical textbook can be duplicated by such patients, plus many combinations not found in any textbook. Generally speaking, the better informed the public is in relation to the function of an organ or system, the more closely will the patient's syndrome approximate a real disease. With this particular reaction pattern, the patient usually worries a great deal about his complaints and is openly and deeply concerned about them.

Another group of physical symptoms without adequate organic basis is characterized by a selective loss of function or normal activity and is usually accepted by the patient with a calm emotional attitude. Several of the more common types are described here. In many instances, the loss of function or activity would seem to the lay person to be caused by neurologic damage or disease.

The partial or complete loss of the ability to speak is a common occurrence in normal stress situations, such as a sudden shock, fright, or the receipt of bad news. A precipitating situation of the same nature may produce speech-lessness in a susceptible person in whom the symptom persists because of anxiety or some unmet need. The physical structures involved continue to function well except for speaking.

A partial or complete loss of appetite is also common in excitement, anger, or conflict. The process of eating has strong social implications, since taking food is usually an experience shared with others and generally means some degree of social acceptance or at least tolerance. It is often a symbolic process indicating acceptance by a chosen group, as in the ritual of communion in the Christian religion. The loss of the ability to eat in emotional disorders is usually related to the symbolic significance of eating and is a form of rejection by the patient. The recovery from this particular form of disorder is not usually dramatic since, once the patient does begin to eat, it requires some time to rebuild the body tissues.

The loss of specific motor activities and the loss of response to sensory skin stimulations are ordinary experiences. People get "frightened stiff" or become paralyzed by danger. Ordinarily painful stimuli may not be felt under such circumstances. In a fist fight or battle, injuries are often sustained that are not felt or realized until the period of immediate danger or fright has ended. When loss of motor activity becomes a major facet of existence, without organic cause for the loss, pathologic behavior is then evidenced. Paralysis may occur in any part of the body—legs, arms, shoulders, or lower half of the body. The distribution of the paralysis may not be neurologically justified, and the loss of activity may relate to only one function. For example, the patient may not be able to walk but may be able to move his legs about quite normally while in bed. Secondary contractures and atrophies may occur if the paralysis persists. Anesthesias that also occur usually have a sharp boundary line and follow lay ideas of functional anatomy. There is no response to painful stimulation in the hand, the arms as far as the elbow, or the leg as far as the knee. In both anesthesias and paralyses, inconsistencies and contradictions in symptoms usually rule out damage to the nervous system as a causative factor.

A symptom particularly likely to show striking inconsistencies is the partial or complete loss of response to visual stimulation. Interference with vision sometimes occurs in anxiety or emotional tension, although one result of anxiety may be increased visual acuity. A more closely related normal phenomenon is the ability to inactivate the function of one eye and exclude its response to stimulation while using the other eye to concentrate on a specimen under a microscope. The degree of loss of vision may vary widely. The sudden, miraculous recovery of sight headlined in newspapers now and then is frequently open to suspicion that the person has one of these personality disorders.

Another interesting loss of function, and one that is usually considered newsworthy, is the partial or complete loss of the ability to respond to stimulation leading to recall or recognition. This loss of memory, or amnesia, may vary in degree from forgetting a few incidents or parts of them through forgetting whole episodes of one's life. Actually, it is much more common for incidents or episodes to be forgotten, without loss of self-identification. The latter does occur, however, and the patient cannot identify himself. Such episodes are exaggerations of the very normal tendency to forget the names of people we do not like, to more easily forget unpleasant experiences, and to leave personal articles at a place to which we wish to return.

Closely related to this latter group of personality disorders is a series in which isolated behavior fragments or episodes appear in an inappropriate environmental context or in opposition to the person's previous behavior pattern. These occur as motor activities of varying degrees of complexity. Tremors, which occur normally in periods of stress or physical weakness, can persist indefinitely and be of a pathologic nature. Tics, or sudden involuntary muscle jerking, may occur; they may involve only a small group of muscles or they may be an elaborate affair involving a considerable portion of the body. These are usually not accompanied by any serious disturbance in the patient's orientation. Other types may cause a complete but temporary break with the continuity of behavior, such as a seizure or convulsion. The pattern of the convulsion is usually the same for each patient but may vary considerably from patient to patient.

The most complex disturbance in motor activity is the occurrence of a multiple personality in which two or more organized systems of behavior alternate in control of the individual, and each system remains unaware of the other or others. This is the ultimate in dissociation. Actually, it is comparatively rare to find patients with clear-cut alternating personalities. More likely to be found is the patient in whom there is a dominant personality system with fragmentary subsystems toward which the dominant is amnesic, that is, is not aware of their existence. The fragmentary system, which takes control of behavior on sporadic occasions, is aware of the activities of the dominant system. This subordinate system is usually childishly immature.

Nursing intervention. No more misunderstood or maligned group of patients exists than those with physical symptoms and inadequate psychophysiologic conditions. They are seldom found in psychiatric hospitals but are more likely to fill the wards of general hospitals. They are not forgotten—they are disliked and abused, and they are the object of contempt and ridicule. Psychoneurotic behavior is acceptable only when it is one's own.

The reeducation of a patient overly concerned with the physical aspect of existence is best promoted in an environment in which the particular needs of neurotic patients can be met without too great a price to others. It is this factor that tends to defeat, under ordinary social conditions, the learning of new skills by hypochondriacs and hysterical patients. Removal from the immediate environment, including close contact with significant persons, is frequently indicated to reduce the pressure on the patient. In a more closely controlled environment, the lessening of demands on the patient is helpful. The pattern of evasion is deeply rooted, thoroughly overlearned, and clung to by the patient even when the behavior pattern defeats its own ends. Environmental adjustments are frequently necessary to make it possible for the patient to learn new methods of behavior.

The environment should be one in which physical illness is not the center of attention and emphasis, yet there should be facilities for a complete physical examination to rule out organic pathology and to have available the negative results of such an examination to reassure the patient once rapport has been established.

Two other factors are important in a psychotherapeutic environment. There should be a routine that permits a balance of work and play, since the recreational needs of these patients tend to be high, and there should be enough pressure of activities to prevent the patient's being alone too much. This would indicate that a general hospital ward may not be the ideal place for the treatment of personality disorders centered around the physiologic aspect of existence. Certainly the general hospital can be effectively used for a thorough physical examination in the initial stages of treatment, but the whole atmosphere and function of such a unit tends to be a handicap in helping the patient to learn new patterns of behavior.

Nurse-patient interpersonal relationships. The greatest single problem in the establishment of healthy interpersonal relationships with this type of patient is the recognition and control of the emotional attitude of personnel toward them. The patient is most commonly viewed as someone who is deliberately malingering and who is perfectly capable of behaving himself if he desires. However, there is definitely something wrong—the patient is sick! In addition, surprising as it may seem, the pain is both real and severe. The patient feels it as much as though actual pathologic disease of tissue structures were present.

To confront the patient with the fact that there is no organic reason for the pain or difficulty does not end the pain. It will continue to exist as long as the patient emotionally needs it. It is *real* pain.

The ability to emotionally accept that fact that these patients are truly sick, that they cannot themselves understand the relationship between their symptoms and their emotional problems, and that they are actually as physically uncomfortable as they say they are is essential for personnel who wish to help them. This tends to be one of the biggest stumbling blocks in the treatment of such patients, since the members of the health team have usually thoroughly overlearned an organic approach to illness and have a mildly spartan philosophy against which they tend to judge patients. The usual definition of a good patient by the persons who care for him is one who accepts anything without complaint. This attitude should be brought out into the open and talked through with someone with a thorough understanding of such disorders the moment one notices a critical and contemptuous attitude toward patients with physical symptoms that do not correlate with organic pathology.

The greatest technical problem in interpersonal relationships is conveying acceptance and a feeling of worth to the patient without emphasizing or paying undue attention to his physical complaints. It is usually wise early in contact with the patient to listen completely and intently to his description and history of his complaints. It has probably been a long time since anyone patiently listened to him. Comments pro or con in regard to complaints should be avoided, and the listening should be done matter-of-factly but with interest. It is easier to avoid commenting than it would seem, for most patients are anxious to pour out their complaints, and they are not too interested in what someone else may think of them. If comments are necessary, they can be limited to repeating the feelings expressed by the patient such as discomfort, fear, anxiety, and worry. After one has listened to all the complaints, it is then wise to avoid leading the patient into a discussion of his physical symptoms. Diversion toward topics that interest the patient should be tried at every opportunity. When later or changing complaints are brought forth, they should be accepted calmly and relayed to the physician for evaluation. Excitement or contempt in regard to symptoms should be carefully avoided. Difficult though it may be from the emotional point of view, it is very important to seek out this patient when immediate routine and procedures do not demand it. This is one of the better ways of convincing the patient that he is a person of some worth.

Early in the patient's experience his pattern of behavior was helped toward fixation by the secondary gain he derived from his illness. This gain is the sympathy received for the presence of the symptoms themselves. While the patient is under treatment, this gain should not be reinforced. Calm acceptance of the patient's complaints and his right to them, without indicating by word or attitude any feeling of pity or of being sorry for him, is the best procedure. One must accept the patient as a person without sanctioning his particular form of maladjustment.

Care should be exercised in discussing medical knowledge with the patient or in his hearing. These patients tend toward suggestibility and are wont to pick up new knowledge and to weave it into the pattern of complaints. Questions asked in regard to specific symptoms of the patient should be limited since they may plant ideas of what else might be expected.

Patients also have a tendency to play personnel against each other, and they usually attempt to discredit anyone who implies by word or look that their illness is not organic in nature. Personnel should avoid being caught in the process by being alert to its appearance.

Reassurance and encouragement should be given the patient carefully and not in relation to physical symptoms if it can be avoided. Positive accomplishments in other areas should be recognized and rewarded, particularly in the ability to develop recreational skills and to participate in activities with others.

Under present conditions, the majority of such patients will be found in clinics, physicians' offices, and general hospitals. Nurses should be able to recognize these patients and to understand what they as nurses can and cannot do for them. In the first place, nurses are not likely to cure or alter the course of events much for the patient unless they can be instrumental in guiding the patients toward psychiatric treatment. This suggestion may best be planted with receptive relatives if there are such. A great deal will depend on each patient's physician and the physician's attitude toward the patient's illness. The one constructive thing nurses can do is to give intelligent nursing intervention during their hospitalization by understanding that their behavior, however annoying it may be, is an expression of their anxiety and self-doubt. If nurses, through their own behavior, can reassure patients as to their own worth and leave them feeling understood and comfortable, a good deal can be accomplished.

Suicide and attacks on others are rare with psychophysiologic patients, although suicidal attempts resulting from unbearable anxiety over a prolonged period of time have occurred. The great protective need of these patients is from panic attacks that can be precipitated by mounting anxiety. The patient's behavior pattern becomes completely disorganized under overwhelming terror. In such a state, injury to self or others is quite possible. Another caution signal is constant verbalization about death or dying. Tactful precautions should always be taken if the patient shows any such preoccupation.

Panic can be avoided by reducing the patient's anxiety and by being careful not to cause the patient further anxiety. A study of the types of situations that tend to increase the patient's tension should be made, and such situations should be avoided if possible. Mounting tension and anxiety should be reported in order that preventive measures may be taken. The patient also needs to be protected from the development of a passive dependence on persons in the environment. Trends in this direction in interpersonal relationships should not be encouraged, no matter how flattering they may be.

Relationships with other patients. These patients, when first introduced into a group, tend to be accepted and sympathized with, but they usually wear out their welcome rapidly and wind up being rejected. Patients on the whole accept them better than personnel. An early and consistent effort to keep them in the group and participating in shared activities often pays dividends. One or two other patients with similar problems can be a help since it gives the patient an opportunity to form a subgroup with them, with a sense of sharing, while remaining a part of a larger group. Isolation from the group should be avoided at all costs. Being alone too much grants many opportunities for concentration on body function.

During the period of convalescence, a very matter-of-fact deemphasis of physical needs and body function should continue. The patient should be very tactfully supervised during routine to prevent fatigue since its symptoms may increase his interest in his body. As the time for discharge nears, a brief exacerbation of physical complaints may be expected and should be taken calmly, without indicating to the patient any anxiety over their appearance.

Social activities, particularly recreational ones, should be encouraged. Patients with psychophysiologic disorders need to learn to play and to enjoy it, and the convalescent period is usually the best opportunity to promote this phase of the patient's treatment.

If the patient wishes to discuss or talk about his illness, he can be permitted to do so. Every care should be taken to show and to encourage the patient to show a healthy attitude toward mental illness. The patient will often need the support of interest in him and his activities while he remains somewhat awkward in his attempts to seek expression of such interest. No attention should be directed toward the patient's awkwardness in interpersonal gestures, but the interest should be expressed freely and without demands attached to it.

COMPULSIVE BEHAVIOR

Ritual, repetition, and magic play a considerable role in modern existence despite the emphasis on changes in the social milieu that is so often stressed. Inflexibility in procedure is a common characteristic of children's play and story-telling activities. Adults also have their rituals in religion, in organizations, and in daily personal routines. Most adults still cherish the magic illusion that a verbal apology wipes out the effects of past behavior and avoids possible consequences. The special virtue of the ritual is its uniformity and sameness, which in effect are a control of the environment and self. The ritual reduces any necessity for a decision and guarantees to some extent the results that follow. This type of behavior, found extensively in normal persons, can become exaggerated to an abnormal degree and can become so marked that it actually interferes with social effectiveness. Behavior becomes pathologically compulsive when an irresistible impulse to say, do, or think some one thing seriously complicates existence and interferes markedly with an adjustment.

Dynamics of development. Compulsive behavior characterized by mounting tension that is temporarily discharged by an indulgence in the compulsive act or thought is closely related to the development of the techniques of self-control in the growing individual. Self-control is a social skill that follows a certain broad pattern of development. Discipline and correction are accomplished in the beginning through outside compulsion, which is brought about by the attachment of unpleasant experience to disapproved acts and by the attachment of pleasure and acceptance to approved acts. Eventually, the child accepts the responsibility for meeting approved standards on his own, in keeping with the values of his parents. This shift of responsibility occurs gradually, and the period of change is marked by ambivalence. The child both reaches for forbidden fruit and chastises himself for his desires and behavior. Emotional experience in the formative years of life that tends to prevent growth beyond the ambivalent period in conscience development provides fruitful soil for compulsive behavior.

Factors important in the early years are closely related to parental patterns of behavior. Compulsive parents tend toward the production of compulsive children, since children so frequently incorporate whole patterns of their parents' behavior. In addition, compulsive parents may carefully train their children in compulsive habits. If the children's compulsiveness is insisted on as a condition of affection or acceptance, the habit will be a difficult one to dislodge in later years. Parents who are not themselves compulsive may train their children in compulsive habits, especially if the parents desire offspring about whom they can brag inordinately to neighbors and relatives. Too much emphasis on detailed procedure and precise end results can establish compulsive work habits. Such patterns, learned in one type of situation and associated with approval, tend to spread to other areas of behavior. Interestingly enough, such methods of education were typical of schools of nursing of the recent past. The procedure was the thing that mattered—the exactness in steps and the precise end result. Understanding of the whys in any given procedure was often lacking, and one was severely chastised if one asked questions. The profession is still peopled with members who heatedly and unintelligently insist that "the way we did this procedure in my school of nursing is the *only* right way to do it!"

In addition to overemphasis on procedure and precise end results, other parental dictates conducive to the development of compulsiveness are burdening children with too much responsibility too early and inculcating too much dread of mistakes and fear of retaliation. Training in guilt attitudes has a marked effect on personality structure. Impressing children with the retribution due immoral conduct long before they are able to understand immorality or ethical problems makes them prone to guilt reactions and confusion about their own thoughts and behavior. When behavior is shared with others, this early training may be overcome, but in all families and in all cultures there are taboos that will continue to produce guilt and conflict when one is trained in guilt attitudes. Relevant to this is our own cultural attitude toward sex. The average individual reaches adulthood having learned far more about sex guilt than sexual function or intelligent sexual expression.

Parental handling of criticism can also be significant in the development of compulsive behavior. The stern and unforgiving parent who withholds affection at the child's slightest deviation from the path laid down for him can easily develop a submissive child who adopts as a ritual the performance that once or twice secures the affection he needs. Generally speaking, children cannot tolerate rejection. A parent who is stern and exactingly demanding of the child builds attitudes of guilt and anxiety that may require ritualistic behavior to overcome.

Early experience and parental attitudes or examples may develop severe anxiety and overmeticulousness in a child. Such a child, constantly threatened by loss of affection over small details and relatively insignificant happenings, needs more than average reassurance and certainty. Security is constantly threatened, and *absolute* security becomes one of the child's emotional needs. By no stretch of imagination is it possible to achieve absolute security in modern existence. The adoption of ritualistic behavior under such circumstances limits free choice of action and serves several purposes. It reduces the number of experiences to which the individual must respond and thereby reduces the number of potential anxieties he must face; its sameness produces a certain form of security, and it becomes a defensive method of self-control. Actually, as an adjustive technique, it is not too successful. The anxiety discharged through compulsive behavior is only a transient relief, since the anxiety builds up again and the compulsion must be indulged again. Such behavior also restricts experience and growth since compulsions and rituals limit the range of experience to which the individual is exposed.

Types of behavior. The forms that compulsive behavior may take all have in common the irresistible urge to do, say, or think some one thing that the individual usually resists, with mounting anxiety, and then indulges with temporary relief from the anxiety.

The compulsion may involve repetition of some significant act or thought. The classic example is compulsive hand-washing, which is a performance that is easy to relate to the underlying guilt, the anxiety it produces, and the necessity to expiate it. In a culture in which cleanliness is next to godliness (and may even precede it!), the connection between cleanliness and lack of guilt is easy to grasp. The patient washes his hands frequently and becomes markedly anxious if the process is blocked. Some patients go through elaborate rituals to keep their hands clean and must wash them every time they come in contact with any object. For others, only one object or types of objects may be the sources of contamination.

The following example illustrates an individual with obsessive-compulsive hand-washing.

A man and his wife were invited to a dinner party at a restaurant by a well-known underworld man, Mr. B. As they approached the restaurant, the wife was informed by her husband, "For heaven's sake, don't offer to shake hands with Mr. B—he *never* shakes hands with anyone." When they entered the restaurant Mr. B. and his bodyguards were waiting for them. Introductions were made (the wife refrained from putting out her hand), and Mr. B., after a brief scrutiny, held out his hand . . . so they shook hands. He turned to his bodyguards and said, "The table is ready. Why don't you go in; I'll be with you in a minute." He then went directly into the men's room, obviously to compulsively wash his hands!

On the way home after the dinner party, the husband said, with amazement in his voice, "Mr. B. must *really* have liked you—he has *never* shaken hands with me!"

The performance of a procedure in an exact order is another form of compulsion. This too can take practically any form that behavior takes. The patient who must dress in exact order is an example. He puts on the right sock, right shoe, left sock, left shoe, and then his coat; if he is not sure that this order was followed, he must undress and start all over to be sure. When the serial order of an act is so rigidly fixed that any slight deviation produces anxiety and requires the act to be done over from the start, the patient is then behaving compulsively. Such behavior requires the close attention of the patient and can absorb practically the whole of his waking time. Such behavior, if severe enough, precludes any possibility of holding an ordinary job or carrying on a relatively normal existence.

Another form of compulsive behavior is compulsive orderliness or cleanliness. The housewife who has this trait to a fairly marked degree usually has an enviable reputation as a good wife and mother in the neighborhood, a reputation that those who have to live with her would be likely to challenge. A meticulously kept house with a place for everything and everything in its place at all times is usually not a comfortable house in which to live. The significant fact in such orderliness or cleanliness that marks it as pathologic is the anxiety and inexplicably strong emotional reaction that any deviation produces.

Self-restraint and asceticism can be compulsive in nature when an individual keeps a rigid and unrelenting iron hand on himself and, all too frequently, on other persons. Rigid rules for conduct and severe penalties for mild infractions are common occurrences in such people. If they have children, the danger of development in a compulsive direction is more probable for those children. Such persons are markedly perfectionistic, with an attention to details and minutiae that makes them a source of severe annoyance to those who must work with or under them.

The indulgence in superstition, magic beliefs, and rituals can also become compulsive in nature. Actually, in the lives of all of us, no matter how scientific and intellectual, there are personal attitudes and beliefs that are not at all influenced by reason. Most of us have some superstitions, prejudices, and magic beliefs that we keep hidden lest we be ridiculed. Magic rituals that produce a marked anxiety when they are interfered with are compulsive. A patient's dependence on magic procedures to allay anxiety can be pathologic. The person who becomes panic-stricken when he walks under a ladder or who is "scared stiff" when a black cat crosses the street in front of him is actually not so far from normal—but he is off the path.

Antisocial compulsions are more common than one would expect, and the epitome of this form of behavior is the urge to kill another person. Although this appears most frequently as a fantasy of doing violence to others that is followed by deep feelings of guilt, it may carry over into overt action. A more commonly seen form of behavior is compulsive stealing that appears to be rather senseless on the surface. The patient usually takes articles for which he has no use or desire, does so only after tension and anxiety have built up, and experiences relief from anxiety when the theft is completed. A milder form, closer to a normal manifestation, is the irresistable urge to shock others verbally with obscene or vulgar comments.

Another form of compulsive behavior is obsessive fear, or phobia. The type of fear, such as fear of heights, darkness, crowds, or closed spaces, is usually related to the patient's past experience. All phobias have in common deep-seated fear of some object or situation which the patient himself cannot explain and which produces panic if the patient is forced into the situation he fears.

Nursing intervention. Ritualistic patients present a difficult therapeutic problem. The long-standing need for absolute security and certainty makes any definite planning for them long range in nature. The restricting effect of their ritual on their range of experience poses problems in dealing with the symptom itself in such a manner as to meet the patient's basic needs.

It is essential in a psychotherapeutic environment for compulsive patients that the patient not be handicapped or punished for his symptoms. To carry out the compulsive act itself is an absolute necessity for the patient during his illness, since it does give transient relief from an anxiety that would otherwise overwhelm him. An environment so adjusted that the patient is not isolated or made conspicuous by the indulgence of his symptoms provides an important element in his treatment.

One of the purposes of ritualistic behavior is to relieve the patient of the necessity for making decisions. Therefore the environment should be sufficiently controlled and the routine consistent enough to tactfully relieve the patient of as many decisions as possible. The consistency in environment and routine also helps to limit the range of experience to which the patient is exposed. New experience carries a threat and should be carefully introduced.

The demands made on the patient in regard to complying with routine and participating in activities should make full allowance for his anxiety, his ritual, and his unrecognized fear of new experience. In other words, the patient needs an environment in which he can be comfortably sick.

Nurse-patient interpersonal relationships. Interpersonal relationships are tools designed to contribute to the ritualistic patient's security, to reduce his anxiety, and to build his confidence in relations with others. The major problems presented by the patient's behavior are his ritualistic activity, his periodic mounting anxiety, his ambivalent attitude, his tendency to integrate situations that produce guilt, and his hostility that he fears to express except symbolically.

The compulsive act must be accepted in a comparatively permissive manner. When possible, its indulgence should be permitted in as constructive a manner as possible for the patient. For example, one patient relieved some degree of his anxiety by thoroughly scrubbing the shower stall after having his shower. When the activity was denied him, he became restless and anxious and was unable to carry on with the activities of the day. Routine was adjusted for him so that he took his shower early in the day, scrubbed the shower stall thoroughly immediately thereafter, and was then able to join the patient group in recreational and occupational therapy. Because the completion of the compulsive act is usually succeeded by a feeling of relief, this period can be used consistently to treat any possible effects of the compulsive acts. In this instance, the problem was the prevention of damage to the skin on the patient's hands, which tended to break down after the vigorous daily scrubbing with strong soap.

Ritualistic behavior is time consuming, and the patient must be allowed adequate time without any sense of pressure or criticism. Attempts to reason with the patient concerning his behavior are useless and will not influence the course of events except destructively. An intellectual explanation leaves the patient with a feeling of inadequacy and of having been criticized for his failure to meet the standards implied for him. The end result is an increase in anxiety and further guilt feelings for his failure. Extreme care must be observed in the attitude of personnel toward the symptom—it should be treated as though it were a completely natural and expected phenomenon. Any hint of criticism, any special attention, or any punitive measures must be carefully avoided in relation to the compulsive act.

When limits must be drawn on carrying out the compulsive act, for example, when it would cause serious interference with maintenance of the patient's health, the limits must be consistently enforced. In addition, the decision as to where the line is to be drawn should be determined for the patient, and any necessary procedures, such as tube feeding, should be carried through quickly and efficiently. Long explanations and coaxing are usually upsetting and increase the psychologic trauma involved.

The patient's anxiety stems from confusingly ambivalent feelings and a deep sense of guilt. Helping the patient control anxiety involves taking full account of these important feelings. A great deal of patience and tact are necessary to avoid any comments or any hint of impatience in attitude or behavior that might increase the patient's sense of failure and his feeling of guilt. For this reason, discussion of the patient's symptom(s) should be only on his initiative. Any judgment in regard to the ritual must be scrupulously avoided. Every effort should be directed toward making the patient as comfortable as possible with and about his ritual.

An ambivalent attitude should be expected and calmly accepted. Alertness for its expression helps one to avoid reacting to ambivalence in a manner that may imply criticism of negative emotional expressions or undue praise of positive expressions. Dislike and hostility may be expected, even though they are not often too openly expressed. More positive emotions may be expressed at the same time or later. In either case, it is wise not to lean too strongly on the positive emotional expression or to expect it to continue indefinitely. An attitude expressing approval of such behavior is a threat to the patient since he is incapable of maintaining the more positive level.

Since therapeutic interpersonal relationships must take account of the patient's reduced and restricted abilities, it is important with ritualistic patients to keep routine and attitudes as consistent as possible. New procedures and variety in established ones carry more threat than stimulation of interest and should be avoided. The pathologic need for absolute certainty should be respected, and every effort should be made to keep the patient as certain as possible about what to expect under any and all circumstances.

Many patients who rely on excessive ritualism show, for lack of a better term, "verbal insight." They are, in the course of their illness, able to express some intellectual understanding of the relationship of their behavior to their feelings of guilt, although they may be unable to indicate why they feel guilty. It should be recognized that only very late in the course of treatment is this insight accepted emotionally so that the patient is able to use his knowledge to influence his behavior. Insight of an intellectual nature that does not influence behavior is partial insight and is extremely painful to the patient. In a sense, he knows enough to be aware that he should be able to control his behavior, but he cannot. The result of such partial insight is to increase the patient's dissatisfaction with himself and to increase his sense of failure. Any expression of such verbal insight should be evaluated as to how it makes the patient feel about himself, and care should be taken in responding not to increase the patient's discomfort. Whenever such verbalization occurs while the patient continues his compulsive act, personnel should not be confused by what the patient has to say. Above all, they must not act as though they expected the patient to behave in conformity with the knowledge his words would seem to indicate. Any compulsive or ritualistic behavior should be tactfully observed and reported and completely ignored as far as the patient is concerned.

Regardless of the particular problem, a carefully planned schedule for the patient's treatment should be carried out. If possible, full advantage should be taken of the fact that the patient's most comfortable period is usually at the completion of the ritualistic behavior.

A more serious problem arising at times is fatigue; this occurs when the patient's behavior is so elaborate and involved that it exhausts him. A plan to guarantee the patient adequate rest should be worked out and consistently carried through.

Patients in this group have two major protective needs: they must be protected from the consequences of their behavior and from the development of panic. Protecting the patient from the consequences of his behavior will depend on the form the compulsive behavior takes. If the patient steals compulsively, for example, no issue should be made concerning the act itself. Rather, careful observation of what is stolen and quiet return of stolen articles would be a wiser procedure. Periodic tactful search for the patient's compulsive acquisitions may be instituted. The principle involved is the avoidance of punitive measures for behavior the patient cannot control.

The avoidance of panic rests upon keeping anxiety at the lowest possible level in the patient. The particular danger point is the compulsive act itself, which should not be blocked or used in any manner to create further anxiety in the patient. The careful avoidance of contribution to the patient's sense of guilt is also important.

Relationships with other patients. The ritualistic patient tries to isolate himself from group contacts, and this tendency is to be tactfully combated at every turn. It can be helpful to adjust routine to permit the compulsive act when and where it does not make the patient conspicuous in the eyes of the group or interfere with group activities. As a rule, a definite effort on the part of personnel to introduce and encourage group activities by the patient is necessary. He also needs support in group activities in which his sense of adequacy is threatened; therefore, it is sound procedure to start him with an activity in which he is already interested and has some skill. A tendency on the part of the patient to do menial tasks for other patients (self-punishment) should be calmly permitted. Unless the compulsive act itself is a sharp handicap, the patient is usually fairly well accepted by a group that does not have too many members like himself. He can often be a fairly constructive group member.

The major emphasis during the patient's convalescence is on satisfactory socialization with others. The patient's tendency to be impatient and to demand much of himself should be recognized, and the necessary support and encouragement should be given. He may often show contempt for the symptom he is losing and may be sharply critical of himself for having been ill. Under no circumstances should personnel agree with any such expression, but they should encourage the patient with the real improvement he has shown.

REFERENCES

Abse, W.: Hysteria. In Arieti, S., editor: American handbook of psychiatry, vol. 1, New York, 1959, Basic Books, Inc., pp. 272-292.

Aguilera, D. C.: Review of psychiatric nursing, St. Louis, 1977, The C. V. Mosby Co.

Alexander, F.: Psychosomatic medicine, New York, 1950, W. W. Norton & Co.

Cannon, W. B.: Bodily changes in pain, hunger, fear, and rage, ed. 2, New York, 1929, Appleton-Century-Crofts.

Chrzanowski, G.: Neurasthenia and hypochondriasis. In Arieti, S., editor: American handbook of psychiatry, vol. 1, New York, 1959, Basic Books, Inc., pp. 258-271.

Dunbar, F.: Emotion and bodily changes, New York, 1954, Columbia University Press.

Edwards, J.: If I touch, will you tell? ANA Regular Clinical Conference, New York, 1967, American Nurses Association, p. 274.

Friedman, P.: The phobias. In Arieti, S., editor: American handbook of psychiatry, vol. 1, New York, 1959, Basic Books, Inc., pp. 293-306.

Horney, K.: Neurosis and human growth, New York, 1950, W. W. Norton & Co.

Kolb, L. C.: Modern clinical psychiatry, ed. 8, Philadelphia, 1973, W. B. Saunders Co., pp. 425-430.

Mirsky, I. A.: The psychosomatic approach to the etiology of clinical disorder, Psychosom. Med. **19:**424, 1957.

Purintun, L. R., and Nelson, L. I.: Ulcer patient: emotional emergency, Am. J. Nurs. **68:**1930-1933, 1968.

Selye, H.: The stress of life, New York, 1956, McGraw-Hill Book Co.

Solomon, P., and Patch, V.: Handbook of psychiatry, ed. 3, Los Altos, Calif., 1974, Lange Medical Publications.

Sullivan, H. S.: Conceptions of modern psychiatry, Washington, D.C., 1947, William Alanson White Psychiatric Foundation, pp. 54-59.

Walike, B. C.: Rheumatoid arthritis: personality factors, Am. J. Nurs. **67:**1427-1430, 1967.

CHAPTER 12

Psychotherapeutic techniques

PSYCHOTHERAPY

Psychotherapy is a systematized professional technique whereby mental symptoms can be ameliorated or disordered behavior brought under control by means of an on-going structured relationship between a trained therapist and a patient. Psychotherapy should be distinguished from many nonprofessional—though often quite effective—ways in which one person can influence or help another, such as kindness, advice, education, persuasion, exhortation, or inspiration.

In this chapter, psychotherapy is presented as a pragmatic technique based on an understanding of the psychodynamics of mental illness but not confined to this. Theoretical considerations are discussed first and then various therapy modalities.

Theoretical considerations. Psychotherapy is used in the treatment of psychogenic disturbances wherever these may occur: neuroses, psychoses, personality disorders, psychophysiologic disorders, and behavior problems, including alcoholism, substance abuse, and delinquency.

Some degree of minor psychogenic disturbance probably afflicts everyone at some time in life. Most people are never seen by a therapist, and, just as most headaches, digestive disturbances, and upper respiratory infections disappear in time without formal treatment, so also do most minor anxiety and depressed states disappear. However, if psychogenic symptoms persist or are severe, a therapist is usually consulted. Many observers have estimated that a large proportion of a physician's time is actually spent in the care of psychogenic illness, and the few good studies available bear out these statements.

Validity of psychotherapy. Research workers have encountered great difficulty in attempting to determine whether psychotherapy actually does what it claims to do. The problems of quantifying and controlling such variables as type and degree of illness, patient motivation, kind of psychotherapy, personal characteristics of the therapist, and measurements of results are almost imponderably baffling. Before the mid-1950s, methodologic difficulties led to little more than confusion, dominated by Eysenck's (1966) contention that neurotic patients did no better when treated than when kept on a waiting list.

Subsequently, more sophisticated studies by Frank (1961), Wallerstein (1966), and Malan (1973) showed that psychotherapy is indeed an effective therapeutic technique with a potential for making the patient either better or worse, depending on how it is used. Extensive studies at the Menninger Clinic, Columbia University, Tavistock Hospital, and elsewhere have also demonstrated that psychodynamically oriented psychotherapy is effective (Malan, 1973).

The patient. The patient usually undertakes psychotherapy because he has decompensated psychologically. He or his family may use the words "nervous breakdown," a phrase widely used to indicate a major disturbance in the patient's ability to cope with life's problems. Evidence of these difficulties appears at work, school, or home or in interpersonal relationships. Internal symptoms center around anxiety, depression, and other forms of emotional suffering.

An important determinant of the outcome of treatment is the patient's motivation to work at psychotherapy as a way of recovering from his illness. Other determinants are age, intelligence, flexibility, type and duration of illness, and reality factors such as family cooperation, geographic circumstances, sociocultural elements, finances, and so forth. It helps for the patient—and the therapist also—to understand early in treatment just what their objectives are and what is *not* expected or desired from the effort.

The therapist. Outcome studies have determined that the most successful psychotherapists are characterized by nonpossessive warmth, genuineness, empathy, and good personal adjustment. Treatment failures occur more often with therapists who are cold and uninterested *or* are so affectionate or demonstrative that they embarrass, confuse, or antagonize the patient. Therapists who exploit patients for their own ends soon generate suspicion and hostility rather than trust—and without trust psychotherapy cannot function. Therapists with psychologic problems of their own may exaggerate or unconsciously overlook similar problems in their patients or otherwise be of detriment to their patients' welfare. Finally, therapists who strive for unrealistic goals for their patients court disappointment and failure.

Mechanisms of psychotherapy. In organic illness, pathogenic and host factors (resistance) play a role. The same dose of toxin or bacteria will make some individuals sick and others not. Treatment in organic illness can be divided into specific therapy for eradicating the offending source, for example, antibiotics for typhoid fever and general management for the acutely ill patient, such as bed rest, fluids, and diet. Much the same can be said for psychogenic illness.

Pathogenic factors in psychogenic diseases are thought to be unconscious emotional blocks or complexes such as fear (of abandonment, loss of love, rejection, punishment, injury, mutilation, castration, or retaliation) or feelings of inferiority or insecurity, rage, jealousy, guilt, shame, ambivalence, frustration, depression, and despair. These pathologic stimuli may express themselves in neurosis, most commonly in anxiety and depression.

> Miss L. was constantly browbeaten by a tyrannical and domineering mother. She was very bright and was an outstanding student, but she was a shy and self-effacing young woman. At age 24, after successfully completing law school and attempting to study for the bar examination, Miss L. became increasingly anxious, distracted, and unable to concentrate on her studies. After a suicidal attempt she was referred to a therapist. In therapy she slowly began to realize that much of her difficulty stemmed from conflicts going back to her mother's rejection and to her own passive acceptance of it.

Pathogenic factors may also express themselves in psychophysiologic conditions, through organ dysfunction. By the mechanism of neurosis and psychophysiologic disorder, almost any medical symptom can be duplicated. The "great imitator" in medicine is no longer syphilis but psychogenic disorders. An example of a psychophysiologic condition is illustrated in the following case study.

> Mrs. R. developed ulcerative colitis when everything in her life seemed to be going perfectly well. She had been married for 5 years to an engineer and they had a good relationship. She was very happy when she found she was pregnant, and all went smoothly during the baby daughter's birth. During infancy, the baby received much attention; she was a beautiful little girl and everyone commented on how lovely she was and everyone adored her. It was at this time that the ulcerative colitis symptoms began.
>
> Mrs. R. was very uncooperative with her gastroenterologist and was referred to a therapist. In therapy it developed that she had had a miserable childhood because of what she regarded as favoritism on the part of her parents toward her younger sister. Her life had become riddled with anger, jealousy, and envy, not only toward her sister but toward anyone who experienced good fortune. She learned to conceal these feelings even from herself, but they eventually came out as hostile, defiling diarrhea.

Psychologic host factors are those basic mental traits or circumstances whose absence or insufficiency contributes to the causation of psychogenic disorder and who presence or strengthening assists in ameliorating or over-coming the disorder. These factors are poorly understood and are usually ascribed to genetic or constitutional influences. Therapists, in an effort to un-cover psychogenic factors, sometimes neglect to give due consideration to inherent tendencies in the makeup of the host.

The term "ego strength" has become widely used to denote the conglom-erate of mental and personality traits that contribute to mental health. Con-versely, "weakness of the ego" has served as an explanation of a patient's failure to improve in therapy. The elements of what constitutes strength or weakness in this context have never been adequately formulated. Kleeman and Solomon (1974) believe that the following mental characteristics—not mutually exclu-sive—are contributory:

1. *Tolerance:* the ability to tolerate—or resign oneself to—the pain of loss, failure, disappointment, frustration, insult, shame, and guilt. This in-volves either neutralization, extinction, or postponement of satisfaction.

2. *Forgiveness:* the ability to forgive and feel sorry for those who have caused an injury or injustice. One must somehow erase pain, anger, and retaliatory impulses and replace them with attempts to understand, to see in perspective, to identify with others to some extent, and thus to feel compassion for them.

3. *Acceptance of substitutes:* the willingness to forego what is not presently possible or expedient and to seek something else in its place; for exam-ple, to give up short-term goals in favor of long-term goals.

4. *Persistence:* the ability to continue efforts with determination despite meager or no early success. It helps to have a long attention span, drive, or what may seem to others stubbornness.

5. *Ability to learn:* ingenuity, creativity, and the ability to be resourceful and innovative may be of value here. Behavior can thus be modified or conditioned by positive or negative reinforcement so that adaptation and change may occur.

6. *Vitality:* a little recognized but important element in life. Individuals vary greatly in the degree to which they have power, energy, or a driv-ing force for generating and sustaining effort and activity.

Most of these—perhaps all—are fundamentally determined at birth, but it is likely that their potential may vary in response to the experiences and vicissitudes of life, increased by good physical health, stimulating activities, and joyous feelings and decreased by physical distress, environmental impover-ishment, and depressed feelings.

Improvement in psychotherapy. Short-term benefits may occur imme-diately and are usually attributed to a ventilation of feelings. The patient may take comfort in the simple fact that he has been given an appointment to come again. So-called transference cures are extensions of this early response and result from the patient's feeling that he has been accepted and forgiven by a respected and admired parent figure. Such cures are fragile and often transient but should not be disdained because they offer a respite from suffering and may represent the first stage of the work of psychotherapy.

Long-term benefits must be sought over a period of months or years. These come through changes in the patient that may be difficult or painful for him to make, changes that represent a healthier attitude toward the realities of his past, present, and future life. To bring them about, some or all of the following may be instrumental:

1. Insight, or understanding of the psychologic disturbances in his personality. Freud thought insight was essential to successful treatment. Now, however, it is considered to be helpful although not necessary or sufficient.

2. Corrective emotional experiences, a "reliving" of traumatic experiences in order to achieve a healthier perspective on the events and on the people involved. These may occur during a therapeutic session, in a dream, or in the course of routine events; or they may not occur at all. Such experiences have emotional cathartic and maturing effects and may be quite useful in therapy, but, like insight, they are neither necessary nor sufficient for success.

3. Reeducation, a change from infantile, pathologic, or maladaptive attitudes to more mature and healthier ones. Both insight and corrective emotional experiences may play important parts in reeducation. So also may the hours of conscious and unconscious learning acquired during the time spent with the therapist. Transference reactions, interpretations, increased objectivity, and some degree of identification with the therapist may all play a part. The therapist joins forces with the healthy part of the patient's personality, and together they attempt to change the unhealthy part.

4. Growth, denoting change with time. This often works in helpful ways to cure emotional problems. Patients in therapy have usually been in a rut and have stopped growing in the sense of making progress toward fulfilling their potential as men and women. Successful therapy removes obstacles to growth and permits the process of self-actualization to continue.

Personality change and maturational growth may be seen in patients in much the same way as they are seen in children, students, and friends. They appear as a broadening and mellowing of outlook, with long-range views taking precedence over immediate problems. The ego boundaries expand to include more outsiders and their needs and welfare. Strengthening of purpose and will power develops as the patient learns to avoid reflex emotional responses in favor of considered intellectual ones.

SPECIAL PSYCHOTHERAPIES

In recent years, scores of special kinds of psychotherapy have sprung up, ranging from primal, behavioral, and conjoint therapies to the therapeutic uses of such philosophies as yoga, Zen, and EST. A few have been espoused for their usefulness in certain kinds of problems, with certain kinds of people, and within the framework of certain practical considerations. Most have been practiced by psychologists and other mental health professionals, while a few have been practiced—at times ineffectively or with unfortunate results—by essentially untrained and unqualified laymen.

Brief psychotherapy. Brief psychotherapy has evolved as a distinct form of psychiatric treatment as a result of the observation that many patients achieve marked relief of symptoms and moderate character changes in a few sessions, whereas continued therapy may produce little further progress. If a patient comes for treatment in a crisis situation, his established defenses and behavior patterns are broken down, and this may prove to be an ideal time to develop healthier defenses and better solutions to conflicts. Immediate therapy in a crisis situation will prevent continuing anxiety, depression, and other symptoms from producing greater disorganization and psychopathology. An acutely suffering patient is better motivated for change than one to whom chronic suffering has become a way of life. The limited time available for clinic treatment, the scarcity of psychiatrists, and financial pressure in private practice have tended to encourage the development of brief psychotherapy, but the chief reason for its emerging importance is that it is more effective than long-term therapy for the management of acute psychiatric problems.

Brief psychotherapy is defined as a mutual undertaking by the patient and therapist to change the patient's perception, thinking, feelings, and behavior within an agreed number of therapy sessions, usually weekly. Agreement on the number of sessions at the outset minimizes the problem of overdependence and motivates the patient to work hard to resolve his difficulties. It differs from long-term therapy not only in the number of sessions but also in its emphasis on the current situation. Character problems are taken up only if they are pertinent. If possible, the patient's feelings for the therapist are kept positive and are not taken up as an issue in treatment, and the therapist is more active in focusing on the problem. Dependence and regression are discouraged.

Brief psychotherapy may be tried for any psychiatric condition, but good results cannot usually be achieved in chronic psychotic illnesses, chronic obsessive-compulsive neuroses, and severe character problems such as sexual perversion or alcoholism. An acute episode of anxiety or depression occurring in a patient with one of the above-mentioned conditions may be treated provided the precise goals of treatment are stated so that the patient is not led to be overoptimistic. The patient with symptoms occurring in response to maturational stress—changing schools, graduation, marriage, increased job responsibility, and so forth—who has a previously sound character is best suited for brief psychotherapy. Others are patients with unexplained emotional or somatic symptoms or neurotic symptoms superimposed on organic illness.

Patients must be motivated for treatment. Features that lead to a good prognosis are (1) a good reality situation, (2) stable relationships with people, (3) an ability to look at themselves realistically, that is, the ability to introspect, (4) no language barrier, (5) at least average intelligence, (6) willingness to accept personal responsibilities for their difficulties, (7) the ability to tolerate anxiety, anger, and frustration, and (8) no significant secondary gains from their symptoms.

The therapeutic factors in brief psychotherapy may be summarized briefly as follows:

1. *Suggestion* is an important therapeutic factor since the very fact that he is in treatment leads the patient to hope for improvement. Therefore he is receptive to ideas deliberately or otherwise implanted by the therapist. Direct advice and guidance may be given, but the results are better if the patient's own ideas, solutions, and insights can be reinforced and authenticated.

2. *Verbalization* consists of putting thoughts, wishes, fantasies, and feelings into words so that they can be examined. The act of putting things into words often makes it possible for the patient to deal with previously unrecognized matters in a therapeutically beneficial way.

3. The *support* the patient receives from the therapist permits him to feel that something is being done for him and gives hope that in the future he will find another person to whom he can relate honestly and from whom he can expect an honest appraisal. While accepting the patient's problems as real, the therapist should also point out the patient's successes in life and not concur uncritically with those of the patient's unjustified self-criticisms. In successful therapy, the therapist will frequently serve as a model with whom the patient identifies.

4. *Abreaction* is the recollection by the patient, with emotional discharge, of previously unconscious experiences and ideas, with the result that

the patient gains awareness of the relationship between the undis-charged emotion and his symptoms.

5. The *corrective emotional experience* in the patient-therapist relationship makes it possible for the patient both to understand and to feel that the people in his present life are not identical with the pathogenic figures in his past life. In some cases the therapist may deliberately assume a role opposite the one the patient has been expecting, for example, being very strict in contrast to the patient's weak, yielding parent.

6. *Clarification* is the restatement by the therapist of previously unconnect-ed facts that were unconscious or preconscious, with the goal of cor-recting misunderstandings.

7. *Interpretation* is the explanation to the patient of his productions, re-sistances, and character defenses. This is best done by demonstrating patterns of responses using examples from the treatment or current reality situation.

8. *Insight*, the intellectual understanding and emotional acceptance of the origin and development of symptoms, will help to protect patients from the repetition of previous conflicts. Patients should be helped to attain it *only* when they are able to tolerate it.

9. In *working through*, the patient puts to use in real-life situations what he has learned about himself in therapy. The satisfaction in mastery of once difficult situations serves as a stimulus to further progress.

Psychoanalytic psychotherapy. Psychoanalytic therapy differs from psy-choanalysis in that it is less intensive and less concerned with unconscious material. It is used for the following reasons:

1. Less time and money are involved per patient treated than in psycho-analysis.

2. Less extensive training is necessary for the therapist.

3. A greater variety of psychiatric disorders can be treated with this tech-nique than are usually regarded as suitable for formal psychoanalysis, particularly the functional psychoses, schizophrenias and affective psy-choses, and the borderline psychoses.

4. More flexibility is permitted in the use of adjunctive or combined treat-ment procedures, for example, the use of tranquilizing or mood elevat-ing drugs, environmental manipulation, and direct suggestion and support.

This type of therapy has the widest application of any of the psychothera-pies. It is useful in nearly all psychiatric disorders that are generally con-sidered to be amenable to verbal treatment: neuroses, functional psychoses, personality disorders, and psychophysiologic reactions. Variations of it may be used with almost any age group from childhood to old age. Because less time and money are involved, it is often a more practical approach than formal psychoanalysis. "Psychologic-mindedness"—the ability to form insight—is, as with psychoanalysis, an important factor in the success of treatment.

The primary goal of psychoanalytic therapy is the relief of symptoms. Undesirable personality traits and defense patterns can often be modified, but the aims are more modest that with psychoanalysis. The patient usually can be helped to handle mental conflicts and anxiety-producing situations in a more efficient manner and with less distressing side effects.

Psychoanalytic therapy usually requires one or two visits a week over a period of 1 to 4 years. It is uncommon to use a couch. The patient usually faces the therapist directly, or chairs may be placed at angles so that the patient need not look directly at the therapist unless he wants to do so.

The length of treatment in psychoanalytic therapy depends on many factors, largely on the goals that the patient and the therapist set for themselves. Often these goals, particularly those of the patient, have to be modified to conform to reality. The important goal is the elimination or great reduction of symptoms. An attempt to modify the characteristic defense patterns is also made. It is hoped that the patient will be better able to tolerate previously symptom-producing stresses and to cope more efficiently with them.

With reasonable selection of patients, psychoanalytic therapy produces essentially the same degree of success, in terms of its somewhat more limited goals, as does psychoanalysis in its more far-reaching goals. This means, roughly, a marked improvement in about a third of the patients and a moderate improvement in another third, with less favorable results in the remainder (Solomon and Patch, 1974).

Group therapy involves processes that occur in formally organized and protected groups and that are calculated to cause rapid improvement in personality and behavior of individual members through controlled group interactions. Methods of group therapy generally have similar counterparts in methods of individual psychotherapy. To a large degree, group therapy is based on the same theoretical principles as individual therapy, but it has new dimensions and addresses itself to problems not always met by individual therapy.

Traditionally, group therapy has been conducted by psychiatrists, psychologists, and social workers. In response to the growing demand for it, many clergymen, nurses, educators, other professionals and semiprofessionals, and even laymen have become involved as leaders of group therapy sessions.

The criteria for success in group therapy are essentially the same as for individual therapy, that is, relief from distress, enhanced personal dignity, insight, and improved behavior and social relations. Individual therapy is sometimes preferable in achieving insight, but group therapy is often more effective. To see ourselves as others see us is a form of insight that groups provide.

The success of group therapy depends to a large extent on the degree of involvement of the therapist and the proper selection of patients. The therapist who considers group therapy to be an inferior form of psychotherapy tends to prescribe it for the least promising patients; if the results are then poor, his prejudice is reinforced.

Economy in money and personnel is perhaps the most obvious advantage of group therapy over individual treatment. This is not the *only* advantage, however, and it may not be as important as others. Group therapy, for example, offers a correction against social isolation engendered by technologic improvements in modern life.

The obvious advantages of group therapy in terms of the therapist's time and cost per person lead some to regard it as a cheap treatment or as diluted individual therapy. The therapist and his patients should both consider how the group can multiply therapy by bringing many minds and viewpoints to bear on each patient's individual problem.

Group therapy offers the further advantage of providing each member with a safe human relations laboratory. Under its protection, one has the opportunity to test various ways of relating to others and to discover how others respond.

The patient's dignity is enhanced when he is a giver as well as a receiver of help. Truly valuable insights and interpretations are often given by one patient to another. Altruism is often fostered, sometimes in people in whom this quality has seemed to be lacking. In the atmosphere of mutual help, the patient also becomes a therapist.

Evocative group therapy. Evocative methods of group therapy are those that encourage spontaneous expression of feelings by patients in an atmosphere of acceptance and of effort toward understanding those feelings. In group therapy the vocative leader promotes mutual interaction among patients in preference to patient-to-therapist (and therapist-to-patient) exchanges. The leader avoids authoritarianism. He does not demand that patients express the *right* attitude; he wants them to feel free to express their *real* attitudes. Generally, in evocative groups, the members and leader should be seated comfortably in a circle; the therapist is not placed in any special position that would make him the focal point of the group's attention.

Directive groups. Directive methods are those in which the leader asserts his authority, especially as an expert on proper attitudes and conduct. Advice and commands may be given. In directive groups the leader stands or sits in a special position, such that he is the focal point of the group's attention, like a teacher before his class or a preacher before his congregation.

For many years, religious groups have been used to inspire a shared sense of meaning and purpose in their members, to reinforce adherence to codes of belief and conduct, and to promote fellowship and solidarity.

Alcoholics Anonymous and Recovery, Inc., are nonsectarian directive groups with a religious flavor, founded by physicians but run by the members. Synanon is a similar group for narcotic addicts.

Didactic groups. Didactic methods aim at educating patients, often with factual knowledge about their problems and what is known about their treatment. There may be an overlap between these methods and directive methods. When there is a distinction, the didactic approach seeks to *educate* whereas the directive approach seeks to *indoctrinate*.

Organized classes and seminars for institutionalized patients with psychoses, sex deviations, and other problems that respond poorly to less structured approaches can be of great value. Patients are taught about the nature, causes, and treatment of their condition. Their intelligence is thus acknowledged and enlisted. Through understanding, fear and hostility toward treatment are diminished and the patient is motivated to cooperate with other types of therapy.

Number of patients. Evocative groups should be limited to four to nine members; optimal would be six or seven. Larger numbers of patients are feasible with directive and didactic groups. One should allow for dropouts and absentees by starting the group at about one third more than the optimal number.

Types of patients. The appropriate types of patients vary with the therapeutic approach. However, in all instances, and especially for evocative groups, careful screening should be done to eliminate individuals so close to a psychotic or suicidal break that treatment of any kind is dangerous.

The most suitable patients for adult and adolescent evocation groups are those suffering from interpersonal maladjustments. Patients may have neuroses, psychophysiologic disturbances, or personality disorders (if they have sufficiently developed consciences). Patients with overt psychotic and antisocial personalities are generally not desirable for evocative groups.

Within the group, patients may vary with regard to sex, age, diagnosis, and other qualities provided that no individual is sharply set off from the others—for example, a solitary male among females, one 50 year old among others in their twenties, one homosexual among heterosexuals.

Ideally, patients should have no previous acquaintance with one another. Exceptions occur with group therapy techniques designed for families, married couples, and certain training groups.

Special indications. Many problems may be more amenable to group therapy than to individual therapy. Some of these include the following:

1. For shy and lonely people the group process of universalization can be very helpful; that is, they discover they are not so different from others after all. Such patients are typically reluctant to enter group therapy, protesting that groups are especially threatening to them. They can be told that this very fact makes group therapy promising.

2. Patients who become too dependent on an individual therapist may resist the idea of sharing the therapist's attention with others. Group therapy helps them to distribute their dependent transference around the group and mitigates their tendency to cling to the therapist.

3. Group reinforcement gives added incentive to overcome phobias. In a group with more than one phobic individual, a healthy competition toward improvement may develop.

4. Antagonism and fear toward parental and authority figures may cause the patient to withhold the expression of his feelings in individual therapy, but he may overcome his reticence in a group, where hostility toward the therapist is more easily verbalized.

5. Patients who have had unsatisfactory experiences with siblings, or no experience at all, may benefit from group interaction.

6. Adolescent girls with confused sexual identification can do well within a group situation.

7. Patients with difficulty in getting along with others (poor interpersonal relationships)—that is, patients spoiled as children, those who tend to demand much and give little, and those who have other unrecognized ways of alienating people (abrasive personalities)—are likely to show their characteristic behavior in the group and to be made aware of it by others.

8. Patients with afflictions seen as shameful or unusual—homosexuals, enuretics, alcoholics, substance abusers, obese persons—can be of great emotional support to one another.

9. Group therapy with three or four married couples is a promising new approach. With two therapists, preferably a man and a woman, five couples may be feasible. It is sometimes difficult for a marriage counselor to maintain an unbiased role when working with one couple at a time. In couples' group therapy, the opportunity to pass the buck to others in the group makes it easier to escape the judgmental role. Furthermore, in couples' groups, members discover that neither they nor their spouses are so peculiar after all. They find that disharmonies they had considered unique to their marriage are often present in other marriages also.

Although the patient may have already acknowledged his need for some sort of psychiatric treatment, he may still be reluctant to accept a recommendation for group therapy. Typical objections are fear of ridicule, condemnation, or rejection by the others, as well as shyness, stage fright, and discomfort in groups and social situations. The therapist may tell the patient that group therapy is especially helpful for such problems. Other concerns may include fear of breach of confidentiality by other members and a desire for the therapist's individual attention. If the therapist is familiar with the indications and contraindications for this type of therapy and is personally convinced that group therapy will have specific advantages for the patient, the therapist can usually persuade him to try it.

Behavior therapy. The behavior therapies have been gaining increasing acceptance as useful techniques for the treatment of a variety of psychiatric conditions. The behavior therapies differ in several important respects from traditional psychotherapeutic procedures.

Perhaps the most important difference is that behavior therapists view disturbed behavior as largely a psychologic rather than a medical problem. Therefore they address themselves directly to the task of modifying maladaptive behavior—the patients' symptoms—rather than attempting to identify the underlying unconscious disease process that most psychotherapists believe "cause" symptoms. For this reason behavior therapists, most often laboratory-trained clinical psychologists or psychiatrists who think of themselves primarily as behavioral scientists, avoid psychodynamic formulations; do not deal with the unconscious, ego structures, or defense mechanisms; and do not employ insight as a prime treatment vehicle. They concern themselves only with maladaptive, inappropriate, or irrelevant kinds of *behavior* that can be measured and observed accurately and modified systematically. For the same reason, behavior therapists select their patients from among those who show a set of circumscribed behavioral difficulties rather than from those whose diverse symptomatology pervades their lives.

The two major types of behavior therapy differ in the kinds of behavior they endeavor to modify and in the procedures they use. The *classic conditioning therapies* employ unlearned, constitutional, physiologic reflex behavior to modify or eliminate unwanted, usually reflex (involuntary) behavior. The *operant conditioning therapies* employ operant (voluntary) environmental procedures to control the consequences of the patient's voluntary behavior; in so doing, they ultimately enable the patient to control the behavior itself.

Behavior therapists consider these techniques to be effective in the treatment of all neurotic conditions, especially the anxiety and phobic reactions, and other functional psychiatric disorders, including the psychoses. They also assert that most behavior therapy is successful; that is, all symptoms disappear within eight to twelve sessions and subsequent symptom substitution rarely occurs.

Classic conditioning therapies. Counterconditioning, subvarieties of which are reciprocal inhibition, desensitization, and aversion conditioning, developed out of the fundamental behaviorist assumption that neuroses are simply persistent maladaptive learned habits associated with persistent anxiety. Carefully controlled experiments by Wolpe (1969) suggested that anxiety could be eliminated by inhibiting its expression with competing responses.

The stimulus most commonly used to countercondition anxiety is the state of deep muscle relaxation. The therapist employing relaxation as a reciprocal inhibitor of anxiety usually spends two to three sessions training patients in keep muscle relaxation. The patient then practices relaxation at home until he can consistently invoke the state on command.

Assertive training—in self-expression, self-control, and self-assertion in interpersonal situations—is given at the same time since successful assertive behavior, like relaxation, is thought to inhibit anxiety. Instruction in assertive training usually begins during an early session of behavior therapy. The patient is asked to emit an assertive response—usually a verbal statement of objection to or comment on someone else's verbal behavior toward him—that he would not usually make. The patient is reassured that an assertive response is not by definition a hostile one. It is, rather, a verbal expression of control and self-confidence, but one that he has not been willing to make of his own accord. The therapist asks the patient to make assertive responses only once or twice a day at first. Gradually, as therapy proceeds and the patient learns that a firm but not necessarily hostile statement of his own opinion about something of importance to him does not meet with counterhostility, he begins to make such responses more naturally. He also learns that assertive behavior and anxious behavior cannot coexist and that if he can be self-confident enough to be assertive, he will have to spend less and less time being anxious.

The desensitization procedure itself is a relatively simple one. After the patient informs his therapist that he has been able to relax completely, the therapist asks him to imagine a neutral control or reference image to serve as a non–anxiety-producing image as counterconditioning proceeds. The therapist then describes that scene in the patient's hierarchy that causes the least anxiety or fear. If the patient—now presumably completely relaxed—can experience this scene in his imagination without also experiencing anxiety or fear, the therapist proceeds to succeeding scenes until the patient indicates that he does feel anxiety. The therapist then stops immediately and either backtracks to images in the hierarchy that the patient can successfully experience without anxiety or terminates the session.

Reciprocal inhibition procedures have also been used to eliminate other unwanted behaviors. Adversive conditioning techniques involve the repeated coupling of a negative stimulus—for example, an electric shock, an emesis-producing substance, a verbal admonition—and the behavioral sequence to be interrupted. They have been used extensively to treat drug and alcohol addiction and some types of sexual deviations. Whenever the patient behaves in an unwanted manner, he is punished immediately by an unpleasant stimulus until he cannot emit the maladaptive behavior without also experiencing the effects of the negative stimulus. The unwanted behavior eventually decreases and, as a rule, ultimately disappears.

Positive reconditioning—the classic conditioning of new motor habits—has become less important as a treatment technique as more flexible operant techniques for generating both voluntary and involuntary behaviors have evolved. Positive reconditioning is still used occasionally, however, to treat nocturnal enuresis. The technique employs an alarm set to awaken the sleeping patient, usually a child, as soon as he excretes the first drop of urine. Coupling the alarm with the first appearance of urine eventually decreases the child's tendency to urinate in response to bladder stimulation during sleep.

Experimental extinction—the classic conditioning therapy—aims at progressively weakening an unwanted motor habit through repeated nonreinforcement (extinction) of the responses that manifest it. Tics and overeating have been most successfully treated in this way. Because this technique requires careful identification of the reinforcers that maintain the unwanted behavior, its utility is limited to fairly simple behavior problems with a limited and identifiable number of reinforces. It should be used only with patients whose inappropriate motor habits are not maintained by nonspecific internal variables like motivational states that cannot be readily extinguished.

Operant conditioning therapies. The complex of therapeutic techniques that go by the generic name *behavior modification* all aim to modify or eliminate inappropriate modes of operant (voluntary) behavior by systematically altering their consequences. All of them require as a first step an accurate frequency (baseline) count of the target behavior or set of behaviors to be modified, along with complete identification of all environmental variables that appear to control (reinforce) them. Although behavior modification techniques are best known for the successes they have achieved in altering psychotic behavior patterns on psychiatric hospital units, they have also been used effectively to treat less formideable behavior and educational problems. Behavior modification techniques are the treatment of choice for many unit management problems and for a variety of other relatively circumscribed learned behavior problems.

One of the earliest reports on the use of behavior modification techniques in an institutional setting involved the psychiatric nurse as a behavioral engineer, since behavior modification procedures in hospitals require that behaviors be under continuous observation and control and depend in large part on the cooperation of the unit nursing personnel. The study by Ayllon and Ayrin (1968) presented behavior modification data on nineteen patients, fourteen schizophrenic and five mentally retarded. Various procedures were employed to alter maladaptive behavior patterns in these patients. One patient, whose frequent visits to the nursing station usually succeeded in disrupting nursing activities, gradually decreased the frequency of these visits over a period of 8 weeks when attention was systematically withdrawn from her each time she appeared. Another patient who consistently produced only psychotic talk was systematically punished by withdrawal of attention whenever she talked "crazy" and reinforced with praise and interest whenever she produced nonpsychotic talk. Over the course of 12 weeks the frequency of the psychotic talk decreased and nonpsychotic talk increased significantly. Other psychotic behaviors modified by operant techniques in this group included psychotic posturing and withdrawal, anorexia, and hoarding. Various procedures were used to effect the systematic withdrawal or modification of the consequences (reinforcers) that had served to maintain these unwanted behaviors.

The behavior of psychotic children has also been treated with operant techniques. Wolf, Risley, and Mees (1964) successfully treated an autistic child's severe temper tantrums, bedtime problems, mutism, and eating problems with a variety of operant techniques. The usual procedure was first to extinguish inappropriate behavior, such as placing the child in a room by himself whenever he began a tantrum. More appropriate behavior was then established by shaping procedures; for example, socially appropriate verbal behavior was instilled at first by rewarding the child with food when he repeated appropriate words, and later when he used words without prompting.

Normal educational problems have also been dealt with successfully by operant conditioning procedures. Efficient study habits were instilled in college students by operant shaping techniques. Of five students chosen for inclusion in the study, two were above and three below the college achievement average. All were required to prepare a careful analysis of their daily study schedules. Inappropriate and maladaptive study habits such as daydreaming, difficulties in concentration, partial learning, and inefficient use of study time were altered by operant shaping procedures designed at first to force the student to concentrate intensively for limited periods on circumscribed units of school work. Only when he could do so was he then scheduled to spend longer and longer periods on a greater variety of material, as he grew able to make more and more efficient use of his time. Four of the five students responded positively to these control procedures by making higher grades the semester following institution of the techniques (Wolf, Risley, and Mees, 1964).

If the extensive confirmatory literature of behavior therapy can be believed —and many therapists have come to believe it—then it is clear that the principal advantage of these techniques is that they succeed where other therapies have failed. The behavior therapists claim consistent success with patients who have been burdened for years with phobias, severe and intractable anxiety, and obsessional thinking. They also report success in the treatment of sexual disorders of all kinds and, with less conviction, in treatment of drug addiction and alcoholism.

Back ward psychotic patients who have been restricted to locked wards for years because they lack elementary social skills and competencies are often able to leave the hospital following behavior modification procedures that teach them the rudiments of these skills. While they may not be able to leave the hospital, they are able to spend their days in much happier circumstances, perhaps sitting under a tree instead of on a ward bench.

Behavior modification procedures are easily taught to persons unsophisticated in psychologic theory and technique. Psychiatric attendants, parents, and public school teachers have been taught the principles of behavior modification with such success that they are able to assume responsibility for treatment with a few hours of instruction. The procedures are clear-cut, unambiguous, and consistent, all qualities that make for ready transfer of skill from professional to nonprofessional therapist.

Another advantage of these procedures over conventional ones is the much shorter period of time they require for a positive outcome. Patients who would have spent years in psychoanalysis are said to be helped greatly by treatment lasting only a few weeks. At the same time, the behavior therapists claim success equal to or greater than that of older procedures, with only rare instances of symptom substitution or reappearance of old symptoms.

Finally, these procedures offer many more opportunities for objective, scientific inquiry into modes of action and degree of therapeutic success than older procedures, notably psychoanalysis, which are relatively inaccessible to such inquiry.

At this point, the major shortcoming of behavior therapy lies in the enthusiasm with which its adherents sell the technique as a cure-all for all the world's ills. In many ways, such dedication to a single therapeutic point of view, accompanied as it is by selective inattention to other methods and points of view, is strikingly reminiscent of the early days of the psychoanalytic movement.

Family therapy. In family therapy, the emphasis is on the family group as a single unit, and the family is treated simultaneously on a periodic and continued basis. Behavior and symptoms are therefore viewed as a result of processes within the family that have an interchangeable relationship with each family member's intrapsychic life, the assumption being that mental disturbance in one member of the family may be an indication of dysfunction within the family unit.

Ackerman (1958) stated that the family becomes a source of sick emotional contagion. Psychiatric patients come from disordered families, and the first family member referred for psychiatric care may be the most or the least sick member██disturbed, it creates an inordinate amount of stress in the other family members.

Several variations or techniques of treatment may be used, with the trend toward including nuclear family members in therapy. Some family therapists also include others who may be significant to the family members, such as girlfriend, boyfriend, or grandparent. After several joint sessions, the children may be terminated from the therapy sessions while the parents continue. The primary focus is toward understanding the family's patterns of interaction and the best method to help them with their problems. Collaborative therapy has been used in some institutions for many years. This technique refers to the parents of hospitalized patients being seen in individual treatment by different therapists. On a periodic and continued basis, all therapists of the family members hold conferences about the problems, needs, and interactions within the family unit. Conjoint therapy in which all the family members meet together as a unit was developed at the Mental Research Institute, Palo Alto, California (Jackson and Weakland, 1968). The technique of network therapy was used by Fleck (1967). In this type of therapy at home, as many as thirty people—including relatives, neighbors, police, priest, and others, as well as family members—might be involved in one session. Several families may also be seen together in groups for treatment.

Members of families are individuals with self-concepts; when other family members give out messages that do not fit with the individual's definition of himself, it destroys his self-concept. Since children are different every day, whatever parents do will confirm or disconfirm their children. Individuals can be taught to see a different world by introducing them to a new concept. Family therapy can introduce a new concept into the family group, and the family members then perceive that they themselves control behavior.

Some families never stay together long enough to talk. In such a situation, the therapist may put all of the family members in a room with a one-way mirror and go to the adjacent room to observe their interaction. The therapist and the family may never agree on the problem within the family but in the process of getting together, talking, and interacting, the family improves. The therapist may use drama, humor, tact, ambiguity, and ceremony to help the family members save face. Ambiguity is part of healthy communication. When there are different premises in people's minds about a situation they are in, the result may be conflict. Some therapists ask each family member in turn for comments; most families have not had this experience before and it can be very illuminating to those concerned to hear their perceptions about each other. The therapist may question, model, and summarize at the end of the ▮▮▮▮▮▮▮▮▮▮▮▮▮▮▮▮▮▮▮▮▮▮▮▮▮▮▮▮▮▮▮▮▮▮▮ on each therapist's orientation. Some therapists insist that all family members come for the assessment interview, while others do not. The work situation of the family may prevent all members from coming unless evening appointments are available. Ackerman believed the home visit was ideal for the diagnostic interview. He also liked to keep the children involved in the therapeutic sessions, whereas other therapists do not. Some therapists talk with each family member alone in the initial interview and at other times during therapy.

The concept of nurses as primary agents in home treatment, assisting with the supervision of patients on medications, conducting individual and family therapy, and supervising the general needs of patients and families is supported by Weiner, Becker, and Friedman (1967). Nurses have entree to families under stress because they are seen in the helper role. Orientation of nurses in this role helps in reaching individuals and families where approaches by other professionals may fail.

Application of the concept of interdependence within families was presented by Hover (1968) in her work with a family with multiple problems. Her first impression was the need for hospitalization of one member. Subsequent visits involved assessing the total needs of the entire family, making a diagnosis of the family problems, setting priorities, and providing help. Busch (1968) describes the use of the home visit with a child and mother in follow-up care after hospitalization and in collaboration with the child psychiatrist and the school nurse.

The following case study illustrates not only the effectiveness of family therapy but also the nurse as a therapist:

Mrs. D. and her 16-year-old daughter Karen came to a community mental health center because Mrs. D. was having problems with Karen. They were seen in a collateral session.

Karen was a slim, attractive, but very sullen 16 year old; Mrs. D. was a quiet, reserved, and bewildered mother. When asked what the problem was, Mrs. D. stated that she didn't understand Karen's recent behavior. When asked specifically: "What behavior?" Mrs. D. replied vaguely, "She won't mind her father." The nurse-therapist sought validation from Karen by asking:

"Do you mind your father?" Karen answered angrily: "Of course—most of the time." In the first 30 minutes Karen related *all* of the "unreasonable" demands her father placed on her. Mrs. D. remained passive and agreed with Karen occasionally and disagreed with her mildly at times.

The nurse-therapist stated that Mr. D. was apparently the bone of contention. Since he was not there to defend himself, Mrs. D. was asked if he would come to the next therapy session. She replied rapidly, and seemingly frightened, "No, he works and can't come in." She was then asked about other family members. Mrs. D. began to smile and said that they had a son, Steven, 11 years old, "who is a delight—*he* doesn't have any problems." This statement was made with a side glance at Karen. Karen muttered, "He is a pain." Mrs. D. meekly said, "Karen—you shouldn't talk like that."

The nurse-therapist said that she would *really* like to meet Steven and Mr. D. and asked what time Mr. D. usually got home from work. Mrs. D. replied, "He gets home at 5:00 P.M.—and we *always* have dinner at 5:30 P.M." The therapist then said, firmly but pleasantly, "Then I could come to your home at 6:30 or 7:00 P.M. and wouldn't disturb your dinner. Shall I come tomorrow night at 7:00 P.M.?" Karen grinned mischievously and winked at the therapist (assuming that she had an ally) and said: "Super!" Mrs. D. looked slightly confused and replied meekly, "Yes, I guess that will be all right." The therapist got directions to their home, shook hands with Mrs. D., tousled Karen's hair, smiled at both, and said, "I'll see all of you tomorrow night at 7:00 P.M."

The next evening promptly at 7:00 P.M. the nurse-therapist arrived at the D.'s modest home in the suburbs. There was a soccer game being played in the street in front of their home, so she parked further down the street. As she approached their driveway one of the soccer players halted the game and ran up. He looked about 11 years old and had blond wavy hair and sparkling blue eyes. She said, "Hi, are you Steven?" He smiled and said, "Yes. Are you the nurse who is coming to see us about Karen?" The therapist answered "Yes, come in and join us—I want to get to know you too." Again a charming smile and "O.K. I want to!" He and the therapist walked to the front door together and discussed soccer briefly. Mrs. D. was waiting at the front door, looking apprehensive, but managed a weak smile and asked the therapist to come in.

Mrs. D., the therapist, and Steven entered the living room (which was immaculate) and Karen came in from her room smiling and said "Hi!" When she saw Steven her face flushed with anger and she said, "I see you have already met the *angel!*" The therapist smiled and replied: "Yes, I've met Steven, but I didn't know he was an angel. In fact, I see a little devil in his eyes." Steven laughed and Karen seemed to relax.

Mrs. D., with Karen's help, served coffee and freshly baked cookies. It was easy for the therapist to comment on how delicious they were, how attractive their home was, and so forth. (Mr. D. had not appeared and the therapist avoided asking where he was.) The coffee table was apparently handmade out of an old wagon wheel. The therapist stated that it was most unusual and whoever made it obviously was quite skilled. Mrs. D. stated that her husband had made it and pointed out other things he had made. Mr. D. appeared in the doorway from the kitchen with a can of beer in his hand (for courage, no doubt). Mrs. D. introduced him to the therapist, who stood up and held out her hand and said: "I'm very happy to meet you, Mr. D.; I was just admiring your coffee table." He came over and shook hands and looked suspiciously at the therapist. They discussed where he had found the wagon wheel, how long it took him to make, and so forth. As he talked he seemed to relax and forget that she was there as a therapist. Karen had said little but seemed fascinated by the interaction. Steven was in and out of the living room repeatedly—grabbing a cookie, bumping Karen's chair (deliberately), and in general trying to be the center of attention. Mrs. D. occasionally would say mildly, "Steven, you shouldn't do that."

When the "social session" was over and everyone, including Mr. D., appeared comfortable and relaxed, the therapist said to Mr. D., "I understand you are having problems with Karen." He replied, "Yes, she has changed—she just won't mind me any more; I don't understand why." She asked for some specifics—what had he asked Karen to do that she didn't? He said that the previous Friday Karen and a girlfriend had gone to the high school football game. "She knows that she is supposed to be home at 9:30 P.M. every Friday and Saturday night—and she came home at 10:00 P.M.!" The therapist asked Karen why she came home at 10:00 P.M. if her curfew was 9:30 P.M.? She replied that no one else had to be home at 9:30 P.M.—her father was too old-fashioned and strict. She also said, "I didn't do anything wrong. We just went and had a Coke after the game."

The nurse-therapist explained to Mr. and Mrs. D. the normal maturational stresses that Karen was undergoing—that is, wanting to be liked and accepted by her peers, needing some realistic guidelines for her behavior and yet enough freedom to enjoy life and seek some independence. She told them that she also had children who were going through the same "growing pains." They seemed relieved that she could relate to how they were feeling about Karen's rebellion.

They then discussed some realistic guidelines—times Karen should be home, what she should do to help around the house, and so forth. They were tactfully told that a 9:30 P.M. deadline on Friday and Saturday nights was a bit old-fashioned. Karen was asked what time *she* thought she should be in. She replied, "On normal Fridays and Saturdays I feel that 10:00 P.M. would be reasonable, but on special occasions I should be permitted to come in at midnight." Mr. D. said he would agree to the 10:00 P.M. but *never* to midnight. By negotiation they managed to get Karen and Mr. D. to accept a 11:00 P.M. curfew for special occasions.

With that problem settled and the time running out, the therapist asked if she could return next week at the same time so they could work on some more compromises. They agreed very enthusiastically. The therapist then added that she also wanted to talk to them about Steven's behavior—that he was, as Karen had said, "a pain" and absolutely spoiled rotten. Mr. D. said to Mrs. D., "You see, I told you that you spoil him rotten!" Mrs. D. looked embarrassed and said, "I guess I do." Karen laughed with glee and Steven glowered. They walked the therapist to the door. She asked Steven if he would walk her to her car. He agreed reluctantly. As they walked they talked. She told him not to worry—"look what Karen got with her compromises"—and that if he were honest he would admit he had been getting away with murder. He grinned sheepishly, with that devilish gleam in his eyes, and said: "You are right—and you are O.K.: Just don't make me give up *all* my fun!" She laughed and said, "See you next week, you little devil!" He laughed and waved good-bye.

The remaining sessions went very well. Mrs. D. would have the coffee pot and cookies on the coffee table and everyone helped themselves whenever they wanted. Mr. D. was always prompt to enter the living room and shake hands when the therapist came. Occasionally they would have to round up Steven; he constantly tested the limits, discussed within the family, on his behavior. Karen seemed to blossom, and Mrs. D. became more assertive with encouragement and support. Mr. D. was able to discuss his reasons for being so strict and was able to modify his behavior regarding Karen. He also began to take over the discipline of Steven, who needed a firm hand. In essence, they became a warm, cohesive family unit, with everyone working on problems as they came up.

Psychodrama. Psychodrama was introduced in the United States in 1925 by Moreno (1959), and since then a number of clinical methods have developed: the therapeutic psychodrama, the sociodrama, role-playing, the analytic psychodrama, and various modifications of them.

The chief participants in a therapeutic psychodrama are the protagonist or subject, the director or chief therapist, the auxiliary egos, and the group. The protagonist presents either a private or a group problem; the auxiliary egos help him to bring his personal and collective drama to life and to correct it. Meaningful psychologic experiences of the protagonist are given shape more thoroughly and more completely than life would permit under normal circumstances. A psychodrama can be produced anywhere, wherever patients find themselves: in a private home, a hospital, a schoolroom, or a military barracks. It sets up its laboratory everywhere. Most advantageous is a specially adopted therapeutic space containing a stage. Psychodrama is either protagonist-centered (the private problem of the protagonist) or group-centered (the problem of the group). In general, it is important that the theme, whether it is private or collective, be a truly experienced problem of the participants, real or symbolic. The participants should represent their experiences spontaneously, although the repetition of a theme can frequently be of therapeutic advantage. Next to the protagonist, the auxiliary egos and the chief therapist play an important part. It is their responsibility to bring the therapeutic productivity of the group to as high a level as possible.

The auxiliary egos are actors who represent absentee persons as they appear in the private world of the patient. The best auxiliary egos are former patients, who have made at least a temporary recovery, and professional therapeutic egos who come from a sociocultural environment similar to the patient's. If there is a choice, "native" auxiliary egos are preferable to professional egos, however well trained the latter may be. Many investigators who have tried to apply psychodrama to different cultural settings have found that the proper choice of auxiliary egos is of prime importance.

Since the task of the auxiliary egos is to represent the patient's perceptions of the internal roles or figures dominating his world, the more adequately they are able to present them, the greater will be the effect on the patient. Instead of talking to the patient about his inner experiences, the auxiliary egos portray them and make it possible for the patient to encounter his own internal figures externally. Such encounters go beyond verbal communication and help the patient strengthen his vague internal perceptions to which he can relate without external aid. These symbolic figures of his inner life are not mere phantoms but therapeutic actors with real lives of their own.

The general rule in classic psychodrama is that the patient can choose or reject the egos portraying the significant roles in his life and vice versa, that the egos are free to choose or reject in their willingness to cooperate with the patient. However, there are exceptions where the patient is exposed to a certain ego in a special role, created without his consent, and, at times, the therapist is instructed to assume a role which he or she does not particularly like to portray. Indications or counterindications are the mental benefits expected to be derived by the patient from such traumatic procedures.

On portraying the role it is expected that the ego will identify himself privately with the role to the best of his ability, not only to act and pretend but to be it. The hypothesis is that what certain patients need, more than anything else, is to enter into contact with people who apparently have a profound and warm feeling for him. For example, if it happens that as a child he never had a real father, in a therapeutic situation the one who takes the part of the father should create in the patient the impression that here is a man who acts as he would like to have had his father act. If he never had a mother when he was young, here is a woman who acts and is like what he wishes his mother to have been. The warmer, more intimate, and genuine the contact is, the greater are the advantages that the patient can derive from the psychodramatic episode.

The psychodramatic method rests on the hypothesis that to provide patients, singly or in groups, with a new opportunity for a psychodynamic and sociocultural reintegration, therapeutic cultures in miniature are required, in lieu of or in extension of unsatisfactory natural habitats. Vehicles for carrying out this project are (1) existential psychodrama within the framework of the community life itself, in situ, and (2) the neutral, objective, and flexible therapeutic theater. The latter represents the laboratory method in contrast to the method of nature and is structured to meet the sociocultural needs of the protagonist.

REFERENCES

Ackerman, N.: Psychodynamics of family life, New York, 1958, Basic Books, Inc.

Aguilera, D. C.: Review of psychiatric nursing, St. Louis, 1977, The C. V. Mosby Co.

Aguilera, D. C., and Messick, J. M.: Crisis intervention: theory and methodology, ed. 2, St. Louis, 1974, The C. V. Mosby Co.

Alexander, F., and Ross, H.: Encouraging the patient to new life experiences outside the treatment. In Alexander, F., and Ross, H., editors: Dynamic psychiatry, Chicago, 1952, University of Chicago Press, p. 34.

Anderson, D. B.: Nursing therapy with families, Perspect. Psychiatric Care 7(1):21-27, 1969.

Ayllon, T., and Ayrin, N.: The token economy, New York, 1968, Appleton-Century-Crofts.

Bandura, A.: Principles of behavior modification, New York, 1969, Holt, Rinehart and Winston.

Barten, H. W.: Brief therapies, New York, 1971, Behavioral Publications.

Bellak, L., and Small, L.: Emergency psychotherapy and brief psychotherapy, New York, 1965, Grune & Stratton, Inc.

Berne, E.: Principles of group treatment, London, 1966, Oxford University Press.

Busch, K. D.: The use of the home visit by the child psychiatric nurse, American Nurses' Association Clinical Sessions, New York, 1968, Appleton-Century-Crofts, pp. 352-357.

Carter, F. M.: Psychosocial nursing, ed. 2, New York, 1976, The Macmillan Co.

Caudell, W., Redlick, F. C., Gilmore, H. R., and Brady, E. B.: Social structure and interaction processes on a psychiatric ward, Am. J. Orthopsychiatry 22:314-334, 1952.

Eysenck, H. J.: Behavior therapy: unlearning neuroses, Med. Opin. Rev. 3:68-74, 1966.

Eysenck, H. J.: The effects of psychotherapy, New York, 1966, International University Press.

Fleck, S.: The role of the family in psychiatry. In Friedman, A. M., and others, editors: Comprehensive textbook of psychiatry, Baltimore, 1967, The Williams & Wilkins Co., pp. 213-224.

Frank, J. D.: Persuasion and healing: a comparative study of psychotherapy, Baltimore, 1961, John Hopkins Press.

Franks, C. M., and Wilson, G. T.: Behavior therapy: theory and practice, New York, 1973, Brunner/Mazel.

Fromm-Reichmann, F.: Principles of intensive psychotherapy, Chicago, 1950, University of Chicago Press.

Hover, D. E.: The theory of the interdependence of family members and its application in an emotionally disturbed family. In American Nurses' Association Clinical Sessions, New York, 1968, Appleton-Century-Crofts, pp. 46-52.

Howard, J.: Please touch, New York, 1970, Brunner/Mazel.

Jackson, D. D., and Weakland, J. H.: Conjoint family therapy: some considerations on theory techniques and results, Palo Alto, Calif., 1968, Science and Behavior Books, Inc.

Kleeman, S. T., and Solomon, P.: Psychotherapy. In Solomon, P., and Patch, V., editors: Handbook of psychiatry, ed. 3, Los Altos, Calif., 1974, Lange Medical Publications.

Kovacs, L. W.: A therapeutic relationship with a patient and family, Perspect. Psychiatric Care 4(2):11-21, 1966.

Malan, D. H.: The outcome problem in psychotherapy research, Arch. Gen. Psychiatry 29:719-729, 1973.

Marmor, J.: The future of psychoanalytic therapy, Am. J. Psychiatry 130:1197-1202, 1973.

Moreno, J. L.: Psychodrama. In Arieti, S., editor: American handbook of psychiatry, vol. 2, New York, 1959, Basic Books, Inc.

Pinney, E. L., Jr.: A first group psychotherapy book, Springfield, Ill., 1970, Charles C Thomas, Publisher.

Satir, V.: Conjoint family therapy, Palo Alto, Calif., 1964, Science and Behavior Books.

Solomon, R., and Patch, V. D.: Handbook of psychiatry, ed. 3, Los Altos, Calif., 1974, Lange Medical Publications.

Stanton, A. H., and Schwartz, M. S.: The mental hospital, New York, 1954, Basic Books, Inc.

Tarachon, S.: An introduction to psychotherapy, New York, 1963, International University Press.

Wallerstein, R.: The current state of psychotherapy, J. Am. Psychoanal. Assoc. **14**:183-225, 1966.

Weiner, L., Becker, A., and Friedman, T.: Home treatment, spearhead of community psychiatry, Pittsburgh, 1967, University of Pittsburgh Press.

Wolberg, L. R.: The technique of psychotherapy, New York, 1967, Grune & Stratton, Inc.

Wolf, M. M., Risley, T., and Mees, H.: Application of operant conditions procedures to the behavior problems of an autistic child, Behav. Res. Ther. **1**:305-312, 1964.

Wolpe, J.: The practice of behavior therapy, New York, 1969, Pergamon Press.

Yalom, I. D.: The theory and practice of group psychotherapy, New York, 1970, Basic Books, Inc.

ADDITIONAL READINGS

American Nurses' Association: Standards of psychiatric-mental health nursing practice, Kansas City, Mo., 1973, The Association.

American Nurses' Association: Guidelines for the Council of Advanced Practioners in Psychiatric-Mental Health Nursing, Kansas City, Mo., 1974, The Association.

Branson, H. K.: The nurse's role in behavior modification, Nurs. Care **8**(12):21-23, 1975.

Bulbulyan, A.: The psychiatric nurse as family therapist, Perspect. Psychiatric Care **7**(2):58-68, 1969.

Caplan, G.: The mental hygiene role in maternal and child care, Nurs. Outlook **2**(1):14-19, 1954.

De Young, C.: Nursing's contribution in family crisis treatment, Nurs. Outlook **16**(2):60-63, 1968.

Dumas, R.: This I believe . . . about nursing and the poor, Nurs. Outlook **17**(9):47-50, 1969.

Lewis, O.: The children of Sanchez, New York, 1961, Alfred A. Knopf, Inc.

Meldman, M. J., Newman, B., Schaller, D., and Peterson, P.: Patients' responses to nurse-psychotherapists, Am. J. Nurs. **71**(6):1150-1151, 1971.

Niemeir, S. F.: Nurses can be effective behavior modifiers, J. Psychiatric Nurs. **14**(1):18-21, 1976.

Ozarin, L. D., and Spaner, F. E.: Mental health corporations: a new trend in providing services, Hosp. Community Psychiatry **25**(4):225-227, 1974.

Reres, M. E.: A survey of the nurse's role in psychiatric outpatient clinics in America, Community Ment. Health J. **5**(5):382-385, 1969.

Rouslin, S.: On certification of the clinical specialists in psychiatric nursing, Perspect. Psychiatric Care **10**(5):201, 1972.

Stachyra, M.: Nurses, psychotherapy and the law, Perspect. Psychiatric Care **7**(5):200-213, 1969.

Stachyra, M.: Self-regulation through certification, Perspect. Psychiatric Care **11**(4):148-154, 1973.

Underwood, P.: Communication through role playing, Am. J. Nursing **11**(6):1184-1186, 1971.

CHAPTER 13

Ego functions, mental status, and current therapies

EGO FUNCTIONS

According to Caplan (1951), the most important aspects of mental health are the state of the ego, the stage of its maturity, and the quality of its structure. Assessment of its state is based on three main areas: (1) the capacity of the person to withstand stress and anxiety and to maintain ego equilibrium, (2) the degree of reality recognized and faced in solving problems, and (3) the repertoire of effective coping mechanisms employed by the person in maintaining a balance in his biopsychosocial field.

The description and assessment of the ego and the strength of its various functions have come to play a central role in the description, diagnosis, prognosis, and treatment of many psychologic disorders.

Some function of the ego is affected in every emotional disorder. Assessment of the strengths and weaknesses of the various ego functions, therefore, tells which functions have been disrupted or weakened by the disease process and which remain relatively unaffected.

Knowledge of ego functions and their disturbances and the ability to evaluate them quickly from historical data are basic requirements for nurses in psychiatric–mental health nursing. Presenting the ego as a single construct neglects the interrelationship between the ego and all other psychodynamics. Despite this, a schematic presentation of ego functions and their disturbances serves a practical value by providing a frame of reference for diagnosis and treatment. Bellak and Small (1965) describe nine ego functions, which are discussed here.

283

Adaptation to reality. This is best viewed in terms of the cultural matrix, as adjustment in the popular sense, getting along in the world, relationship to family, school, employment, marriage, crisis, and the like. Appropriateness of role-playing in real life is a concomitant of appropriateness of behavior and is an essential aspect of assessment.

Disturbances in the adaptive capacity lead to maladjustment both to the people and to the tasks in an individual's life. They are manifested by varying degrees of inappropriate behavior, accompanied by subjective and objective difficulties. The individual with a decreased adaptive capacity is easily disturbed by departures from normal routine. Often such persons protect themselves by retreating to a limited activity that demands few of their resources and little of their energy. Conversely, others move about from one situation to another, displaying great instability in their search for an arena of functioning that they can tolerate.

Reality-testing. This function is an integral part of real-life role-playing, involving perception, judgment, and intelligence. Despite these components, reality-testing primarily involves the ability to differentiate external data from internal determinants.

Disturbances in reality-testing are reflected in distortions in the individual's perception of his role and the role of others. At the extreme, the schizophrenic projects, denies, distorts, rationalizes, and otherwise twists reality in the service of his own dynamics. The processes of rationalization, denial, and distortion are also observable in lesser disturbances. Individuals prone to acting-out behavior reflect not only poor impulse control but also a deficiency in reality-testing, denying the consequences of their behavior.

Sense of reality. As an infant develops he must differentiate between *himself* and the *rest of the world* in terms of person, place, and time, creating in the process ego boundaries or self-boundaries. A good sense of reality is reflected in the absence of conscious awareness of the self, just as there is not awareness of other well-functioning, healthy parts of the individual. Where the sense of reality is intact, there is no intrusion of the self as either a subject or an object.

Disturbances in the sense of reality range from very minor to very severe, but almost all of them are accompanied by anxiety. Depersonalization, a state in which the body image is often involved, is probably the most frequently observed form of disturbance in the sense of reality. Many physiologic disturbances contribute to the sense of unreality; feelings of light-headedness may arise in severe fatigue or as a result of hyperventilation; emotional and physical isolation produces disturbances in the sense of reality; and déjà vu may occur under stress in normal people, although it is excessive in schizophrenic persons. Usually disturbances in the sense of reality are generated by unconscious hostility.

Control of drives. The ability to regulate instinctual drives develops both from learned patterns of behavior accompanying the socialization of the child and from internal maturational phases involving drive increase, drive decrease, and control. Observable differences in drive intensity may be a result of the genetic endowment of the individuals involved. However, environmental factors may either intensify or decrease the strength of drives. The ability to regulate drives depends both on the intensity of the drive and on acquired methods for dealing with drives. Tolerance for frustration and anxiety is an important feature in the control of instinctual drives.

Early evidence of disturbance of control includes temper tantrams, bedwetting, tics, and nail-biting. Neuroses, character disorders, and psychoses are their later equivalents. At the end of the range are catatonia and mania, catatonic rigidity, the psychomotor retardation of depression, and various other psychotic mannerisms.

Discrepancies in drive regulation are the most frequently encountered disturbance among the ego functions. These are observable in the delusions and hallucinations of psychotic individuals as well as in their motor behavior. They are also observable in depressions, hysteria, and experiences of depersonalization.

Object relations. Object relations have usually been described qualitatively, such as oral, anal, phallic, and sadistic. Pathologically, they are sometimes described as phobic, obsessive, hysterical, schizoid, ambivalent, and hostile. Clinically, the intensity of object relations may be observed most accurately in terms of the distance between himself and others the patient finds most comfortable. Some people need complete closeness, others require great distance. Marital partners often control the intensity of their relationship to each other by limiting the frequency of their contact, by using separate bedrooms, by always going out with other couples and never being alone with each other, by taking separate vacations, and so on.

The disturbances in object relations are many. Symbiotic object relations are frequently encountered in adult schizophrenic patients, who in treatment attempt to merge with the therapist. Such a patient cannot conceive of the other person as having an existence outside of the relationship to the patient. These patients exhibit excessive clinging; they expect that their thoughts can be read by the other person and that their needs will be recognized and satisfied without expression on their part.

Thought processes. The perceptions of the infant are at first diffuse. Increasing differentiation takes place slowly—visual, spatial, and temporal, as well as in all other sensory modalities. As clear conceptualizations are formed, the secondary process is gradually established, developing out of the primary process. In essence, the successful development of the secondary process implies the ego's ability to scan selectively and to avoid contamination by inappropriate material. As long as the thought process function is sound, the secondary process prevails; when it fails, the content and form of the primary process reemerge.

Although not among the first to emerge, disturbances in the thought process are perhaps the most sensitive indicators of serious ego disturbance. More generally in the development of an acute schizophrenia, anxiety in relation to the loss of impulse control and labile uncontrolled affect emerge earlier than thought disturbances.

Defensive functions. Ego defenses serve as a barrier against both external and internal stimuli of a threatening nature. More specifically, the defenses enable one to deal *selectively* with internal and external stimuli. Repression, the first defense mechanism described by Freud, has come to be accepted as an important, normally present aspect of the mind. Repression is part of directed thinking or action, of selectively scanning and focusing, and of purposeful behavior.

By and large, the earlier a defense emerges the more primitive it is likely to be and, consequently, the more pathologic its consequences in the adult life of the individual. Extensive denial and projection are probably the most seriously pathologic because of their effect on the individual's adaptation to reality.

Impairment of defensive functions overlaps with the concept of failure of the synthetic function of the ego; if repression fails and the primary process emerges, the patient seems unable to "hold together"; there is inability to concentrate, memory is impaired, and general efficiency is greatly decreased. In such cases it appears that so much energy is being used in the barrier function of the ego that little is left for adaptive, spontaneous functioning.

Failure of repression may result in déjà vu experiences, in minor impairment of control, or in the lack of control. Overcontrol is another indication of impairment in defensive functioning, since it interferes with the general adaptation of the individual. Overcontrol may be noted in relationship to affect, ideation, and motor functioning, and in many cases it may constitute a last-ditch fight against the breakthrough of a psychosis. In some patients the weakening of the defensive functions may manifest itself only or particularly at those times when the ego is normally weakened, such as in times of physical illness or when an object loss has been suffered.

Autonomous functions. The concept of autonomous ego functions includes perception, intention, object comprehension, thinking, language, productivity, and various phases of motor development. These are defined as functions of the conflict-free sphere of the ego.

In schizophrenia some autonomous ego functions may be affected whereas others are not. Unsophisticated persons are often surprised to find among schizophrenics very intelligent or proficient individuals, skilled in art, languages, mathematics, or other fields. Sometimes an autonomous function such as mathematical ability is developed in lieu of object relations of a less abstract nature and may constitute a substitute for contact by language.

Adolescents present some difficult diagnostic problems both because of the increased drive apparent in them and because so many of the autonomous functions are placed at the service of the increased drive and the defenses against them. It is frequently difficult to decide whether the impairment of the ego function in the adolescent deserves the schizophrenic label or whether a less serious diagnosis may be justified.

The synthetic function. The synthetic function is the ego's ability to unite, or bind, and to create. This can be interpreted as the ego's ability to form *gestalten* or wholeness. The synthetic function is probably the aspect that most overlaps with all other ego functions and is most highly correlated with the general concept of ego strength, much as the vocabulary is most correlated with general intelligence.

The synthetic function, in short, describes the individual's ability to maintain the necessary functions of life and adaptation. When the synthetic function is weak, the ego splits off certain activities or functions because of this weakness.

MENTAL STATUS EXAMINATION

The major components of the mental status examination include:

1. General appearance and behavior
2. Characteristics of speech
3. Mood or affect
4. Content of thought
5. Sensorium functions
6. Insight and judgment

General appearance and behavior

Appearance. Much can be gained by observing a patient's physical appearance: dress, the state of body hygiene, and grooming. Are they appropriate to the person's position? For example, the teacher who comes from his office unshaven and dirty and does not seem to recognize the inappropriateness of his appearance would be evaluated differently from a construction worker with a similar appearance.

One should observe facial expressions, body and limb movements, and mannerisms, noting particularly how they change when the topic of conversation changes. Staring into space, as if preoccupied, with sudden head or body movements, may be the first hint of hallucinations; this gives the nurse the opportunity to ask whether the patient is listening to something. Strange postures, stereotyped movements such as grimacing or tics, apparently spontaneous emotional outbursts, rigidity of expression, and physical withdrawal should be noted.

When a patient will not or cannot communicate verbally, all inferences of mental status may depend on observations of his nonverbal behavior.

Behavior. One should observe the general manner in which the patient approaches the nurse and how he reacts to the interview. Is he cooperative, frank, open, fearful, hostile, or reticent? Does his general attitude change during the interview? A certain initial anxiety is to be expected, but is it unusual in intensity or duration? Is the patient's general manner congruent with the demands of the situation? Does he try to take over the interview in an inappropriate way?

Characteristics of speech

Abnormalities of speech may be quantitative or qualitative or both. Quantitative abnormalities range from incessant speech, as if there is a pressure of ideas to be expressed (the so-called flight of ideas in manic illnesses), to scant, almost monosyllabic talk found in some forms of depression and mutism. Qualitative abnormalities include such things as (1) circumstantiality, needless peripheral detail, (2) talking past and around the point, (3) perseveration, the repetition of and constant return to some particular idea, (4) irrelevance, a statement rational in itself but not germane, (5) incoherence, a statement without sense in any context, (6) word salad, a meaningless jumble of words, (7) jargon talk, and (8) senseless punning and mere animal-like sounds. More general abnormalities of form, such as affectations, talk that is incongruent with the patient's level of education, and strange inflections and impediments such as stammers, stutters, and lisps should be noted. Whenever possible, adequate samples of abnormal talk should be recorded verbatim. Change in form of speech is often a valuable guide to progress in certain illnesses such as the manic phase of manic-depressive psychosis.

Mood or affect

The level of and changes in feeling are a very sensitive index of emotional illness. There are many possible moods: depression, elation, euphoria, anger, suspicion, fear, anxiety, panic, hostility, calm, happiness, sadness, grief, and a combination of these. The object is to be able to describe in a precise way *how* the patient is feeling and not to be content with conventional one-word labels such as "hostile" or "sad."

Two factors that should be evaluated to determine the patient's feeling state are: (1) Is the mood appropriate to the thought content? (2) Is it at a reasonable level of intensity?

Bizarre, inappropriate moods may be observed in some patients suffering from schizophrenia. Depressed patients may show a mood that is appropriate in direction but excessive in degree. Patients with organic brain damage may show wide fluctuations in mood in response to seemingly trivial stimuli; this is called mood lability. Blunted or flattened affect may be seen in a wide range of conditions, including simple schizophrenia and some types of brain damage, especially to the frontal lobes.

While the mood of some patients may be very obvious, careful questioning is necessary to determine the true state of affect in others. For example, smiling depression will be missed unless the nurse specifically inquires about feelings of sadness, depression, and ideas of suicide, since the patient may wear a euphoric facade. Anger, rage, and hostility are usually well concealed by patients because they fear rejection.

Content of thought

In recording abnormalities of thought, it is necessary to distinguish between what is directly presented and what is inferred. The nurse should always note the bases for the inference. All delusions or hallucinations should be described exactly. For example, "patient believes that the FBI is out to kill him" is much more descriptive than simply recording that the patient has paranoid delusions.

Thought content abnormalities may be bizarre and obvious, or they may be quite subtle and not readily revealed by the patient, particularly if he has encountered a hostile response previously while trying to say what is in his mind. The patient's general attitude and behavior may offer clues. A patient who appears to be listening to something or who speaks as if replying to a voice should be asked a deliberately leading question—for example, "Can you tell me what the voice just said to you?" rather than, "Are you hearing voices?" which often prompts a false negative reply.

Hallucinations and illusions. These may affect any of the senses. Their vividness and degree of reality should be described and the circumstances when they are the most and least prominent noted. Does the patient develop delusional explanations to account for them? Can he start them or stop them voluntarily? Do they have an "out-there-ness," or does the patient recognize their inner origin? Illusions or faulty perceptions are often recognized as such by the patient, but insight is rare in true hallucinations, which are almost always pathologic.

If auditory hallucinations are prominent, schizophrenia should be suspected. Visual and tactile hallucinations are most often encountered in toxic states such as delirium tremens, drug intoxications, and deliria. Hallucinations of the other senses are relatively rare and suggest the possibility of organic brain disease such as temporal lobe epilepsy or tumor.

Delusions and misinterpretations. The distinction between frank delusions and giving exaggerated meanings to events is often the result of personality characteristics rather than mental illness. *Paranoid* delusions include ideas of persecution, suspiciousness, or megalomanic or grandiose notions. Depressive delusions concern ideas of guilt and unworthiness. Patients having *somatic* delusions have ideas of bodily changes, such as believing that their internal organs have turned to stone, their bowels have disappeared, or rats are eating up their brain. Ideas of reference ("I could see them talking about me") or of influence ("My thoughts control the President") are also delusional. Care should be taken in interpreting the delusional nature of logically possible ideas, for example, the unfaithfulness of a spouse.

Obsessive and phobic ideas. In phobias, the patient's own testimony about his symptom can be taken as valid. If he can avoid something outside himself to escape anxiety, he has a phobia. If he is fearful of his own inner thoughts or impulses, he has an obsession. The nurse must try to determine how distressed the patient is. A distinction should also be made between being compulsive about something and merely being concerned. In compulsiveness the patient makes no differentiation between trivial and important matters and feels excessive anxiety in either case.

Sensorium functions

Disorders of the sensorium are most often a sign of organic brain disease. They may be transient, as in toxic states, or more or less permanent, as in dementia. However, it may be impossible to assess the status of the sensorium in an extremely excited, hostile, depressed, or psychotic patient because of the functional disorganization of other mental processes. An acutely paranoid patient may be quite well oriented but refuse to answer questions. A manic patient may have an excellent memory but be unable to concentrate long enough to achieve recall.

Orientation. Three areas of orientation are usually tested: person, time, and place. The sense of personal identity is usually the last to be lost in organic brain damage, but its loss is the presenting complaint in hysterical amnesia. The distinction should be made between practical orientation (the ability to find one's way in familiar surroundings, awareness of the passage of time sufficient to eat and sleep appropriately) and what for some persons—for example, a retired person leading a simple life—may have no "survival value," for example, the name of a city or state. Many elderly people appear much more disoriented in unfamiliar surroundings, such as when they are first admitted to the hospital, then they would be in their normal situations.

A fourth area of orientation is situational orientation. Does the patient sense his circumstances and surroundings? Is he able not only to say where he is, who he is, and when it is but also to behave congruently with his replies?

Memory. Memory may be by rote or by a process of logic. Rote memory of heavily overlearned material such as the multiplication tables, nursery rhymes, or prayers may persist long after the ability to grasp the meaning of what is repeated is lost. Some patients, aware of defects in memory, will attempt to mislead others by reciting irrelevant material. The patient's account of his life, especially when it can be compared with that given by others, will be a general guide to past memory. In general, events that the patient did not personally experience will be forgotten before experienced events, and recent events will be forgotten *before* remote ones.

A simple memory test consists of asking the patient to repeat numbers of three digits, four digits, and so on. The digits should be given slowly, about 1 second apart, then the patient is asked to repeat the numbers backward. The nurse can illustrate this first by doing it. Most people can repeat numbers of five or six digits forward and three or four backward.

Attention and concentration. Can the patient's attention be aroused and sustained? The nurse must record what seems to distract the patient. Telling the months of the year or the days of the week in reverse order is a very good test of concentration for patients with a deprived educational background.

Information and intelligence. Tests of general information should be geared to the patient's experiences, interests, and level of education. As with memory tests, some standard questions can be developed. For example, "Can you name the President?" "Who was the President before him?" "And before him?" "Who is the Governor?" "What are the capitals of France, England, Spain, West Germany?" "Can you name the five largest cities in the world?" "What can you tell me about any event currently in the news?" A gross measure of the patient's intelligence can be derived from his account of his history, general knowledge, and reasoning powers. When under great strain patients with borderline intelligence may manifest anxiety, frustration, fear, and behavior that resembles psychosis.

Insight and judgment

Insight does not, in this case, mean a deep understanding of the unconscious processes that cause symptoms. In the context of a mental status examination, a patient has insight if he sees himself as "sick", as having mental, nervous, or emotional problems, or as needing some sort of help or treatment or if he understands that his symptoms or difficulties may be based, at least in part, on concerns and disturbing emotions within himself.

As tests for judgment the nurse may ask, "What would you do if you were lost in the woods?" ". . . if you were in a movie theater and you were the first to see a fire break out?" " . . . if you found a letter on the street, and it was addressed, sealed, and stamped." A lack of sound judgment does not necessarily indicate mental illness. However, deterioration in judgment is an important diagnostic clue, and the level of judgment may influence treatment programs and the prognosis.

APPROACHES TO PATIENTS

Talk person-to-person, not interrogator-to-patient. If you are informal, the patient may open up to you.

Be good-humored and avoid looking grim and determined even if you feel that way. A pleasant remark or two may help you both to relax.

Suit your manner to your patient. You should be direct and straightforward with most patients, but you may have to be more gentle and delicate with more sensitive and reticent patients. Do not be high-brow to the low-brow or vice versa. Talk to the patient's level of language.

Trust yourself. Develop a technique that comes naturally to you. There is no right or wrong way; no two interviewers act the same. Be aware of the patient's behavior, speech patterns, and hesitations. If you feel like asking a question or making a remark even if you are not sure why, go ahead. Explain if you like. If you show some human feelings, the patient is more likely to do the same.

Avoid leading questions that can be answered yes or no unless they are intentional. For example, avoid questions like this one: "Since the accident have you felt anxious?" Instead ask: "How have you felt since the accident?" It is often best to ask questions such as, "What was it like?" "How did you feel?" "What went through your mind?" or to say, "Tell me about it."

With rational and cooperative patients, it is usually best to begin with routine questions that carry little emotional charge, such as identifying data, their name, address, telephone number, and the like. As the patient settles down, you can then say, "Now tell me your problem."

During the discussion of the presenting problem, mention is usually made of a parent, sibling, or other family member. This is a good opportunity to interrupt and ask about the family background.

To check the patient's orientation you can ask: "Is your memory pretty good?" "Do you remember what day it is today?" "What day of the month and year?" and so forth.

To check delusions ask: "Do you ever get so nervous that you almost imagine things?" ". . . that people have a grudge against you?" ". . . that they talk about you?" ". . . that you have a special role to play in life?" Also: "Do you believe that supernatural things can sometimes happen?" "Have you ever experienced something supernatural, or something that was hard to understand?"

About hallucinations you can ask: "You think deeply, don't you?" "Do you sometimes think so deeply you can almost hear your thoughts aloud?" "Do you ever hear a voice when there is nobody there?"

About suicide you can ask: "Have you ever felt so down or depressed you almost wished you were dead?" "Did you ever think you might do something about it?" "What?" "How?" "Have you taken any steps to prepare for it?" "What?" "Tell me about it." Assess the lethality of the threat. Is the patient merely thinking about it or does he have a specific plan and time and place?

Other useful questions are: "Do you sometimes feel that you know things nobody else knows?" "Do you ever have thoughts that bother you?" "Do you think that your emotions are normal?" "Are you afraid of things more than you ought to be?" "Are you depressed or do you feel empty inside?" "Do you cry a lot?"

Emotionally charged areas. When the assessment is about to deal with potentially emotionally charged material, the best attitude is to be keenly interested but nonjudgmental. You can laugh with the patient, but never cry with him. A moderate degree of sympathetic concern is all right.

As long as new material continues to appear, let the patient take the lead. When progress stalls and you begin to see why, wait until you are certain of the reason and then point out the block. Try to study its origins, possible causes, and different modes of expression.

Silences should not disturb you. It is a good idea to let a silence develop at least once in every interaction. Let the patient break it, since what he then says spontaneously may be of special interest. If silences seem to embarrass the patient you can say, "You don't have to talk every second. This isn't an ordinary conversation. If you want to stop and think for a while, it's all right." If you think the patient could use a little help, you can say, "What are you thinking of?" or "Just say whatever comes to your mind." If silences become troublesome, you can investigate their possible meaning by asking, "Is there something that you find difficult to say?" Or, to be more specific: "Are you silent because of some feeling toward me that you don't want to express?" Or even, "Are you angry with—disappointed in, or upset about—me?" Patients' feelings toward you should not be avoided, but they should not disturb you either.

COMMON SOMATIC THERAPIES

Physical (somatic) methods of treatment of the mentally ill are treatments administered to the patient's body in order to produce changes in his behavior. In the widest sense they include electroconvulsive therapy, sleep therapy, body restraints, and drugs. In common usage, however, the term "somatic therapy" has come to mean either drug therapy or electroshock therapy, since these treatments are most commonly used; the others are becoming mainly of historic interest.

It should be stated explicitly that the modes of action of all the physical methods of treatment are largely unknown. Those who claim that the physical methods of treatment are more scientific than psychologic are correct only in the sense that it is easier to apply statistical methods of analysis to their results. One can easily measure and record a drug dosage or the amount of electric current used for shock treatment, whereas quantitation of the "dose" of psychotherapy is impossible.

Electroconvulsive therapy

Electroshock therapy (EST)—now usually called electroconvulsive therapy (ECT)—is the most widely used of the physical therapies with the exception of drug therapy. Originating with the mistaken observation that epilepsy and schizophrenia never occured in the same patient and the false conclusion that convulsions might eliminate the symptoms of the illness, efforts were made in the early 1930s to induce convulsions as a form of treatment. Camphor injections, pentylenetetrazol (Metrazol) injections, and, more recently, flurothyl (Indoklon) have been used for this purpose. However, the method of producing convulsions introduced by the Italian psychiatrists Cerletti and Bini in 1938 (passing an alternating electric current through the head and brain) has proved the most reliable, convenient, and effective.

ECT can now be given to patients or selected outpatients with a minimum of preparation. It is customary to give three treatments a week until substantial improvement occurs and then another three or four treatments to complete the course. A minimum of six treatments, an average of nine treatments, and a maximum of twenty-five treatments are considered normal limits for a course of treatment.

All depressions other than neurotic depressions tend to respond favorably to ECT. Depressive components of other illnesses are likely to respond as well. Acutely suicidal patients and patients in a state of manic or catatonic excitement may respond at least temporarily. Some psychiatrists believe that ECT is the treatment of choice for acute schizophrenia, but intensive drug therapy with phenothiazine should be tried first.

Character disorders, neurotic states, and chronic schizophrenias do not themselves respond to shock therapy, but an excited, depressed, or suicidal phase may develop in the course of any of these illnesses and may best be treated with ECT.

The only absolute contraindication to ECT is brain tumor, since in this condition the increased intracranial pressure that occurs during the convulsion may have dire consequences.

When the decision is made to give ECT, the patient must be told, even though he is psychotic. He should also be told that a transient period of impaired memory may persist for nearly a month after treatment. If the patient is told that he will be put to sleep, will receive a treatment, will feel no pain or discomfort, and will wake up before an hour has passed with no recollection of what has happened, it is likely that he will be reassured and cooperative.

The usual sequence of events is as follows: (1) The patient receives nothing by mouth for at least 4 hours before treatment (to avoid the complications of vomiting). (2) Atropine sulfate, 0.8 mg, is given subcutaneously 30 minutes before treatment to decrease salivation and bronchial secretions. (3) Pentothal is given intravenously to induce sleep. (4) Just before the shock is delivered, an intravenous muscle relaxant such as succinylcholine (Anectine) is given to prevent violent muscle contractions.

Because the muscle relaxant paralyzes the muscles of respiration, it is usually necessary to assist respiration mechanically and through the use of oxygen during a brief period of postconvulsant apnea. *An anesthetist should be in attendance*, since prolonged apnea or respiratory arrest may occur.

During the recovery phase, an experienced nurse must be present until the patient is awake and able to care for himself. If he is left unattended, he may roll from the recovery bed or stumble around the recovery room during waking confusion. Because of the period of impaired memory associated with ECT, the patient receiving a course of treatment should be advised against making important business decisions until fully recovered. Also, if he is receiving treatments on an outpatient basis, he should be under someone's supervision while traveling back to his home after treatment.

Nursing intervention. Patients receiving electroshock therapy need a great deal of reassurance because of the marked memory defect that accompanies the treatment and because of the general tendency of persons to fear the loss of consciousness. There is usually some apprehension in regard to the convulsion as well, since most patients know that it will occur.

The preparation for the treatment is both physical and psychologic. Breakfast should be either very light or completely withheld. All dentures should be removed, and nothing loose should be in the patient's mouth during the convulsion. All metal objects, such as bobby pins and clips, should be removed from the patient's hair. Clothing should be loose. The most common psychologic problem is the patient's apprehension in regard to the treatment. Pleasant surroundings in which to await treatment and agreeable diversion to keep the patient occupied should be provided.

Nursing care during the actual convulsion consists of control of the patient's body to prevent fractures or other injuries. The shoulders should be gently held in place and the pelvis loosely so. During the clonic phase of the convulsion, the arms and legs should be permitted rather free motion but should be guided to prevent adduction from the body plane. Tight restriction of body movements during the convulsion may contribute to fractures. A mouth gag, preferably of soft rubber covered with gauze, is kept inserted between the teeth during treatment. If the patient refuses to bite down on the gag before the treatment is started, it is usually possible to insert the gag during the tonic phase of the convulsion when the patient shows the characteristic tonic yawn. Upward pressure should be applied to the chin to prevent dislocation of the jaw or swallowing of the tongue. As soon as the convulsion ends, the patient's head should be turned on one side since breathing is stertorous and mucus tends to collect in the back of the throat.

The patient should be closely observed following the convulsion to prevent injury and to give reassurance as needed. Some patients are extremely restless and overactive and can injure themselves seriously while thrashing about. The pattern of behavior postconvulsively is usually typical for each patient so that it is fairly easy to know which patients need the closest observation. When the patient is able to answer simple questions, he can usually be helped out of the treatment room.

The patient is then returned to his unit, where is he showered, dressed, and fed. Because of his confusion and memory defect, he will probably need reassurance. The regular program of activities should be followed for the rest of the day. During the course of treatment the patient is likely to become more accessible; this period should be thoroughly exploited to establish good relationships and to give the patient a sense of being with interested and understanding company.

Continuous sleep therapy

Since 1922, when Klaesi, a Swiss psychiatrist, first used drugs to induce long periods of sleep in psychiatric patients, sleep therapy has enjoyed occasional vogue. Patients have been maintained in deep sleep for over a week at a time, being awakened only for feeding and elimination of wastes.

The results of sleep therapy seem to be no better than those of ECT. Consequently, sleep therapy is little used in the United States, although it is still enjoying some popularity in Europe, particularly in Russia.

Body restraints

Since Pinel removed the shackles and chains from his patients, physical restraint of disturbed psychiatric patients has gradually been discarded. Straightjackets are no longer standard equipment in mental hospitals, although some police departments still use them to control violent behavior. A patient may be stimulated to even more violent, disruptive behavior rather than quieted by the application of restraints. It has been found that patients who are deprived of their freedom in a locked ward become more regressive and assaultive than when the doors are unlocked and the ward left open. The same seems to be true of patients who are physically restrained.

Acupuncture

Acupuncture is an involved technique in which the operator inserts needles into specific points in the skin of patients for the purpose of effecting either relief of symptoms of a wide variety of illnesses or generating preoperative anesthesia. Most physicians see in the growing popularity of acupuncture another public fancy comparable to mesmerism, dianoetics, and scientism. Chiropractors, hypnotists, and others have been quick to exploit the possibilities of acupuncture as a cure for illnesses not readily amenable to treatment by accepted medical procedures. Although some claim that chronic psychotic states (largely schizophrenia and depressions), neuroses, drug addiction, alcoholism, obesity, and behavior disorders are sometimes curable through acupuncture, there is no evidence to justify such claims.

Considering the ideologic background of acupuncture (in China) and its spectacular features, it is likely that the powers of suggestion, persuasion, and hypnosis-like conviction play a large part in any benefit claimed by patients. Like hypnosis and psychotherapy of any sort, acupuncture has great potential to motivate a patient in a desired direction. The dangers lie not in the method but in its improper use. As part of a rational system of psychotherapy, acupuncture may find a useful place in some hands.

Psychosurgery

Psychosurgery has often been understood to include, by definition, all operative interventions on the organically intact brain of severely disturbed mental patients. In a broader sense, psychosurgery includes any operation on brain tissues that is undertaken for the principal purpose of improving or eliminating disturbed behavior. Thus operations for tumors cannot be termed psychosurgery even though they may result in striking improvement of behavior.

A surgical approach to the treatment of mental illness was begun by Egas Moniz, a Portuguese psychiatrist, who reported the use of prefrontal lobotomy in 1935. The next year the procedure was introduced in the United States by Freeman and Watts. The use of psychosurgery has decreased with the advent of the tranquilizing drugs.

In prefrontal lobotomy, the association fibers between the frontal lobes and the thalamus are severed. Although the specific functions of the frontal lobes are not clearly understood, there is general agreement that the thalamus is the place where emotional responses are invested in ideas and sensations. The surgical procedure is thus an effort to detach the emotional component of the psychosis to enable the patient to live more comfortably. The operation is performed through burr holes in the skull, and the association fibers are cut in the plane of the coronal suture. The behavioral effects of radical frontal lobotomy have been much debated. It is now generally agreed that this drastic procedure is neither desirable nor necessary.

Other surgical procedures, based on the same principle, have been developed. Topectomy consists of the removal of areas of cortex in the frontal lobes. In thalamotomy, an electric needle is inserted in the thalamus to destroy some of the tissue and thus reduce the patient's emotional tension. Transorbital lobotomy consists of severing the association fibers from above the eye. This procedure, introduced by Freeman and Watts, is probably more extensively used than any other.

Patients who retain a strong emotional reaction to their illness and to their psychotic ideas have responded best to psychosurgery. Patients with agitated depressions, withdrawal, and projective patterns have tended to show improvement. However, while psychosurgery may result in the patient's being able to return to the community, he is very likely to show some deterioration from his prepsychotic level of behavior as a result of the operation. Unpleasant traits are likely to be magnified, social inhibitions may be somewhat lessened, and the ability to carry out complex tasks may be reduced. Nevertheless, when all other forms of treatment have been tried and have failed and the patient is markedly uncomfortable in his illness, psychosurgery offers a hope of some improvement.

The issues underlying the use of psychosurgery have been debated recently. An article in *The New York Times* (Brody, 1973) pointed out the following:

> At the center of the controversy is a debate over the purpose, effectiveness, side effects—indeed the very nature—of psychosurgery, a modern technique by which tiny portions of tissue deep in the brain are destroyed through surgery, electricity, radiation, or sound. . . . 400 to 600 such operations are done annually . . . for the purposes of treating . . . uncontrollable epilepsy, violent behavior, schizophrenia, severe depression, and destructive hyperactivity.

The psychosurgery technique of the past left many individuals with the existence of vegetables. Today's operations are said to be more refined and exacting.

The issues raised by this article have important implications for psychiatry, law, and medical research.

> Can the state indefinitely detain so-called insane and dangerous persons in mental institutions without a realistic hope for adequate rehabilitative treatment?
>
> If such persons are released without treatment, or if they are treated, released and then relapse, who will protect society?
>
> Can an involuntarily hospitalized or mentally ill patient or a prisoner give truly "informed, voluntary" consent to experimental procedures or radical treatments?
>
> What are the relative roles played by societal ills and organic brain disease in causing mental illness, and what does this mean for methods of treatment?

The proponents of psychosurgery point out that psychotherapy is not realistically possible for all who need it and particularly for those with mental illnesses of long duration. Although there are efforts toward prevention of mental illness and maintenance of mental health, the long-term mentally ill continue to need some hope for treatment and cure; psychosurgery may be the only recourse for some. Some authorities advocate strong controls for the use of psychosurgery. A national activist group, the Medical Committee on Human Rights, advocates the strong control or banning of psychosurgery. Their opinions include the fear that psychosurgery would be used as a weapon of control for political antagonists, institutionalized patients, and violent prisoners. They fear that the incentive and motivation to continue every effort to correct the factors causing mental illness and the provision for psychotherapy would be diminished. These issues should be of concern to both professionals and the public.

It is regrettable that psychosurgery has been made a political issue. Patients have been depicted as helpless, perhaps not-so-sick victims of mutilating procedures. Any and all neurosurgical procedures that modify behavior have been dumped into the same basket of blunting operations. These are obvious distortions, though there is some truth in the statement of a universal effect of psychosurgical procedures. However, this criticism has led to much soul-searching by investigators in the field as well as pressure for legislation to abolish these procedures.

The judicious placing of a psychosurgical lesion has undoubtedly proved to be helpful in a number of selected cases. As long as our knowledge of effects is uncertain, these procedures must be done not only with proper ethical safeguards and in cooperation with knowledgeable psychiatrists, but also with detailed and prolonged follow-up studies.

Nursing intervention. The immediate postoperative nursing care of patients with a prefrontal lobotomy is surgical in nature. Temperature, pulse, respiration, and blood pressure are checked at frequent intervals. Danger signs are pulse rate below 60 or above 120, temperature over 102° F, sudden drop in blood pressure or a rise in systolic pressure over 150, continued vomiting, failure to regain consciousness in 3 or 4 hours, and, after the return to consciousness, marked restlessness followed by drowsiness or unconsciousness. After reacting, the patient is likely to be confused and disoriented and will need reassurance and tactful encouragement to refrain from pulling at his bandage or removing it. Ordinarily the patient is allowed out of bed briefly the day of surgery or the first postoperative day, and every effort is made to get the patient ambulatory as soon as possible. While the patient does remain in bed, crayons and drawing paper, bright objects, rag dolls or teddy bears, building blocks, or similar articles are used to keep him occupied, to keep his bandage intact, and to combat masturbatory activity.

Following the operation most patients are regressed, some to a greater degree than others. The major task in nursing care is resocialization through habit training. Incontinence, which is exceedingly common, gradually comes under control through regular toilet periods. Feeding habits are poor, and training in table manners is necessary. The biggest difficulty in the habit-training program is encountered in the patient's inertia, procrastination, and complete lack of regard for time. It becomes necessary to initiate activity for the patient and to help him carry through. Negativism also frequently presents a problem and must be met firmly. The convalescent period for a patient who has undergone psychosurgery is a period of growing up again, a period of reacquiring all the basic social skills. It is quite important during this period that the patient have a planned schedule of activities and adequate supervision designed to encourage his assumption of responsibility for his own activities.

Narcoanalysis

The use of various drugs in the treatment of mental illness dates as far back as the history of psychiatry. One particular use of barbiturates—the intravenous injection of sodium amytal and pentothal sodium—received a tremendous impetus during World War II and resulted in making the procedure known as narcoanalysis a respectable and effective adjunct to psychiatric therapy. In addition to barbiturates, simple narcotics, and anticonvulsants, sodium amytal and pentothal sodium are now used in establishing contact with suspicious and inaccessible patients, in shortening therapy by overcoming resistance, and as a first-aid measure in traumatic situations. The barbiturates are central nervous system depressants and have some effects comparable to hypnosis. Patients' inhibitions are often lessened, and the patients are able to discuss material that they could not otherwise. They may also be able to recall experiences that have been repressed. They may become receptive and accept reassurance and constructive interpretation of what has happened to them.

Narcoanalysis consists of the very slow intravenous injection of sodium amytal or pentothal sodium. The dose required to produce results varies widely, and the amount given is determined by the degree of relaxation and the accessibility of the patient. The needle remains inserted in the vein during the treatment so that further medication may be given to maintain the patient at the desired level. The physician then directs questions or conversation to sensitive areas, either to elicit desired information for his own use in planning therapy or to permit the patient to recall painful experiences. Reassurance and suggested synthesis of the experience for a more constructive attitude on the part of the patient are given before the treatment ends. A very definite attempt to establish rapport with the patient is integrated into the procedure. The treatment may be used only once or a few times with a patient, or a series of injections may be given.

Nursing intervention. In narcoanalysis, nurses should be alert to the opportunity to establish rapport with the patient. They should also recognize the patient's increased receptiveness and be careful to maintain a positive and reassuring attitude. Indecision and doubt on their part immediately following the treatment may unsettle the patient. Particular care should also be taken in regard to material discussed by the patient. The choice of bringing up topics should be left to the patient and not referred to unless the patient himself mentions it.

Psychopharmacology

The distinctiveness of the effects of the antipsychotic or phenothiazine tranquilizers from those of the sedatives was first clearly recognized by French surgeons and psychiatrists in 1951 and 1952. The impact of the tranquilizers on psychiatric practice has been truly revolutionary, and their effectiveness has stimulated much research in psychopharmacology.

The related antidepressant drugs have reduced the need for electroconvulsive therapy. The availability of new sedatives, some of them drugs whose sedative action was not formerly recognized, and the more permissive attitude toward drug therapy engendered by the success of the tranquilizers have encouraged the use of drugs in the symptomatic relief of anxiety.

Sedatives. The sedative drugs are useful for the induction of sleep and for the relief of anxiety and feelings of tension. These two uses represent a great need and market, and the proliferation of compounds is correspondingly great. Improper application of the term "tranquilizer" to refer to this class of drugs has led to confusion.

It is not necessary or feasible to separately evaluate each of the drugs avail-

Table 1. Dosages of commonly used sedatives

GENERIC NAME	TRADE NAME	ORAL DOSE	
		FOR SLEEP (SINGLE DOSE)	SEDATIVE (3-4 TIMES A DAY)
Short-acting			
Chloral hydrate	Chloral hydrate	0.5-1 gm	
Chlorobutanol	Chloretone	0.5-1 gm	
Ethchlorvynol	Placidyl	0.5-1 gm	
Ethinamate	Valmid	0.5-1 gm	
Flurazepam	Dalmane	30 mg	
Hexobarbital	Sombulex, Evipal	250-500 mg	
Methaqualone	Quaalude, Sopor, Parest	150-300 mg	
Methyprylon	Noludar	200-400 mg	
Paraldehyde		12-16 ml	
Phenobarbital	Nembutal	100-200 mg	
Secobarbital	Seconal	100-200 mg	
Intermediate-acting			
Amobarbital	Amytal sodium	100-200 mg	15-30 mg
Aprobarbital	Alurate	120 mg	20-40 mg
Butabarbital	Butisol	100-200 mg	8-60 mg
Diazepam	Valium		5 mg
Glutethimide	Doriden	500 mg	125-250 mg
Heptabarbital	Medomin	200-400 mg	50-100 mg
Meprobamate	Miltown, Equanil		200-400 mg
Vinbarbital	Delvinal	100-200 mg	30 mg
Long-acting			
Chlordiazepoxide	Librium		16-60 mg
Chlorazepate	Tranxene		15-25 mg
Mephobarbital	Mebaral		30-60 mg
Oxazepam	Serax		10-20 mg
Phenaglycodol	Ultran		200 mg
Phenobarbital	Luminal	100 mg	15-30 mg

able, since drugs can be placed in groups. The most useful classification of the sedatives is based on their duration of action (see Table 1).

The sedative class of drugs, exemplified by the barbiturates, has been used for the relief of anxiety and the induction of sleep since about 1903. These drugs should not be confused with the antipsychotic tranquilizers, which do not relieve anxiety. Each of the drugs listed in Table 1 as a sedative will diminish anxiety. If given in progressively larger doses, sedation, excitement, disinhibition, ataxia, general anesthesia, and, ultimately, respiratory and vasomotor depression and death will occur. With repeated or continuous use, the sedatives are anticonvulsant and habituating. They cause physical dependence (and a withdrawal state when use is discontinued suddenly) and are voluntary muscle relaxants and spinal cord depressants.

Antipsychotic tranquilizers. All of the drugs classified in Table 1 as sedatives are useful in the treatment of anxiety. They cannot, however, alter the symptoms of a psychotic episode or dependably quiet a manic patient without inducing a state of anesthesia. A separate class of drugs, the antipsychotic tranquilizers, is effective in controlling psychotic behavior. Even when huge doses are used, the patient can still be aroused.

Table 2. Antipsychotic tranquilizers

GENERIC NAME	TRADE NAME	EQUIVALENT ADULT ORAL DOSE (3-4 TIMES A DAY) (mg)	TOXICITY
Chlorpromazine	Thorazine	25-50	
Chlorprothixene	Taractan	25	
Prochlorperazine	Compazine	5-10	
Promazine	Sparine	50-200	
Thioridazine	Mellaril	10-25	
Triflupromazine	Vesprin	10-20	
Acetoprenazine	Tindal	10	Cause less sedation
Butaperazine	Repoise	5-10	but more likely
Carphenazine	Proketazine	25-50	to produce
Fluphenazine	Permitil, Prolixin	1	extrapyramidal
Haloperidol	Haldol	0.5	side effects
Perphenazine	Trilafon	2-4	
Piperacetazine	Quide	10	
Thiopropazate	Dartal	5-10	
Thiothixene	Navane	1-2	
Trifluoperazine	Stelazine	1	
Promethazine	Phenergan, Remsed	25-50	Comparatively greater degree of sedation

The term "tranquilizer" is not precisely defined, and in common usage it is applied to many of the sedatives. Confusion can be avoided by referring to tranquilizers as antipsychotics, antipsychotic tranquilizers, or phenothiazine-type tranquilizers. The antipsychotics most widely used are phenothiazine derivatives. The most common antipsychotic tranquilizers, with adult oral dose and toxicity, are listed in Table 2.

Reserpine and related Rauwolfia alkaloids. Reserpine affects behavior as other tranquilizers do, and the drug was used briefly in the treatment of psychotic states. However, it is now regarded as an antihypertensive drug, and the behavioral depressant effect is regarded as a side effect.

Phenothiazine tranquilizers. The phenothiazines may be classified according to the nature of the side chain that bears the tertiary amine function.

Nonphenothiazine tranquilizers. The phenothiazine part of the tranquilizer molecule is not essential and may be replaced by some other bulky chemical group. Chlorprothixine (Taractan) and haloperidol (Haldol) are quite similar in their effects to chlorpromazine. Others (such as hydroxyzine) are qualitatively similar to the phenothiazine tranquilizers but are less potent in the sense that the greater atropine-like side effects limit the size of the dose that can be used.

Related drug groups. The antihistamines, including those used as antiemetics, and the parasympatholytic drugs have central nervous system effects comparable to those of the antipsychotic tranquilizers. Conversely, the antipsychotic tranquilizers have parasympatholytic and histamine-blocking properties.

Lithium. Lithium ion, administered in the form of lithium carbonate, is used as an alternative or supplement to the major tranquilizers in the control of the manic stage of manic-depressive illness.

Lithium is distributed more evenly between intracellular and extracellular

Table 3. Antidepressants that resemble tranquilizers

GENERIC NAME	TRADE NAME	INITIAL DOSE (3 TIMES A DAY) (mg)	MAXIMUM DAILY DOSE (mg)
Amitriptyline	Elavil	25	150
Desipramine	Pertofrane, Norpramin	25	200
Doxepin	Sinequan, Adapin	25	300
Imipramine	Tofranil	25	200
Nortriptyline	Aventyl	10	100
Protriptyline	Vivactil	5-10	60

spaces than is sodium or potassium; that is, lithium behaves at the cell membrane somewhat like both sodium and potassium. How this property relates to the mechanism of action of lithium is as yet undefined.

Therapeutic doses do not have gross effects comparable to those of the tranquilizers or the sedatives. The onset of action is delayed for several days after the drug is started, and 6 to 10 days elapse before the peak effect is reached. The drug is well absorbed after oral administration and is excreted by the kidneys.

Lithium should *not* be used in the presence of impaired renal function or cardiovascular disease or in any situation that involves a restricted diet, diuretic drugs, fluid loss, or inadequate fluid intake. It should *not* be used during the first trimester of pregnancy or when facilities for the determination of serum lithium levels are not available.

Antidepressants and central nervous system stimulants. The drugs that are most commonly used in the treatment of severe depression should be classed as a subgroup of the antipsychotic tranquilizers. They are treated here as a separate group to conform to current, but changing, clinical thought. The major antidepressants that resemble tranquilizers, with initial and maximum dose, are listed in Table 3.

Antidepressants that resemble tranquilizers. Drugs such as amitriptyline (Elavil) or imipramine (Tofranil) are the most widely used antidepressants. Their properties are quite similar to those of the antipsychotic tranquilizers.

Sympathomimetic amines. Amphetamine and related drugs are comparable to ephedrine.

Monoamine oxidase (MAO) inhibitors. The MAO inhibitors are no longer widely used in the treatment of depression, but great interest in their mechanism of action remains. They have central nervous system stimulant properties that are qualitatively similar to those of amphetamine.

Amphetamine and related sympathomimetic stimulants. These drugs are variants of the ephedrine class of sympathomimetics and were selected because they exhibit relatively more potent central stimulant effects and relatively less potent cardiovascular effects. Table 4 lists the amphetamine and related stimulant amines along with the usual oral daily dosage.

Common side effects of the amphetamine and related stimulants are tremulousness, anxiety, awareness of heart action, dry mouth, and alteration of sleep habits such as increased insomnia or increased dreaming. The side effects are usually not troublesome after a few days of continued use, but some patients are unable to tolerate the stimulation of any amphetamine.

The amphetamines, like other drugs with a potential for misuse, are abused to different degrees by different users. Amphetamines may be used episodi-

Table 4. Amphetamines and related stimulant amines

GENERIC NAME	TRADE NAME	USUAL ORAL DAILY DOSAGE (mg)
Amphetamine	Benzedrine	5-15
Benzphetamine	Didrex	25-50
Chlorphentermine	Pre-Sate	65
Dextroamphetamine	Dexedrine	5-15
Diethylpropion	Tenuate, Tepanil	24-75
Fenfluramine	Pondimin	40
Mazindol	Sanorex	2
Methamphetamine	Desoxyn, Methedrine	5-15
Methylphenidate	Ritalin	10-30
Phendimetrazine	Plegine	35
Phenmetrazine	Preludin	25-75

cally as "spree" drugs to improve performance, defer fatigue, or prolong an alcoholic binge. They may be used intermittently over a long period but in moderate dosages for their euphoriant or antidepressant effect.

The principal adverse result of amphetamine abuse is the loss of productive activity imposed on the individual by his preoccupation with obtaining the drug. In some individuals large doses precipitate a toxic psychosis so that they are admitted to mental hospitals as emergencies, often diagnosed as schizophrenic. Those who are inclined to abuse drugs (drug addicts) or alcohol (alcoholics) are now more correctly referred to as substance misusers or substance abusers.

Nursing intervention. It is important to realize that these psychopharmacologic compounds have been in use for a relatively short time. The consequences of their long-term use is not known conclusively. Many patients whose mental illness is controlled by these drugs may have to take the medication throughout their lives, as diabetic persons must take insulin. Knowledge of the intricate function of these drugs within the tissues of the brain and body is based primarily on indirect evidence. The nurse should know these factors and should give the greatest attention to the administration of the medication and to the effects it has on each individual patient.

The dosage of the drug is based on the individual's susceptibility. It may be some time before changes in behavior are noted following the administration of the medication. The nurse should not anticipate changes based on previous experiences with other patients and other medications. Each patient has his own reaction to the drug and dosage, and adequate time should be provided to try the drug before concluding that it is ineffective for a particular patient.

Flexibility in dosage should be used, particularly in the beginning, for progress to the high dosage the patient may require for maintenance at the optimum level. This factor is particularly significant with the major tranquilizers.

Knowledge of the drug and of the side effects that may result from toxicity is essential for anyone administering these drugs. Elderly and debilitated patients should be considered carefully, and a low dosage may be indicated to prevent overdosage. The nurse's responsibility for the supply and administration of these drugs is of particular importance in preventing misuse or abuse of these drugs.

Alert observation and accurate recording of drug effects on the hospitalized patient will facilitate effective adjustment of the prescribed medication to his needs. Any sensitivity or toxic reaction should be reported immediately, since reactions can have serious consequences.

It is not unusual to find that some patients complain of loss of appetite and nausea, particularly at the start of drug therapy. Attention should be given to the patient's symptoms in order to make proper adjustments in medication or food preparation. If constipation is a problem, fluids and roughage in the diet should be increased. An accurate report of the nutritional intake is necessary to protect physical stamina.

When drowsiness, inattention, and inactivity are evident, particularly in the early part of the drug therapy, the nurse should note and report this so that an adjustment in dosage may be made or a supplementary medication added. Light-headedness or weakness may be signs of hypotension.

Since the drugs tend to modify the patient's disturbed behavior, the patient is capable of participating in a constructive routine and in many therapeutic activities. Patients who were unapproachable without drugs may now be amenable and accessible to personnel and the environment. The environment must of necessity be conducive to improvement and must provide the opportunity to reeducate the patient to some degree of self-reliance. Nurses and other personnel need to consider the total plan to rehabilitate the patient toward a more normal and independent existence and, where possible, toward his eventual return to his family and the community.

Perhaps the most bewildered people in the whole sequence of events are the patients' families. Many are being called on to assume responsibility for their relative-patient. The nurse will be called on to explain the patient's change after years of unapproachable behavior. The family's fears and hostility are often evident, since this responsibility may alter their way of living. Nurses may be the innocent recipients of family hostility growing out of guilt, fear, or frustration. They have an important role to play in helping the family to plan for the patient's return. They should consider referral to a community mental health center to help the patient and family during the adjustment period and for follow-up.

Today, community mental health facilities are being developed more extensively than ever before. Many types of professional and nonprofessional personnel, as well as multiple agencies, are cooperating in the preventive and maintenance aspects of psychiatric care. The nurse in the community has an important role in seeing that the patient continues with the proper dosage and proper medication needed to sustain him at home. Well-meaning families may take it upon themselves to reduce or stop the medication because the patient is doing so well, or they may feel that the medication may result in harmful side effects. This has been one of the major factors in the revolving door syndrome, the pattern of recurring discharge and admission. Teaching the family and patient the importance of uninterrupted drug therapy is an essential task for nurses in the hospital and in the community.

In the early stages of administration of certain antidepressants, nurses need to keep in mind that the patient may become more active and less inhibited before the antidepressant action affects the mood. Despondency with over-activity may lead to tendencies of aggression and self-destruction, possibly resulting in a well-executed suicide. Without a doubt, nurses and other personnel need to exercise careful supervision of these patients to prevent any suicidal attempts.

It seems appropriate to refer to remarks made by Dr. Ayd (1965a) as the closing statement for nursing care on psychopharmacology:

> It is true that we need more research to discover even more effective and safer drugs for the mind. But equally necessary are more nurses prepared to care for psychiatric patients; nurses who respect the personal dignity of those patients and are aware of their responsiveness to compassion, understanding, patience, and an attentive ear—needs for which there are no chemical substitutes.

REFERENCES

Aguilera, D. C.: Review of psychiatric nursing, St. Louis, 1977, The C. V. Mosby Co.

Ayd, F. J., Jr.: The antidepressants, Am. J. Nurs. **65:**78-84, 1965a.

Ayd, F. J., Jr.: The chemical assault on mental illness: the major tranquilizers, Am. J. Nurs. **65:** 70-78, 1965b.

Ayd, F. J., Jr.: The minor tranquilizers, Am. J. Nurs. **65:**89-94, 1965c.

Bellak, L., and Small, L.: Emergency psychotherapy and brief psychotherapy, New York, 1965, Grune & Stratton, Inc.

Brody, J. E.: Psychosurgery will face key test in court today, The New York Times, March 12, 1973, pp. 1 and 25.

Caplan, G.: A public health approach to child psychiatry, Ment. Health **35:**235-249, 1951.

Clawson, G.: Nursing care of psychiatric patients receiving insulin therapy; for patients who are ambulatory during treatment, Am. J. Nurs. **49:**621-623, 1949.

Crary, W. G., and Crary, G. C.: Depression, Am. J. Nurs. **73:**472-475, 1973.

Freeman, W.: Psychosurgery. In Arieti, S., editor: American handbook of psychiatry, vol. 2, New York, 1959, Basic Books, Inc., pp. 1521-1540.

Freeman, W., Watts, J., and Ewald, F.: Psychosurgery: the nursing problem, Am. J. Nurs. **47:** 210-213, 1947.

Goth, A.: Medical pharmacology, ed. 8, St. Louis, 1976, The C. V. Mosby Co.

Horwitz, W. A.: Insulin shock therapy. In Arieti, S., editor: American handbook of psychiatry, vol. 2, New York, 1959, Basic Books, Inc., pp. 1485-1498.

Kalinowsky, L. B.: Convulsive shock treatment. In Arieti, S., editor: American handbook of psychiatry, vol. 2, New York, 1959, Basic Books, Inc., pp. 1499-1520.

Kalinowsky, L. B., and Hoch, P. H.: Somatic treatments in psychiatry, New York, 1961, Grune & Stratton, Inc.

Kline, N. S., and Davis, J. M.: Psychotropic drugs, Am. J. Nurs. **73:**54-62, 1973.

Kolb, L. C.: Modern clinical psychiatry, ed. 8, Philadelphia, 1973, W. B. Saunders Co., pp. 620-655.

Lynn, F. H., and Friedhoff, A. J.: The patient on a tranquilizing regime, Am. J. Nurs. **60:**234-240, 1960.

Man, L. P., and Bolin, J.: Further exploration of unilateral electroshock treatment, Dis. Nerv. Syst. **30:**547-551, 1969.

Morgan, M. M., and Denny, M. F.: Retraining after a prefrontal lobotomy, Am. J. Nurs. **55:**59-62, 1965.

Solomon, R., and Patch, V. D.: Handbook of psychiatry, ed. 3, Los Altos, Calif., 1974, Lange Medical Publications.

ADDITIONAL READINGS

Branson, H. K.: The nurse's role in behavior modification, Nurs. Care **8**(12):21-23, 1975.

Niemeir, S. F.: Nurses can be effective behavior modifiers, J. Psychiatric Nurs. **14**(1):18-21, 1976.

ORGANIC BEHAVIOR PROBLEMS

CHAPTER 14

Characteristics of aging and organic behavior disorders

Gerontology is the study of the aging process, while geriatrics focuses on the disease processes of old age. Senescence, the term associated with the process or state of growing old, is one of the natural, developmental phenomena of man. Like childhood, adolescence, and middle age, it is a normal state that has its rewards and its accompanying problems. Various conditions present in society form particular stress situations for the elderly, as they do for each age group.

NORMAL AGING

To establish on a normative scale a cut-off point at which one moves out of adulthood to old age is impossible. However, most investigators and authorities in developmental psychology and some in physiologic research use age 65 as the focal point for considering the physiologic, psychologic, and sociologic aging changes in man. This arbitrary but generally accepted age has become more fixed as we consider social forces that impose changes in our life-style, such as retirement with its change in work productivity and economic return. There is as great a variability among persons age 65 with respect to physical stamina and intellectual ability as, for example, there is among adolescents age 16 and adults age 30. Until recently, developmental psychology has focused on children and young adults rather than individuals 65 years and older. Population census and statistical predictions of the Department of Health, Education, and Welfare with respect to age groupings show that more people will be living longer and so there will be a larger proportion of individuals age 65 and older within the population.

313

Volume II of the five volume series developed from the Gerontological Society and published by U.S. Department of Health, Education, and Welfare (1970) is entitled *Biological, Psychological and Sociological Aspects of Aging.* This interesting and important publication opens with a Perspective.

> Almost 1 in 10 Americans is 65 or older, nearly 20 million persons. This exceeds by a million the total population of our 20 smallest states.
>
> . . . [B]y 2000, about 30 million will be aged. These figures clearly foretell part of the need for comprehensive services for the aged.
>
> The fact that there are increasing numbers of persons 65 years of age and older has become common knowledge in recent years. But what has not been as widely recognized is the fact that people are living more often into the oldest ages. . . .
>
> Half of all people now 65 and older are about 73 or older; 6 per cent are 85 or older—more than 1 million persons. In the years ahead, the increase will be particularly great at the oldest ages. With the population 65 and older projected to rise 50 per cent between 1960-85, the population 85 and older may double.

Because of the physical changes characteristic of most people 65 years and older, certain adaptations are evident in their patterns of living. An early student of human development, Havighurst (1953), identifies the following as the developmental tasks of late maturity: adjustment to decreasing strength and health, adjustment to retirement and reduced income, adjustment to death of spouse, establishment of more meaningful relationships with one's age group, ability to meet social and civic obligations, and establishment of a satisfactory living pattern.

The physical changes consistent with old age include impairment of senses of hearing, vision, taste, and smell; loss of teeth; decline in muscle and motor strength; osteoarthritic changes; connective tissue changes; wrinkling of skin due to inelasticity; and changes in the functions of internal organs, often with the evidence of organic illnesses, such as heart disease, hypertension, and diabetes.

The person's psychosocial response to the aging process is related to his self-image and his basic personality. His past ability to deal with life's experiences and stresses will serve as the framework for dealing with old age. The identification of the common psychosocial problems is for the convenience of study. The presence of these in the elderly varies from person to person in number and intensity. It is important to emphasize that these characteristics are normal and not symptomatic of mental illness.

The intellectual level of the person can vary considerably. When a person's livelihood depended primarily on intellectual skills rather than on manual skills, the intellect has been known to continue productively into old age. Very often changes are not seen until there are situations where the person needs to use abstract reasoning rather than to draw on past experiences. Memory becomes altered for recent events rather than those of the past. Many of us readily acknowledge we are getting older when we find we are repeating ourselves because we have forgotten what we had mentioned before.

The circumstances surrounding old age often contribute to the characteristic of narrowing interests with a tendency toward reclusiveness, suspiciousness, pessimism, melancholy, rigid adherence to old ways, rejection of new ideas, and hostility toward people, very often close members of the family. The elderly are not able to accept changes in their physical condition—good or bad. If their pattern of life included neurotic traits, such as hysteria or hypochondriasis, these continue to be manifest and at times become exaggerated.

It has been found that people who have thought and prepared for old age and who have provided for possible dependencies are rewarded with the relief from past pressures of work, ambition, and social responsibilities. They find that this part of their lives provides time for contemplation on matters previously pushed aside, time for hobbies, and time for relationships with family and groups that were not possible in previous years. For these individuals it is often a fulfillment of some important life ambitions.

The growing dependencies, financial, physical, and psychosocial, are bases for much concern. Individuals who were breadwinners for most of their lives are threatened by their lack of an adequate income and their dependence on Social Security. Often it is not enough, and they resent this act of government charity. Today, many have small retirement pensions that help to defray living costs. When they need to resort to assistance from the family, this creates a basis for conflict. The elderly person's self-esteem suffers, and the lack of alternatives, because of his physical inability, can result in difficult behavior. It is not unusual for these individuals to recount all that they have done for family and others in the past or to become aggressively hostile as a means of asserting their independence. There are times when it is extremely difficult to give to an elderly person directly. Tact and diplomacy can go a long way in establishing a give-and-take relationship.

Despite the various behaviorisms typical of old age, these individuals are important to our society. Like all of us, they need love, affection, interest, support, and interdependence. There are significant roles they can play in the family constellation, if we take time to plan and work these out. All too often, the middle-aged children are too involved with their own problems and activities to be concerned about their parents. It is not unusual to find better communications and relationships between grandparents and grandchildren. When elderly parents need to live with their children, it is often a situation of great conflict for both parties. The elderly prefer to live alone within easy access to family and friends. Maintaining their independence is a crucial factor in their lives.

The stresses encountered during old age are dealt with by each individual in his own way, drawing on his past experiences and present resources. Depression is common, particularly when the person has a lonely existence or has lost a spouse or a close friend. Suicide is a frequent occurrence among the elderly. The inevitability of death is constantly in their awareness.

Kübler-Ross (1969) has been most influential in calling attention to the dying process, particularly among professionals, physicians and nurses. She describes five stages of the dying process:

1. Denial
2. Anger
3. Bargaining
4. Depression
5. Acceptance

The consideration of death and dying is not necessarily the concern only of the aged, although there is evidence of such preoccupation. The ability to consider these aspects of life has meaning for everyone and in particular those in any age group who may be imminently facing this phase because of illness or those related to someone who is dying. (See Chapter 2, p. 61.)

Since most of the elderly are and will continue to be a significant part of the community, the nurse's involvement with their problems is essential. Community-based facilities for the aged should be encouraged and supported politically and financially. Maintaining their health and supporting their shortcomings are important responsibilities that the public health nurses and office nurses must meet. Knowledge and association with the elderly in the neighborhood, in the church, and in other community centers provide the nurse the opportunity to share as a good neighbor and a friend. Often, friendly conversations, advising ways and means of dealing with problems, can bring about better results than formal counseling can. The true nurse does not stop nursing after working an 8-hour tour of duty or after leaving the hospital. Specialization in a nursing area does not preclude the ability to help people of all ages to stay well. When illness or symptoms of mental disorders become apparent, the specific therapeutic resources should be utilized.

The nurse as a member of a community can use the frequent opportunities of teaching and assisting friends and neighbors to care for and maintain elderly parents or relatives. Sensitivity to and understanding of the needs of the elderly in their activities of daily living involve consideration of psychologic, sociologic, as well as physical factors.

Being able to understand what an elderly person feels and how he perceives things and situations around him requires the ability to empathize with him. A student of 20 or a nurse of 30 needs to do some conscious introspection to understand with the eyes and heart of an older person.

The strong need for the elderly to remain independent can be the basis for a variety of problems. Dependence on their children for housing and subsistence can be a serious blow to their self-esteem. This may become manifest in cantankerous, critical remarks and attitudes toward the children (now adults), or the elderly may internalize their shame by withdrawing and avoiding social contact with family, friends, church, and community. Their sense of worth is demoralized. Nurses can contribute a great deal by discussing and teaching family members to understand the reasons underlying their parents' behavior and help plan a way of including the elderly member as a participant in the family's life. This is not an easy task. The nurse needs to move slowly and with increasing knowledge of the family members and their relationships to one another.

A prevailing fear with respect to losing one's independence and concomitant ability to care for one self is the threat of illness. Health care as provided by Medicare is minimal. Other public programs are equally inadequate, particularly with respect to ambulatory services. A small segment of the elderly population has supplementary health insurance. The pain of the thought of being a charity case is overwhelming. For these and other compelling reasons, health services for the prevention of illness and the maintenance of health are very important for the elderly. Neighborhood facilities can take many forms: the family doctor, the public health nurse, the independent family nurse practitioner, a mobile health unit making regular stops at specific areas, store-front clinics, satellite units of hospital centers, and the like. Creative and imaginative forms of health care services must replace the traditional hospital and specialist care. Family nurse practitioners, with their special preparation and ability to function independently, could do much to assist the elderly in both their physical needs and their psychologic comfort.

Ebersole (1976) describes reminiscing as a "common activity for most aged people. . . . reminiscing is a tool of aging as natural and useful as sexual fantasies are in adolescence." She points out:

> A nurse can use the natural tendency of the aged to reminisce to learn about a client's past life, his struggles, his concerns, his habitual coping mechanisms, his losses, his strengths, his fears, and his triumphs. Talking about the past is one way of looking at the client's past coping mechanisms. Often these can be applied to current problem solving. Most important, probably, is that when an old person perceives his memories are valued, an empathetic communication process begins. Such a relationship has therapeutic value.

In his column in *The San Francisco Examiner* on September 28, 1976, Guy Wright printed a poem entitled "An Old Lady Has The Last Word," obviously directed to nurses.

What do you see, nurses, what do you see?
What do you think when you're looking at me?
A crabby old woman, not very wise,
Uncertain of habit, with faraway eyes,
Who dribbles her food and makes no reply
When you say in a loud voice, "I do wish you'd try,"
Who seems not to notice the things that you do
And forever is losing a stocking or shoe
Who resisting or not, must do as you will,
Is that what you're thinking, is that what you see?
Then open your eyes, nurse, you're not looking at me.
I'll tell you who I am as I sit here so still,
As I do your bidding, as I eat at your will.
I'm a small child of ten with a father and mother,
Brothers and sisters who love one another;
A young girl of sixteen with wings on her feet,
Dreaming that soon now a lover she'll meet;
A bride soon at twenty—my heart gives a leap,
Remembering the vows that I promised to keep;
At twenty-five, now I have young of my own
Who need me to build a secure, happy home;
A woman of thirty, my young growing fast,

Bound to each other with ties that should last;
At forty, my sons have grown and are gone.
But my man is beside me to see I don't mourn;
At fifty, once more babies play round my knee;
Again we know children, my Loved one and me.
Dark days are upon me, my husband is dead.
I look to the future; I shudder with dread.
For my young are all rearing young of their own,
And I think of the years and the love that I've known.
I'm an old woman and nature is cruel.
'Tis her jest to make old age look like a fool.
The body it crumbles; grace and vigor depart.
There is now just a stone where I once had a heart.
But inside this old carcass a young girl still dwells,
And now and again my battered heart swells.
I remember the joys, I remember the pain,
And I'm loving and living life over again.
I think of the years, all too few, gone too fast,
And accept the stark fact that nothing can last.
So open your eyes, nurses, open and see
Not a crabby old woman; look closer—see ME!

ORGANIC BEHAVIOR DISORDERS

Organic behavior disorders are characterized by the evidence of brain damage (found by laboratory testing) and the following symptoms:

1. Defects in orientation
2. Impairment of memory
3. Impairment of intellectual functions, such as comprehension, knowledge, and learning
4. Impairment of judgment
5. Lability and shallowness of affect

Acute disorders result from temporary, reversible impairment of brain functioning and thus have a good prognosis. Chronic disorders are caused by relatively permanent impairment of the brain and thus the prognosis is limited with regard to return of previous levels of adjustment. The acute disorders are usually attributed to the presence of toxic factors, and treatment and care are so directed. Careful diagnosis and recognition that psychologic responses have their origin in the toxic condition are important in order not to confuse the condition as being chronic in nature with the subsequent loss of identity among the vast numbers of state hospital patients. The nurse's responsibility for careful observations and the maintenance of proper treatment is essential. In acute organic disorders the onset is rapid and reversible, while the chronic disorders are insidious in onset and progressive in nature. Butler and Lewis (1973) point out that acute organic behavior disorders may be distinguished by the following: (1) a fluctuating level of awareness, (2) visual hallucinations, (3) misidentification of individuals, and (4) extreme restlessness. Acute organic disorders may be caused by drug reactions, physical illnesses undiagnosed or out of control, nutritional deficiencies, electrolyte imbalance, head injuries, high fevers, and many others (Libow, 1974). In the chronic organic disorders the usual causative factor is cerebral arteriosclerosis, although other factors, like primary brain disease, are also found. Nurses should be careful to assess the presence of depression and anxiety in the elderly; these may be considered prodromal symptoms to chronic organic disorders. Frequently subtle changes in behavior are not detected until the condition progresses to a morbid stage. Early detection by the nurse of changes in behavior in individuals could mean early treatment and possibly prevent a chronic condition.

It is not unusual to find that the basic personality of the individual determines the kind of behavior he will develop in illness. Exaggeration of the basic personality is common and may be attributed to unresolved emotional conflicts and repressed experiences that surface as the patient's behavior becomes disorganized and previously maintained controls are weakened. For example, a person who tended to be reserved and somewhat withdrawn will most likely develop a more withdrawn, seclusive pattern of behavior, while a person who tended to be suspicious in his association with people may develop frank paranoid tendencies.

Morris and Rhodes (1972) indicate that in organic confusion there is more memory impairment for recent events than remote; there is disorientation as to time, place, and person within a framework of the patient's lifetime and familiar factors; hallucinations are visual and vivid and usually involve animals or insects; illusions are common; delusions center on persons and situations in their immediate environment; and, there are periods of confusion (more pronounced at night) with periods of clearing.

The nurse's concern for and care of this group of patients involve a blending of psychologic and physical care. Burnside (1976) emphasizes the geriatric nurse's challenge "for creative nursing interventions and for nursing management." The overall considerations for the care of the elderly are implicit in the care of patients with organic behavior disorders.

Acute organic behavior disorders

Somatic pathologic conditions. The ability to function adequately as a social being depends on the possession of an organic equilibrium that makes organization of behavior possible. In particular, the five senses and the central nervous system permit the individual to be aware of his environment, to interpret it and its significance including his own relationship to it, and to behave in response to environmental stimuli in an appropriate manner. The disorganization characteristic of behavior disorders may be precipitated by organic damage that leaves the individual with reduced powers to cope with his surroundings.

The reaction of the patient to his illness is quite significant, since the behavior disorder is not a necessary corollary of any disease that involves the central nervous system, any more than it is an inevitable accompaniment of pneumonia or heart disease. The patient can compensate for his failings and inadequacies and learn to live with them. Senile changes in the brain structure do not always mean senile psychosis. A great deal can be accomplished by a psychotherapeutic approach to the problems presented in the organic behavior disorder. This requires recognizing the importance of the patient's reaction to his illness as a major factor in the resulting behavior disorder and using this knowledge to help the patient accept and live with his reduced mental capacity. Psychotherapy is as important in the treatment of syphilis of the central nervous system as chemotherapy.

Toxic reactions. The toxic reaction, characterized particularly by delirium, consistently shows the postmortem finding of brain edema. It is believed that the severity of the delirium may be related to the degree of brain edema.

The course of the reaction is initiated with confusion and impairment of consciousness. The patient becomes restless, does not correctly interpret his environment, shows a recent memory defect, and is disoriented. Hallucinations frequently occur, and the patient's behavior is strongly influenced by them. The hallucinations, misinterpretation, and misunderstanding of the environment produce an emotional response of fear and apprehension. Although the patient's behavior may appear bizarre and inappropriate, it is frequently not so when it is understood in relation to the hallucinations. The patient may be trying to escape from threats against him when he attempts to jump out a window. He may persistently try to get out of bed because he thinks it is full of insects or animals. In any case the patient's seemingly irrational behavior is related to the disordered content of his thinking. In view of this fact, the patient should always be considered to be a potential danger to himself and to his environment.

Although fear and apprehension are the predominant mood characteristics, lability and irritability may also be seen in rapid flashes. Speech may become rambling and incoherent and in severe stages may consist of completely unintelligible muttering. Stupor or coma may finally appear and death may result. Although they almost always precede death, stupor and coma do not always presage its occurrence.

Physically, the patient looks acutely ill. Vasomotor instability is shown in flushing, pallor, excessive perspiration, rapid pulse, and fluctuating blood pressure. Respirations show a deviation from normal. The temperature fluctuates and may be either very high or very low, depending on the toxin and the patient's response. Tremors of the fingers, hands, lips, and facial muscles are common. During lucid intervals the patient complains of headache and weakness.

Toxins producing the described syndrome are numerous. Overdoses of barbiturates, prolonged ingestion of bromides that accumulate in the bloodstream, and buildup of heavy metals such as lead and mercury acquired through occupational exposure are examples. Infectious diseases causing a high temperature, toxemia, and exhaustion are also accompanied by delirium. Pneumonia, cardiorenal disease, acute nephritis, rheumatic fever, and malaria are examples.

Treatment of such reactions is based on detoxification and then rehabilitation of the patient's personality, if this is indicated. A patient whose toxic condition is caused by occupational exposure to industrial poisons may present no or few problems in rehabilitation unless there is a residual reduction of physical or intellectual ability. On the other hand, a patient whose toxic condition is produced by reliance on the continual use of bromides, barbiturates, or other drugs to help him through his emotional crises is definitely in need of personality rehabilitation to enable him to discard his emotional crutches.

The process of detoxification is adjusted to the nature of the particular toxin. In bromide poisoning, for example, large doses of sodium chloride are indicated since the chloride ion replaces the bromide ion and makes its elimination from the body easier. Fluid intake should be increased and elimination vigorously promoted. Intensive vitamin therapy is used to promote the metabolic efficiency of the body. Since the function of the brain is related to adequate carbohydrate metabolism, the administration of intravenous glucose and insulin is frequently indicated. Sedation is avoided if possible, but, if needed, it is used cautiously with full consideration being given to the chemical nature of the offending toxin. Careful supervision of the patient during the delirious period is necessary to protect him from injury and to allay his apprehension. The environment should be as nonstimulating as possible.

Once the acute stage is over and the patient is relatively free of toxin, reassurance in regard to the episode is usually needed. Rehabilitation is directed toward self-understanding and self-acceptance with an encouraging attitude toward the future.

Traumatic psychoses. An acute reaction may occur in response to a head injury, which, incidentally, does not always mean brain injury. A severe enough blow may produce mild confusion, with intellectual dulling, amnesia for a brief period, and mild ataxia without resulting in unconsciousness. The usual outcome is rapid and complete recovery unless the incident happens to be a precipitating factor in the development of a behavior disorder in a susceptible individual. Trauma to the head and the brain may be severe enough to produce unconsciousness. As recovery takes place, the patient is ordinarily confused, dull, and ataxic when he becomes conscious, and in some instances he may show a typical delirious reaction such as previously described. Such a reaction is the exception rather than the rule, and its occurrence has not yet been demonstrated to be related to the extent or location of the brain injury. If traumatic brain injury occurs, it may leave permanent residuals that may result in impaired performance of the individual.

Nursing intervention. The nursing care of patients with acute organic reactions requires a blending of the arts of medical and psychiatric nursing. The use of one without the other complicates the picture in both areas. Poor medical care increases the psychiatric problem, and poor psychiatric care increases the medical problem.

Psychotherapeutic milieu. The patient with acute cerebral incompetence needs an environment in which control of both the patient and the environment is possible. Because he is a potential danger to himself and his environment, the patient needs constant observation. Since restraint produces apprehension and fear, particularly in persons who are unable to grasp and understand current events adequately, there must be someone readily available to prevent the patient from getting out of bed, trying to jump out of the window, assaulting other persons, or otherwise endangering himself or others. Since the patient is apprehensive and tends to misinterpret his environment, stimulation should be reduced to a minimum. In connection with this, it must be remembered that sensitivity to what the patient is experiencing is necessary to effectively reduce stimulation. For example, if a toxic patient sees frogs jumping from a picture on the wall, the picture may be removed. Whenever possible the particular sources of stimulation to the patient should be carefully analyzed, and an attempt should be made to reduce stimulation from that source. The essence of a therapeutic environment for an acutely toxic patient consists of three elements: the necessary physical equipment for care, reduction of stimuli to which the patient is sensitive, and adequate protection for the patient.

Interpersonal relationships. Interpersonal needs of an acutely toxic patient center primarily around his apprehension and fear. Constant reassurance in a firm and positive manner is necessary, along with the realization that reassurance will need almost constant repetition because of clouded sensorium, disorientation, and memory defect. If the patient fears insects in his bed, he should be assured there are none. A brief demonstration may be given, and a positive declaration that the fear will soon disappear should be made. This should be repeated as often as necessary without impatience or irritation. When the patient is indecisive, decisions should be made quickly and firmly for him.

A confrontation technique may be employed as a means of making the patient respond to the reality around him. It is not unusual for patients with delirium to respond to their internal thoughts and stimulations rather than to their environment. The nurse should address questions that demand his attention, thought, and response directly to the patient. The approach and tone in such instances should be kind and supportive and show interest in the patient. The questions and statement should reflect hope in the patient's ability and improvement. These conversations are intended to encourage and to provoke the patient to regulate his behavior instead of resorting to dependence on his illness. A thorough plan for this approach should include all members of the psychiatric team.

Considerable ingenuity is required to secure the cooperation of the patient; force should be avoided if possible. Full advantage may be taken of the patient's memory defect, distractibility, and short attention span. Lucid intervals should be watched for, recognized, and treated as such.

It is wise to limit the number of persons to whom the patient is exposed during the acute period. Seeing the same nurses, who are familiar with the patient's psychotic content and reactions, day after day can reduce to a minimum the threats the environment may carry for the patient.

Physical needs. The patient in a toxic delirious state needs constant nursing care directed toward physical comfort and elimination of the offending toxin. Fluids should be forced, but this must be accompanied by increased elimination since an increase in fluid in the tissues may increase brain edema. Accurate records of intake and output should be kept. Skin care is important since the patient perspires profusely and is likely to be restless, thus increasing the danger of skin breaks and infections. A bath is sometimes needed more often than once a day, bed linen should be changed often to keep the patient clean and comfortable, and drafts (to which the patient is susceptible) should be avoided. Particular attention should be paid to physical comfort through such measures as maintaining oral hygiene, keeping bed linen smooth, adjusting pillows to the patient's comfort, and ensuring adequate ventilation of the room.

As soon as possible the patient should be encouraged to eat, and an intake high in both vitamins and calories is indicated. Fluids should continue to be forced until the patient's toxic condition is past.

Any signs or symptoms that would indicate focal areas of cerebral embarrassment should be promptly reported. The presence of unequal pupils or an indication of paralysis or hyperesthesia constitute examples.

Since the patient needs constant physical attention, the nurse should carry out procedures as quietly and efficiently as possible, making every effort to secure the patient's cooperation in order to avoid stimulation. Quiet reassurance should mark everything the nurse does for the patient. Indecisiveness should be avoided because it may upset the patient, who needs an environment on which he can depend.

Protection. A delirious patient needs someone to accept complete responsibility for him. In his confused state he is incapable of protecting himself from injury or of being aware of injury caused to others if he becomes assaultive. The things and persons he fears should be thoroughly known to those persons who care for him, and he should be carefully protected from injury. Sideboards may be necessary to keep him from falling out of bed, the bed may need to be well away from windows or doors, and the patient should have assistance if he is out of bed for any reason.

Group relations. During the delirious state, the patient's contacts with other people should be as limited as possible. When the patient is up and about, he should be encouraged to join other patients and should be permitted to freely exchange experiences if he wishes. Because of the relative intellectual clearness that accompanies the recovery from a toxic period, even in acutely psychotic patients, the patient may well be a valuable group member. Any tendency to withdraw or stay alone should be discouraged. It is particularly important to establish group contacts as early as possible if the patient is left with a residual handicap.

Convalescence. During the convalescent period, much will depend on the type of toxic infection, the residual handicap (if any), and the patient's basic personality. Problems will be related to these three factors, and their balance will indicate the points of emphasis. If the patient has been dependent on the use of toxins to adjust, he will need encouragement to develop independence and to accept his illness without leaning on it as an alibi or a means to gain sympathy. If the patient is left with some permanent brain damage, he will need help in accepting his new limitation. Careful study of the patient to help him effectively use his strengths and to improve or accept his weaknesses is indicated.

The convalescent period should not bore the patient with inactivity or tire him out. An interesting occupation adjusted to his physical ability is important in shortening the period of recovery to full potential. The attitude of personnel toward the patient's illness should avoid either ridicule or citicism. The temptation to show amusement concerning the patient's inappropriate or bizarre behavior during the acute phase should be carefully assessed against his genuine feeling about the matter. Few persons like to be laughed at, even though they may pretend they do.

Chronic organic behavior disorders

Senile psychoses. Behavior disorders in the senile psychoses are caused by changes accompanying old age that result in an increasing inability to adjust and to adapt to the environment. The brain shrinks, cortical areas atrophy, with a loss of cells, and areas of destruction called senile plaques (which can be demonstrated microscopically) are formed. Fat is markedly increased throughout the brain. Reflecting the loss of functioning cortical cells, the patient shows behavior changes to which he may or may not be able to adapt.

The usual onset of a senile behavior disorder is so gradual that it is often not recognized until some rather startling or shocking failure on the part of the patient calls it sharply into focus. The patient shows increasing forgetfulness and disturbance in orientation. As the patient's grasp of current events begins to slip because of difficulties with retention and recall, interests narrow and new ideas and activities are more difficult to accept. Habits become both more rigid and more deteriorated. Caution becomes suspiciousness, and order-liness becomes compulsiveness. Those with less contact with reality show a reduced capacity to respond with habits of personal cleanliness. Mood becomes labile, and the capacity for depth and continuity of affection for others is re-duced and may eventually be lost. The course of the illness is progressive, and intellectual ability may become so impaired that the patient retains merely a few stereotyped responses from his past experience. He will then exist on a vegetative level until death occurs.

The form of behavior displayed when the patient becomes psychotic will express the basic personality plus his reaction to his failing abilities. The re-action may be predominantly aggressive, depressive, projective, agitated, or withdrawn, depending on the individual. In any instance the behavior will not be specific for the cerebral areas involved.

Treatment for patients with senile changes is aimed primarily at helping the patient accept his reduced capacities through psychotherapy and, when possible, by reducing environmental demands and threats. The course is a steadily progressive one, and the cerebral damage that occurs is not reversible.

Behavior disorders with cerebral arteriosclerosis. In cerebral arterio-sclerosis, behavior disorders occur as the result of an inadequate blood supply to the brain that impairs effective function of cerebral cells. Since arterio-sclerosis occurs in persons in the same age group as persons with senile reac-tions and since the same somatic areas are involved, arteriosclerotic patients present much the same type of picture. For all practical purposes the only dif-ferences are a somewhat more acute onset, a tendency to periodic remissions, a greater personal awareness of physical changes in the early stages, and the occurrence of cerebral accidents in arteriosclerotic patients. Otherwise the general picture of increasing cerebral incompetence, plus the patient's reaction to it, is present.

Medical procedures designed to lower blood cholesterol have been em-ployed in the treatment of cerebral arteriosclerosis, but their value has been controversial. Reduction in cholesterol and a cholesterol-free diet have been tried, and thyroid, iodides, cortisone, and ACTH have been administered. Nicotinic acid and nicotinamide do seem to improve cerebral circulation. Other measures used include shock therapy for depressions and agitations and group therapy as an aid in adjustment to limited abilities.

Senile and cerebral arteriosclerotic behavior disorders have become an important social problem in recent years. The increasing life expectancy has kept alive a greater number of people to succumb to the particular difficulties of old age. The trend toward urbanization of the population has added to the prob-lem, since urban life offers greater hazards to the aged and the pattern of life in cities makes less provision for them than does that of life in rural areas. Social facilities adapted to the needs of older persons have not yet been extensively developed, and as a result, large numbers of older persons are finding their way into state psychiatric hospitals.

General paresis. General paresis is a syphilitic infection of the meninges and encephalon and is most marked in the cerebral cortex of the frontal and parietal regions. Why some patients develop syphilis of the central nervous system whereas others do not is a moot question.

The serologic and neurologic findings in general paresis are nearly always adequate for diagnosis. Neurologically, pupillary changes occur, and the pupils may be unequal, dilated, or contracted. The Argyll Robertson pupil, which reacts to accommodation but not to light, is a common finding. Progressive weakness and incoordination of voluntary muscles is shown in tremors of the tongue, hands, and face, in disturbance of speech, especially slurring, and in changes in handwriting. The lack of coordination of tongue muscles is shown in the patient's inability to enunciate accurately such test phrases as "Methodist Episcopal" and "third riding artillery brigade." Deep tendon reflexes are affected and may be exaggerated, diminished, or lost. Because of the nerve cell damage, the facial muscles may be relaxed and smoothed out, resulting in a younger but somewhat vacant expression.

Serologically, the blood and spinal Wassermann tests may be positive if the patient's syphilitic infection has not been treated. Spinal fluid pressure is usually increased, lymphocytes and proteins are well above normal limits, and globulin is present in the spinal fluid. The Lange colloidal gold curve shows positive findings.

In regard to the behavior aspect, the early symptoms are usually slowing of the mental processes, memory defect, irritability, and increasing loss of judgment and social skills. As the disease progresses, the organic indications of reduced intellectual capacity become more obvious, and the behavior disorder that follows will be in accordance with the patient's personality and experience. He may be expansive and elated, or he may be agitated and depressed. The form of the behavior deviation that develops is specific for the patient but not for general paresis.

Prompt and adequate treatment of general paresis may halt the disease at any stage and prevent further damage. Treatment undertaken in the early inflammatory stages of the infection before actual degeneration of cortical cells has occurred may result in complete recovery for the patient. The earlier treatment is instituted, the greater the organic equipment the patient may retain. By way of caution, not all patients respond to treatment although the majority of them do, nor is the complete physical recovery of the patient an absolute guarantee that the behavior disorder will disappear. The behavior disorder may outlast the illness that precipitated it.

By far the most effective treatment of general paresis is intensive penicillin therapy. Large doses of penicillin, up to 15 to 20 million units, are indicated. The treatment is effective, rapid, inexpensive, and practically free of risk.

It has been noted statistically that there has been an increase in the number of cases of syphilis. This may result from an increase of sexual freedom with lessening of restrictive values and from the ease of treatment. However, the social stigma of venereal disease continues to restrain young adults and others from reporting and seeking treatment quickly. A continuous educational campaign for young people should be an essential component of every school's health program. Youth's folly can result in painful and serious consequences in old age.

Behavior disorders with convulsions. Convulsive phenomena may occur as a symptom of cerebral irritation in organic brain disease or in any illness affecting the central nervous system. Thus they may be a symptom of paresis, meningitis, cerebral arteriosclerosis, uremia, lead poisoning, or any other toxic condition. Convulsive phenomena are also an indication of idiopathic or essential epilepsy. The actual convulsions or their equivalents occur as evidence of the disordered function of the rate-regulating mechanism of the brain. Electric currents are produced in the brain, and the electric discharge ordinarily takes place at a regular rhythmic rate. During the period of a convulsion or its substitute, the epileptic patient shows a marked variation in the rate of discharge as measured by the electroencephalograph. What happens during a convulsion is known, but what initiates the event is unknown.

Epilepsy occurs as a grand mal, petit mal, or psychomotor episode, although a patient not uncommonly shows a mixture of types. All are characterized by a disturbance in consciousness. A grand mal seizure follows a definite pattern. An aura or warning may or may not occur, but it is usually specific for the individual patient and is related to one of the five senses. The patient may see a bright light or a vision, hear something, smell a peculiar smell, or experience some indication that an attack is on the way. The convulsion is initiated with a tonic spasm involving the entire body and is accompanied by a loss of consciousness. The body is then involved in a series of jerking motions, lasting one-half to a whole minute or slightly more. The convulsion is followed by a period of stupor of varying length, and confusion ordinarily accompanies the return to consciousness. A petit mal attack is a momentary loss of consciousness often accompanied by localized muscular twitching. The loss of consciousness is so brief that the patient does not fall.

Psychomotor attacks, or epileptic equivalents, cover a variety of types of behavior, including episodes of overactivity, furors of violent frenzy, and periods of amnesia. Persons with convulsive disorders can and do lead perfectly normal lives and adjust well to their handicap. Some of them, however, do require institutionalization and some show severe behavior disorders. The behavior disorders center around (1) mood disturbances marked by ill humor, cruelty, sickly sentimentality, and marked emotional lability, (2) periods of confusion that may include hallucinatory experiences, and (3) deterioration. Whether the deterioration is a result of the disease, the medication given for the disease, or the social isolation that all too often accompanies epilepsy is uncertain. Fortunately, a psychotic development in the course of epilepsy is the exception rather than the rule.

The treatment of behavior disorders with convulsive phenomena is based on medication to control seizures, regulation of diet, and environmental adjustment. Phenobarbital, phenytoin (Dilantin), mephenytoin (Mesantoin), and primidone (Mysoline) are commonly used in the treatment of grand mal and psychomotor attacks. Trimethadione (Tridione), paramethadione (Paradione), and phensuximide (Milontin) are administered in the treatment of petit mal attacks. Dosage is an individual matter and must be worked out for each patient.

Individuals with epilepsy or convulsive disturbances but without psychoses, as is the case for the majority, need psychologic assistance in knowing how to help themselves. After stabilizing the seizures by the proper medication, physicians should introduce the patient to the nurse or the counselor for assistance in his activities and adjustment to daily living. Without some support and reassurance a sensitive person may resort to isolation as his solution to fear and embarrassment related to his symptoms. The nurse's or the counselor's role in these cases is vital and should begin as a means of sustaining the person with an intentional goal for his early independence. These people are usually seen in the physician's office and at clinics rather than in hospitals.

Huntington's chorea. Huntington's chorea is an unusual behavior disorder for two reasons. First, its occurrence is not common, and, second, it is one illness that is nearly always accompanied by incapacitating behavior changes in which heredity can be demonstrated as the chief etiologic factor. It reveals its presence in middle age and results from gradual degeneration of specific areas in the brain. The physical symptoms are quite striking. Jerky, clumsy, and irregular movements, beginning in the upper extremities and slowly but surely involving the entire body, render the patient quite conspicuous as well as unable to carry out normal activities. Understandably, the patient becomes irritable, emotionally labile, and quite suspicious. Attention, memory, and judgment become quite impaired. Custodial detention usually becomes necessary as dementia progresses.

Postencephalitic behavior disorders. Epidemic encephalitis, a viral disease, takes many forms and often has a residual effect in postencephalitic behavior disorders. At one time Parkinson's syndrome was believed to be solely a belated result of the acute form of epidemic encephalitis, which may also result from other causes. The acute form has no specific course, so the residual behavior disorder has no specific form when it does occur. Any inflammatory disease of the brain may precipitate a behavior disorder of almost any hue and may also leave chronic brain inflammation or damage that may precipitate a behavior disorder.

One of the most interesting postencephalitic behavior disorders is Parkinson's syndrome, which is characterized by listlessness, avoidance of experience, mask like facies, and pill-rolling movements of the fingers. In Parkinson's syndrome, the patient presents a typical physical appearance that is important in diagnosing this behavior disorder. The voluntary or skeletal muscles are tensed, and the resultant appearance and behavior show drooling, slow and monotonous speech, and slow and shuffling gait; the trunk is bent forward, and the arms are flexed before the trunk. The thumb and fingers combine in a characteristic pill-rolling motion. A tremor of the fingers, hands, feet, and head develops progressively. This shaking palsy with its marked intention tremor is seen as a sequel to brain infections and usually produces a marked reaction in patients who undergo the experience. These symptoms will be enhanced or minimized by the patient's reaction to them. In any instance, the encephalitis of whatever origin and its sequelae are often precipitating factors in this behavior disorder.

Drugs to control the physical symptoms of Parkinson's syndrome have been used for some time. Among the oldest, and still useful, are atropine and hyoscine. Rabellon (a combination of hyoscyamine, atropine, and scopolamine) has been effective in some persons. Caramiphen (Parparnit) and orphenadrine (Disipal), which have atropine-like reactions, have received favorable reports. Newer drugs include trihexyphenidyl (Artane), cycrimine (Pagitane), ethopropazine (Parsidol), cyclizine (Marezine), and diethazine (Diparcol).

Nursing intervention. The nursing care of patients with progressive cerebral incompetence offers a real challenge. Until recently the attitude toward such behavior disorders has been so completely hopeless that they have been considered to be an area in which little could be done. A beginning realization has dawned concerning how much can be done in guiding the patient to live effectively and constructively with his handicap. The field is of particular interest since many behavior disorders of organic origin occur in older persons who have previously been constructive members of society. Patients who develop behavior disorders in conjunction with progressive cerebral incompetence represent human resources well worth the effort of conservation.

Psychotherapeutic milieu. The environment must be adjusted to the patient's limitations, depending on the degree of incapacitation of physical and intellectual capacities. Patients who have only a few stereotyped responses left for adaptive purposes may depend completely on the continuity of the environment for any continuity of behavior. For such patients a routine that remains exactly the same in minute detail from day to day is essential. Progressive brain destruction makes it increasingly harder to cope with present and new experiences, so increasing reliance is placed on past habits, successes, and interests. Failing abilities cause an insecurity that accentuates this trend. Therefore an important principle in environmental control for patients with chronic nervous system diseases accompanied by behavior disorders is careful rigidity in routine and reduction of new experiences to the lowest possible level. If the actual damage is relatively small, the patient's experience can be gradually broadened as he profits from the security of a thoroughly dependable daily routine. The patient can then be encouraged by slow steps to the highest level of activity of which he is capable.

The environment should also take into account the potential dangers in failing of such physical capacities as vision, hearing, and muscular coordination. Although the physical surroundings should be pleasant and cheerful, furniture should be sturdy and placed where the danger of falling over it is reduced to a minimum. Extra rugs and small bits of furniture such as magazine racks and footstools should be used with caution, if not eliminated. Only essential equipment should be used, and it should be kept in the same place consistently.

Interpersonal relationships. The problems in interpersonal relationships with patients with progressive cerebral incompetence center around loss of abilities, reduced level of adaptability, and the insecurity stemming from these two sources. The behavior disorder that develops, if one does, will be colored by the patient's prepsychotic personality so that the syndromes of withdrawal, aggression, projection, and preoccupation with somatic function and ritualism will also be seen. In such instances, the principles of the nursing care previously outlined will be applicable.

The central objective is to build the patient's confidence and self-esteem as a person with whatever handicap he has acquired. While constancy in physical environment is important, consistency in attitude and behavior toward the patient is equally essential. His routine should be tactfully manipulated until he learns to depend on it, and then encouragement toward improvement should be instituted. If the degree of intellectual impairment, the probable shortened attention span, the potential irritability, and the explosive emotional response are taken into full account, the patient should be encouraged to undertake responsibilities and activities in which success is a reasonable expectation and failure a remote one. Liberal praise should be given for accomplishment, and criticism avoided. Physical handicaps, such as memory defects, should not be made conspicuous nor should they be ignored. Rather, calm matter-of-fact verbal and emotional acceptance of their existence makes it easier for the patient to accept them. The patient should be helped to develop emotional control and encouraged to develop perseverance.

One area that is often a sensitive one for personnel is the patient's tendency to be less subtle than usual in regard to moral and ethical questions in both speech and behavior. The nurse should be prepared for such expressions of the loss of social graces and recognize them as symptomatic. As the patient improves in behavior, he may be helped to control this particular trait as well.

Physical needs. The physical needs of patients with progressive cerebral incompetence are numerous. Personal hygiene needs constant attention, and the establishment of health habits should be promoted. Elderly patients, for example, are frequently not too enthusiastic about a bath and a change of clothing. Routine that is very much the same from day to day helps, and quiet firmness is another aid. Attention should be paid to oral hygiene, skin care, elimination, and diet. It is usually not wise to attempt to change the eating habits of a lifetime, and if supplements are needed, they can be given medicinally.

Exercise adjusted to the patient's ability is a definite need. Although a patient may no longer be capable of active exercise, whatever he can do safely should be carried through. Exercise also helps with the problem of insomnia. Many patients with this type of disorder are restless at night, and keeping them interested and active in a daily routine helps promote a natural end-of-day weariness and sleep.

Convulsions do occur in diseases of the central nervous system. When a convulsion occurs, the patient should be left where he is until the convulsion ends unless he has fallen where injury is apt to occur. If possible, something should be placed between the teeth to prevent tongue-biting. Clothing should be loosened around the throat and chest, and the head should be supported to prevent injury against the floor. No attempt should be made to restrict the motion of the patient's body. When the tonic phase ends and the patient begins to breathe, the head should be turned gently to one side to prevent the aspiration of mucus, which collects rapidly. At the end of the convulsion the patient should be placed in a low bed, with protection against falling, and should be allowed to remain until he is intellectually clear. A patient who is restless, confused, excitable, or assaultive following such an episode should be closely observed and protected from injuring himself or others. A careful and detailed descriptive report of the convulsion should be charted, including the following information: any incident preceding the convulsion, parts of the body involved, sequence of events, duration, any injury, and behavior after the convulsion.

Protection. The protective needs of patients with progressive cerebral incompetence tend to be rather high and are related to two factors—failing physical abilities and lack of emotional control.

Patients must be protected from self-injury caused by poor vision, poor muscular coordination, and poor memory, among other defects. Protection from drafts or extremes in temperature, careful supervision in the bathroom to prevent falls, care in the application of heat and cold to skin surfaces, observation in the dining room to note such problems as difficulty in swallowing, and assistance up and down stairs and into and out of bed are all measures to be adopted when necessary. Nurses should be alert to the greater possibility of retention of urine and feces in patients with disorders of this type. In other words, nurses should make themselves tactfully responsible for the prevention of any injury and realize that the possibilities for such happenings are much higher than usual.

The other particular threat to the physical safety of such patients is their explosive emotional responses; assaultiveness and excited episodes are fairly common. Close observation and tactful approach, allowing the patient free verbal expression but no more, usually make the management of such episodes easier. Distractibility, poor attention span, and the briefness of such outbursts should be considered during the period of excitement. The patient should be kept away from situations that repeatedly result in difficulties.

Group relations. Patients should be encouraged to join group activities with other patients who have handicaps of similar origin. Supervision should be directed toward avoidance of failure, support when failure happens, and alertness to the possible consequences of irritability and explosiveness. The major problems usually center around getting the patient interested in activities and maintaining his interest. Persistence pays dividends since habits can be established through consistent efforts. Patients with postencephalitic behavior disorders tend to depend more on habits than is usual.

Convalescence. Usually, convalescent care of patients with chronic behavior disorders is not oriented to complete recovery but toward readjustment of the patient to his new status. Therefore, as the severity of the patient's behavior disorder subsides, the major tasks are to determine his greatest potential in terms of his probable future and to help him reach for that level. It is important not to burden him with aspirations beyond his abilities. Attaching importance to the things he can do, making these abilities seem worthwhile in the eyes of others, and encouraging the development of skill in their practice will help the patient to live within his limitations. Considerable tact is required, and the single fact to keep constantly in mind is that the convalescent period should give the patient opportunity to develop skill and security in the types of activity that will constitute his life.

REFERENCES

Baltes, P. B., and Goulet, L. R.: Exploration of developmental variables by manipulation and simulation of age differences in behavior, Human Dev. **14:**149-170, 1971.

Bühler, C.: The developmental structure of goal setting in group and individual studies. In Bühler, C., and Massarik, F., editors: The course of human life, New York, 1968, Springer.

Burnside, I. M., editor: Nursing and the aged, New York, 1976, McGraw-Hill Book Co., pp. 148-164.

Butler, R. N., and Lewis, M. J.: Aging and mental health, St. Louis, 1973, The C. V. Mosby Co.

Ebersole, P.: Reminiscing, Am. J. Nurs. **76:**1304-1305, 1976.

Erickson, E. H.: Identity: youth and crisis, New York, 1968, W. W. Norton & Co.

Havighurst, R., Jr.: Human development and education, New York, 1953, Longmans, Green & Co., pp. 277-281.

Jung, C. G.: The stages of life. In Campbell, J., editor: The portable Jung, New York, 1971, Viking Press.

Kimmel, D. C.: Adulthood and aging, New York, 1974, John Wiley & Sons, Inc.

Kübler-Ross, E.: On death and dying, New York, 1969, The Macmillan Co.

Libow, L. S.: Interaction of medical, biologic, and behavioral factors on aging, adaptation, and survival: an eleven year longitudinal study, Geriatrics **29:**75-85, 1974.

Morris, M., and Rhodes, M.: A guideline for differentiating the organically confused from the functionally confused patient for the psychiatric or medical surgical nurse, Am. J. Nurs. **72:** 1630-1633, 1972.

Neely, E., and Patrick, M. L.: Problem of aged persons taking medications at home, Nurs. Res. **17:**52-55, 1968.

U.S. Department of Health, Education, and Welfare: Working with older people, vol. II, P.H.S. publication No. 1459, Washington, D.C., 1970, U.S. Government Printing Office.

ADDITIONAL READINGS

Burnside, I. M.: Touching is talking, Am. J. Nurs. **73:**2060-2062, 1969.

Calnan, M. F., and Hanron, J. B.: Young nurse—elderly patient, Nurs. Outlook **18:**44-46, 1970.

Fowler, R. S., Jr.: Adapting care for the brain-damaged patient, parts I and II, Am. J. Nurs. **10:** 1832-1835, **11:**2056-2059, 1972.

Markson, E.: The geriatric house of death: hiding the dying elder in a mental hospital, Aging Hum. Dev. **1:**37-49, 1970.

Wilkiemeyer, D. S.: Affection: key to care for the elderly, Am. J. Nurs. **72:**2166-2168, 1972.

PATIENTS WHO DEPEND ON EMOTIONAL CRUTCHES

CHAPTER 15

Patients who depend on alcohol

HISTORICAL OVERVIEW

Alcoholism has been a problem of society since biblical times. In several places the Old Testament makes reference to inebriation. Alcohol was recognized for its medicinal use, while at the same time recognized as the cause of various physical illnesses and mental disturbances.

As people developed a taste for wines and alcohol, as well as enjoying the pleasurable effects that accompanied them, those individuals who became abnormal drinkers or who reacted differently under the influence of alcohol became a growing concern. Since the attitude during these early times was that alcoholism was a moral problem and a weakness of character, the responsibility for cure was in the hands of the church and the law. If the church failed—which was more often than not—and the condition progressed, the law would then attempt to enforce change in the alcoholic. The alcoholic now became a culprit and an outcast, leading him further into a social deviate role.

The temperance movement was an attempt by society to remedy the increasing problem of alcohol and its effects on humans. Total abstinence became the goal, an attitude still focusing on the idea that the intake of alcohol was controlled by character and willpower. The Prohibition Act of 1918 became law but after 15 violent years was repealed, leaving the consumption of alcohol further ingrained into the social customs of most races and countries.

Various scholars began to publish their theories on alcoholism. Probably the first person to define excessive drinking as a disease was Thomas Trotter (1788). At about the same time, Rush suggested that excessive drinking resembled a physical disease. V. Bruhl-Cramer published a monograph in 1819 introducing the concept of drinking mania, making reference to some emo-

337

tional factors in precipitating the illness. Hufeland proposed dipsomania as a general term for all forms of pathologic drinking. In 1839 Rusch stressed the importance of environmental factors and temperamental types. In Russia, Korsakoff (1887) described a disease which he called cerebropathia psychica toxaemica—now generally known as Korsakoff's psychosis.

There still remains a controversy over a universally accepted definition of alcoholism. The concepts vary, depending on the frame of reference, from the physiologic, sociologic, psychologic, or religious point of view.

The World Health Organization (1952) describes alcoholics as: "Excessive drinkers whose dependence upon alcohol has attained such a degree that it results in noticeable mental disturbance, or in an interference with their bodily and mental health, their interpersonal relations, and their smooth social and economic functioning—or those who show the prodromal signs of such developments."

From a sociological frame of reference, four facets of behavior set the alcoholic apart from his fellow drinkers. First, his use of alcohol regularly deviates from the typical drinking standards of his key social groups: home, neighborhood, and job. Second, the performance of his role in these key institutions is impaired. Third, he suffers from emotional and physical damage from his regular excessive use of alcohol. Finally, he shows an inability to stop drinking once he starts, even though he may know his drinking impairs his life; thus, his use of alcohol is beyond his conscious control (Trice, 1966).

English and English's *Psychiatric Dictionary* (1958) gives the following:

> 1. Alcoholism—alcoholic poisoning; the effect of excess intake of alcohol. 2. Chronic alcoholism—addiction to alcohol; considered one of the personality disorders or disturbance. A patient is considered to suffer from chronic alcoholism if (1) his use of alcohol is of such extent as to interfere with successful physical, personality and/or social functioning, and (2) he is either unable to recognize the deleterious effects of his habit or, recognizing them, he is nonetheless unable to curtail his alcoholic consumption and continues in an almost compulsive way to drink heavily.

STATISTICS AND STUDIES OF ALCOHOLISM

The number of individuals involved as sufferers from alcoholism in the United States alone is at an all-time high of approximately 10 million. Another 20 to 30 million individuals feel the destructive impact of the illness. Another shocking statistic is the growing consumption of alcohol by the youngsters age of 12 or 13.

Many studies have developed throughout the years justifying the various concepts on alcoholism. Physiologic research has so far tried to attack the problem of etiology but has dealt mainly with advanced alcoholism, giving important information regarding the effects in the human body.

Sociologic studies have compared incidences between men and women, between different cultures and ethnic groups, between social classes, between countries, and others. For example, in comparing the incidence of alcoholism in Jewish and Irish immigrants in the United States, Bales (1946) found that a ritualistic attitude toward drinking among the Jews made alcoholism a rarity. The Irish had a mainly convivial attitude toward alcohol, using it as a means of relieving their acute emotional needs.

From the frame of reference of heredity, Jellinek (1952) points out that it is very difficult to know when seemingly inherited alcoholism may really be based on direct biologic transmission and when it is an expression of imitation and identification processes taking place in a family atmosphere in which young children are constantly exposed to alcoholic behavior in one or both parents.

Jellinek has formulated a comprehensive account of the development of addiction based on a study of 2,000 alcoholics.

1. The prealcoholic symptomatic phase lasts from several months to 2 years. It is characterized by the gradual change of socially motivated drinking into a means of relieving personal tensions, accompanied by an increased tolerance for alcohol.

2. The prodromal phase lasts from 6 months to 4 or 5 years. It is first characterized by a sudden onset of blackouts, with gradual symptoms of surreptitious drinking, preoccupation with alcohol, avid drinking, guilt feelings about one's drinking behavior, avoidance of reference to alcohol in social conversations, and an increasing frequency of blackouts.

3. The crucial phase is initiated by a loss of behavioral control. Drinking becomes conspicuous, getting reprovals from parents, wife, friends, and employer. One may lose one's job and friends, and greater strain is placed on a marital relationship. A decrease of sexual drive, alcoholic jealousy, malnutrition, guilt feelings, and more all contribute to the further sinking into the use of alcohol as the only coping mechanism, which then leads into the last stage.

4. The chronic phase of alcohol addiction shows marked ethical deterioration, impairment of thinking, alcoholic psychoses, drinking with anyone regardless of social level or personal characteristics, as well as drinking anything that contains alcohol. There comes a loss of alcohol tolerance, probably related to a decreased ability of the liver to accomplish oxidation. Other symptoms are indefinable fears, tremors, psychomotor inhibitions, obsessive thinking, and the development of vague religious desires. At this point the addict is at his lowest and admits defeat, which makes him accessible to treatment.

These sequences described by Jellinek are true for many alcoholics; however, the rate one goes through these sequences is individualistic.

Studies dealing with psychologic and personality theories are quite extensive. Glover (1932) related addiction to sadistic drives and oedipal conflicts. Rado (1933) suggested that alcohol addiction is mainly a means of relieving a problem of depression, the alcohol producing a pharmacologic sense of elation that the patient craves. Menninger (1938) emphasized the self-destructive drives of the alcoholic and termed alcoholism as chronic suicide. Knight (1937) considered that the addictive alcoholic suffers basically from a character disorder distinguished by excessive demands, an inability to carry out sustained effort, and feelings of hostility and rage, with alcohol utilized to satisfy and pacify the alcoholic's frustrated needs.

A study by Kogen and Jackson (1963) on role perception found that alcoholic husbands perceived their wives as dominant, insecure, and unwilling to change themselves and characterized by defenses such as denial, rationalization, and protection. Wives of alcoholics perceived their husbands as being socially undesirable, lacking in emotional growth, and irresponsible and characterized by traits such as gloomy, distrustful, bitter and resentful. In research dealing with marital relationships mention was made of a high probability that a man with alcoholic problems would marry a woman older than himself, in search of having a relationship he had or didn't have with his mother.

Dependence on the consumption of alcohol is considered a symptom or a disease and may be both. Specific etiologic factors are not clearly understood. Persons who are lonely, who have feelings of inferiority, who are anxious, who have fears they cannot verbalize or identify, or who have strong passive dependent needs that are not acceptable to them may become alcoholics. Other personality characteristics generally attributed to persons who resort to alcohol are low tension tolerance, inability to wait for delayed satisfactions, tendency to do everything to excess, impulsiveness, and resentment toward responsibilities. However, such persons may also become withdrawn, aggressive, or neurotic. What determines the particular choice of alcohol as a method of adjustment is uncertain. Some persons drink because of social pressure and some because of inner needs. In either case, if the drinking thus started occurs in a personality with strong emotional conflicts that remain unsolved, the possibility of the development of pathologic dependence on alcohol is present. Drugs are resorted to similarly, as an alternative choice.

One of the first effects of alcohol is to depress the inhibitory centers or areas in the frontal lobes and thereby reduce self-criticism and judgment and produce a more comfortable feeling of sureness and self-confidence. The reduction of inhibitory control over the self permits the free expression of strong emotions that would ordinarily be suppressed. When a person is under the influence of alcohol, deep resentment and hostility, for example, which burn him inwardly will be openly expressed, and he will experience some relief. When he sobers up, however, tension is usually increased by the feelings of guilt and fear of retaliation that follow the expression of hostility, and alcohol becomes necessary again to release the tension. This pattern approximates one of the vicious cycles found in projective behavior disorders. In this sense, alcoholic indulgence to a pathologic degree may be a symptom of basic personality maladjustment. Alcoholism may be substituted for a projective behavior disorder, may delay its appearance, or may precipitate the disorder more quickly. In the same fashion, alcoholism may be a symptom of a neurotic or psychopathic disorder or another form of maladjustment. Alcoholism of this type may be considered secondary to an underlying disorder and is a symptom of that disorder. These disorders are most often associated with aggressive, projective, psychoneurotic, and socially assertive patterns of behavior.

The so-called disease of alcoholism develops in persons who show no characteristic premorbid personality but have difficulties in adjustment. When they are exposed to the effect of alcohol, these persons resort to it regularly as an aid to adjustment. These persons go on to become completely dependent on alcohol even when its destructive effect on social adequacy becomes evident. In many instances, drinking appears compulsive in nature—the person *must* drink and becomes increasingly tense until alcohol is available.

There is one distinction in the field that is of therapeutic significance. Individuals whose personality difficulties are obvious at an early age and whose drinking becomes a problem very early in life are the most difficult to treat. Individuals who have made an adequate social adjustment until 35 or 40 years of age and whose transition from social drinking to alcoholism takes place gradually at that age are more hopeful therapeutic prospects.

The profitable effect of alcohol for persons who are uncomfortable is twofold. It blurs the sharp edges of reality and makes the individual feel more competent to deal with reality. In persons who tolerate anxiety poorly, alcohol is a quick and effective solace. And, in the beginning, it is a socially acceptable form of behavior. However, why the alcoholic individual uses alcohol as an escape rather than some other defense mechanism, why he cannot stop when alcohol ceases to be a help and becomes a problem, and why he continues to drink while knowing the consequences are all questions to be answered.

The prolonged use of a toxin such as alcohol as a definite effect on the central nervous system and its function. The immediate result of acute intoxication is well known. Motor activity is lessened and becomes poorly coordinated, speech is slurred and becomes incoherent and unintelligible, physical strength is reduced, judgment and intellectual activity are impaired, memory is less sharp, and stupor or coma may be the end result. In patients who drink constantly and heavily, a milder but chronic form of such symptoms may be seen. In fact, it may be necessary to know the person rather well to recognize the lowered motor activity, reduced physical strength, mild memory defects, and poor judgment. Prolonged use of alcohol may also produce organic behavior disorders of a rather severe form.

Pathologic intoxication may occur; this consists of an episode of sudden excitement usually accompanied by anger and rage, assaultiveness that may be homicidal, hallucinations, and confusion. The patient is almost always amnesic for the period. Such episodes are precipitated by the ingestion of relatively small amounts of alcohol. The dynamics, either physical or psychologic, of such episodes are not understood, and they may well be wrongly classified when considered alcoholic behavior disorders.

Delirium tremens is a typical acute toxic reaction occurring in patients who have used alcohol heavily over a prolonged period. Motor restlessness, visual hallucinations, great apprehension, marked tremors, and ataxia occur in a severe delirium. Delirium tremens is extremely painful, and in response to his symptoms the patient may accidentally harm himself physically or commit suicide. Constant observation of the patient is essential during this time. The delirium usually terminates rather abruptly in a few days.

Acute hallucinosis may occur in patients who use alcohol excessively. Hallucinations, most commonly auditory, that produce extreme fear are typical features, along with an unusual retention of clearness of the sensorium. Signs of physical illness are less marked than in delirium tremens.

Korsakoff's psychosis or syndrome is a chronic disorder in which permanent damage to the nervous system has followed prolonged and excessive drinking. Its pattern is that of a chronic organic behavior disorder. The most striking symptoms are severe memory loss and marked confabulation. As the illness progresses, there is a tendency to lose contact with reality. Peripheral neuritis or polyneuritis usually accompanies the disorder. Early and intensive treatment with vitamin B may prevent foot drop, with shuffling gait, and other neurologic complications that, in the past, were rather common.

Chronic alcoholic deterioration occurs after years of excessive drinking that may or may not have been punctuated by episodes of hallucinatory experience or delirium tremens. Emotions become labile, suspiciousness and irritability are common, and the emotions gradually show a loss of depth. Ethical sense and judgment suffer. Evidence of an organic memory defect is finally shown, and intellectual ability deteriorates. Patients exhibiting such behavior can be included in the classification of chronic organic behavior disorders.

The treatment of alcoholic disorders has not been satisfactory. Various methods of approach to the problem of therapy seem to show good results in approximately one third of the patients treated. Recently, research, study, and education have been intensified, and it is to be hoped that an increase in knowledge concerning alcoholism will result in better therapeutic techniques. At the present time, three broad approaches are being used, although all methods have much in common.

Alcoholics Anonymous, a lay organization, has contributed a great deal to the rehabilitation of alcoholics. The founders and workers are all former alcoholics, temporarily or permanently under control, who approach alcoholic persons and offer them help. These workers prefer to call themselves, more realistically, alcoholics who do not drink. The basic tenets are that the individual is unable to manage himself and needs to depend on divine help and group support in order to control his drinking, and that once he is a member of the group and under control, the individual can be a useful society member and can help others. Meetings are held at which experiences are freely discussed; this gives the patient both emotional catharsis and group acceptance. When and if the patient slips and begins to drink again, individual help is available during the epidsode from other members of the group.

AA has been more widely accepted in recent years and has received the cooperation of the community. Business and industry have provided the means for using AA to help their workers since alcohol has been found to be the cause of a large percentage of loss in work hours. Psychologic services have been added to industrial health services. AA, in its experience with the complexities of the alcoholic's problems, has developed and expanded its activities to serve the teenagers and the wives of alcoholics. Both of these groups can use this support and assistance to better understand and help resolve the alcoholic's problems.

Community-centered clinics for alcoholics and their families have been established with greater visibility than ever before. The nurse's role in such centers demands knowledge of psychosocial and economic factors relating to the racial, ethnic, and cultural makeup of the community, as well as psychologic, psychiatric, and nursing expertise. Community-centered nursing is a rapidly developing trend and already has greatly influenced the traditional model of nursing practice. This trend has also been followed in community-centered clinics for other substance abusers.

A conditioned reflex method of treatment is also used and is more effective when accompanied with psychotherapy. After the alcoholic has had a few drinks, he is given an intramuscular injection of emetine hydrochloride (or a similar substance), which causes severe vomiting and retching. The injections may be administered two or three times a week following the ingestion of a drink; this treatment results in a vomiting experience. The aversion process takes hold, and the patient is found to gag even at the sight or smell of alcohol. Obviously, this method does not help the patient resolve his problems, but it does render him sober to pursue his work activities and participation in psychotherapy. The patient may need reinforcement of this conditioning treatment from time to time.

Disulfiram (Antabuse) and cortisone are also being used in the treatment of alcoholism. Antabuse, an effective type of therapy for some patients, destroys the taste for alcohol. After taking it, the patient becomes ill if alcohol is ingested. Current thinking estimates that the greatest value of Antabuse is as an adjunct in the treatment of patients who wish to control their drinking but who are unable to do so without help. Cortisone is used in the treatment of acute intoxications, including delirium tremens. It rapidly brings physical symptoms under control. When the patient is in good physical condition, he is discharged and referred to a local unit of Alcoholics Anonymous or is treated as an outpatient in psychotherapy.

Reports on the use of tranquilizing drugs in the treatment of alcoholism are available. These drugs are particularly effective in the treatment of alcoholic delirium, although they are also being used freely to help control the basic anxiety experienced by alcoholics. The most commonly used tranquilizers are derivatives of mepazine.

Psychotherapy is directed toward guiding the patient in understanding himself and his problems, in facing what he is trying to escape, and in learning to live comfortably with himself as he is. He must also learn to abstain completely from the use of alcohol, since most therapists are convinced that alcoholics cannot successfully stay at the level of social drinking. In order for psychotherapy to be effective, it is necessary for the patient to wish to help himself or to develop within a controlled environment the wish to help himself. Reports on treatment vary a great deal, and pessimism is often noticeable. However, there is general agreement that treatment should not stop with the removal of the physical signs and symptoms but must be directed toward personality rehabilitation.

NURSING INTERVENTION

Chronic alcoholism presents a serious nursing and social problem. A negative attitude toward alcoholism has persisted over the years and it affects treatment or nontreatment on the part of the community hospital and its personnel. Acceptance of alcoholism as an illness appears to be at an intellectual level, leaving the study and understanding of this illness as a mere mention in the curriculums of most professional schools of medicine, nursing, and social work.

It is essential that all individual's in the helping professions examine their own attitudes about alcoholism. General and intellectual knowledge about the disease does not prepare them to cope emotionally without feelings of disappointment when identified alcoholic patients continue with the problem for their many varied reasons. A positive and understanding attitude is the first step toward fulfilling the nursing role in helping the alcoholic patient regain his self-respect so that he may function to his greatest potential.

Identifying and counseling the alcoholic individual are summed up by Mueller (1974) in the role of the nurse in counseling the alcoholic. The five C's of counseling are:

1. *Contact.* The nurse must make a therapeutic contact. A recognition of *clues* in possible relationship between alcoholism and admitting diagnosis, observations written by medical staff, and comments by patients or family members is vital. The nurse must have an awareness of the symptoms of withdrawal: tremors, nausea, vomiting, diarrhea, weakness, perspiration, fever, anorexia, insomnia, visual or auditory hallucinations, disorientation, possibly convulsions. Also, the nurse must be alert for those individuals requiring more than or less than the usual sedation.

2. *Concern.* This is most essential in counseling. Demonstrating interest in and caring about the patient as a person are of great importance to the alcoholic, who is dependent, with a deeply embedded low self-esteem.

3. *Communication.* A nonjudgmental and understanding attitude by the nurse of the pain, shame, and despair the patient has gone through may allow him to open up. The patient should be allowed to communicate how he sees his situation. The nurse can provide factual information about the illness, including the progression and danger signs of pathologic drinking. If the patient concedes a possible connection between the present illness to alcohol, exploration can go further. If the patient denies a problem, the nurse must react accordingly.

4. *Confrontation.* The alcoholic develops an elaborate defense system to protect his drinking behavior. The patient should be confronted with discrepancies between what he is saying and what the reality of his situation seems to be. Cause-and-effect interpretations can be presented in a more realistic perspective. The nurse should emphasize the patient's strengths when he is communicating only a feeling of weakness or, conversely, point out his resistance in resolving an immediate problem. This tool must be used honestly, constructively, and with integrity, for confrontation may precipitate a crisis. However, often through crisis the alcoholic begins to take steps toward seeking recovery.

5. *Community.* Information regarding references available on an outpa-

tient basis should be provided. An additional strong reinforcement is a follow-up by the nurse or a social worker. Nurses have a greater opportunity to be in contact with patients in the hospital and in the community, and they can provide a strategic force in influencing change in this problem area.

It is vital in counseling the alcoholic patient to include his significant others as an added support, to help set realistic perceptions of the situation, and to set realistic goals, as well as anticipatory planning for the future. Counseling can be on an individual, conjoint, family, collateral, or group basis. The wives who become active participants in counseling benefit greatly and, ultimately, through awareness and growth, find that *they themselves* cannot force their partners to give up drinking. Once accepting this they can give more consideration to their own needs.

The nursing intervention of patients with alcoholic behavior disorder is ordinarily as difficult as their psychiatric therapy. They are persons who tend to be charming and likable but who do not wear well and are constantly disappointing. The situation created by constant disappointment in the patient is rife with attitude difficulties for personnel.

Because of their inability to tolerate anxiety and their customary reliance on the anxiety-solvent properties of alcohol, patients often need a well-controlled environment for a period of several months in the initial stages of their treatment. If the behavior disorder is sufficiently bizarre, as in delirium tremens or Korsakoff's syndrome, hospitalization is definitely indicated for treatment during the acute stage. Should the treatment of any alcoholic disorder stop with detoxification, however, the only accomplishment is a patient who is in better physical shape to continue drinking. Treatment must be oriented to personality rehabilitation. An environment in which the patient cannot secure alcohol and in which a full program of activities is available when the patient is ready is ideal.

Interpersonal relationships of a therapeutic nature are one of the alcoholic patient's greatest needs, but the establishment of such relationships is not easy. The major obstacles are the patient's inability to face his own problems and fears, his skillful rationalization and minimization of his drinking, his extreme sensitivity, his characteristic ambivalence, and his critically rebellious attitude toward hospitalization that develops a month or two after his admission.

The patient usually comes for treatment in poor physical condition. After a period of prolonged drinking, he is concerned about himself and anxious to be helped. He may be a little ashamed and sensitive about his drinking, so special care is indicated to keep from reinforcing such feelings about himself. As he improves physically, which occurs fairly quickly, he is grateful, congenial, and obviously enjoys feeling physically well again. It is here that personnel most often make the mistake of accepting the patient's explanations and reassurances at face value and letting the patient know that they expect much from him. The patient's minimization of his difficulties and his rationalization of his behavior at this stage are a clever camouflage. A neutral attitude of understanding without being overly sympathetic should be followed. No criticism or judgment, expressed or implied, should be indulged. The patient seems so rational that it is difficult to avoid the temptation to reason him out of his alcoholism. Although the patient will talk extensively, careful listening will indicate that there is also much that is not being told, and that which is not being told is the more important of the two. The patient may brag about episodes that should be listened to calmly and without comment. As soon as possible the patient should be encouraged to participate in a daily program of activities, even though he may be able to convince the nurse that it is not necessary for him since he is quite well, has learned his lesson, and will be all right forever. Behind the patient's smooth facade is a lonely and fearful individual who is unable to look at his fears or admit his problems.

When the patient begins to feel physically well, he will want to go home, stating that he is able to deal with life again. Any suggestion that he begin to come to grips with his problems brings forth evasiveness and negativism. The patient becomes rebellious and critical, turning on everyone associated with the institution. This behavior should be accepted without criticism or disciplinary or emotional retaliation, particularly from the accused personnel. The patient is threatened by the prospect of facing himself and the motives for his alcoholism. Anxiety becomes apparent, and considerable resentment and hostility are expressed in words and in actions. This critical period for the patient requires much understanding, interest, and support on the part of nurses and other personnel. The hostility toward personnel should be accepted matter-of-factly, and its outward expression should not be discouraged. Once this phase begins to subsiae, the patient may be expected to show improvement with a more positive outlook toward psychotherapy.

Most alcoholic patients are ambivalent in their emotional reactions to other people, and evidences of this are to be expected and calmly accepted. It is part and parcel of the patient's problems and is best expressed in the neutral atmosphere the patient needs.

Alcoholic patients need careful attention to complete physical rehabilitation. A diet high in vitamin content and with an above average caloric intake helps in the initial stages to promote recovery. Attention should be paid to all phases of personal hygiene, since most patients have neglected it prior to admission. Not only should physical cleanliness be promoted but also particular efforts should be directed to the cultivation of personal appearance for its psychologic aspect. As the patient's physical condition improves, he will need all his assets in the difficult period of readjustment.

As soon as possible the patient should be placed on a regular routine emphasizing health habits, including exercise. Any defects or infections should receive prompt attention. Disfiguring scars that may have been acquired on a spree should be corrected, if possible.

The patient's protective needs are related to the stage of his illness during hospitalization. When he is confused, disoriented, and restless, he may injure himself unintentionally and should therefore be constantly observed to prevent injury. As he recovers, if any depression is evident, the danger of suicide is present. The patient should be closely observed, kept active if possible, given an outlet for his hostility, and given the emotional support of personnel through interest and attention.

When the patient becomes rebellious, he needs observation to prevent an escape from the hospital. He may also try to injure himself in an attempt to convince his family and hospital personnel that home is the best place for him.

The alcoholic patient tends to be in but not of groups. He will need tactful direction to participate, will need help in toning down his superior attitude toward those he thinks are sick, and will need encouragement to accept any responsibility for group activities. Any particular talent or ability the patient has should be promoted in group activities. Careful supervision to determine which other patients, if any, are upset by his comments during his critical period should be observed. When the patient's behavior is detrimental to others, free ventilation before personnel may help to tone him down with others. If the patient shows a tendency to associate with personnel and not with other patients, he may be brought into group activities through participation with personnel in the group.

The following case study illustrates some techniques one may use when working with patients who are dependent on alcohol.

> Tom M., a 52-year-old male, was admitted to a large general hospital after receiving a stab wound during a brawl in a bar. After he had received care in the emergency room for his wound, he was sent to the psychiatric unit because he was intoxicated. Treatment was started to detoxify him.
>
> The next day, while changing the dressing on his wound, a nurse noted that his fingernails were quite long and that he was nervously picking at the cuticles. She asked if he would like to have his nails trimmed. He looked startled and replied, rather sheepishly, "Yes, I would, I just haven't had time." The nurse said that she would return later and trim them.
>
> Approximately an hour later the nurse returned with a basin of warm soapy water, scissors, hand lotion, and towels. She smiled and asked, "Are you ready for your manicure?" He replied, "Yes" and stared intently at the nurse as she put the items on his bedside table. She placed a towel and the basin on his

lap and asked him to put his hands in the basin to soak, explaining that it would be easier to trim his nails if they were soft. He did as she asked and she sat down in a chair by his bed. She jokingly said, "I'm not the greatest manicurist in the world, but you will have to settle for me—since I'm the only one available."

Tom smiled slightly and said, "I appreciate your taking the time to do this." The nurse stated that she was happy to be of help. He looked at the nurse and asked quietly, "You know I am an alcoholic?" She answered, "Yes, I know— why do you ask?" He began to tell her of his many bad experiences in hospitals with staff who treated him "like a piece of dirt." She listened and let him ventilate his feelings regarding his previous hospitalizations. Afterward he appeared to relax.

The nurse began to trim his nails and asked him to tell her about himself, and why he thought he abused alcohol. Tom, apparently sensing the nurse's interest and genuine concern, began telling her about his life. He stated that he was the oldest of four sons and had grown up on a farm in the middle west. He described his childhood as one of "work, work, work . . . and beatings by my father." The nurse asked what his mother was like. He said she was very passive, completely dominated by his father, and very undemonstrative to her children. He was asked, "Did you feel that she loved you?" Tom answered bitterly, "No, how could she? She never stopped my father from making us work like dogs—or beating us!"

He was asked when he had started drinking. He replied, "As soon as I could; I think I had my first drink when I was 13." He stated that he had run away from home when he was 16 and had never been back. He continued, saying that he had lied about his age and joined the Army, where he *really* began drinking as often and as much as he could. He stayed in the Army for 8 years because he had nothing else to do.

After the Army he moved to the city where he got a job as a used car salesman, which he really enjoyed, and he did quite well financially. When asked if his drinking pattern changed when he was working, he said that he continued to drink after work and on his days off, but not as much as he did when he was in the Army. He was asked if he was still working and he replied, "I got fired 6 weeks ago, and Mary, my wife, moved out. She took our two children and every stick of furniture 3 weeks ago." The nurse expressed her concern over both incidents and asked why he had been fired.

Tom said that he and Mary had been arguing about his drinking for the past 3 months—"all she did was nag, nag, nag"—and he had gone to work drunk. A customer had complained and he had been fired. He was asked why Mary had left him and he stated that she had said she was sick of his drinking and did not think it was good for the children to see him drunk most of the time. He was asked about his children and tears flooded his eyes. He said, "I love them so much I don't want to live without them. I know I shouldn't drink, but I can't help it. It's too late now."

The nurse said, "Tell me about your wife—what is she like?" Tom said that Mary was a wonderful woman and a great mother, was well liked in her job as a hairdresser, and was 5 years older than he. He said they had been married 12 years and that the first years of their marriage had been wonderful. Their children, Joseph, age 11, and Lillian, age 9½, were marvelous. He added ruefully, "I have to give Mary all the credit—she really kept us all in line."

The nurse asked what *he* had tried to do to stop drinking and he replied, "Nothing, really." He was then asked if he really did want to stop drinking and he replied, firmly, "Yes, very much. I want Mary and the children back." He was asked if he knew about Alcoholics Anonymous. He said he had heard about it but didn't know anyone in it. The nurse said she could have someone from AA come to the hospital and discuss their program with him if he wished. He said he would like to talk to someone about the program.

The nurse called AA and told them about Tom and his problem, and two members came the next day and talked with him. They continued to visit him during the 10 days he was in the hospital. The nurse called his wife and told her that Tom was talking with members of AA and that it was possible he might start attending their meetings when he was released from the hospital. She was told that AA also had groups to lend support to the wives and children of alcoholics. Mary reluctantly agreed to visit Tom in the hospital "just to talk" and to meet with the members of AA who were visiting Tom.

After Tom's discharge from the hospital the nurse talked with the members of AA at intervals and was told that Tom was a very active member, that he was working again, and that he and Mary were back together. Approximately 4 years after Tom's hospitalization, the nurse requested AA members to visit a young alcoholic, and one member was Tom! He looked well and very happy.

While this case study illustrates that Alcoholics Anonymous was effective with a patient who was dependent on alcohol, it is not our intent to imply that it would be successful with *every* patient.

REFERENCES

Aguilera, D. C., and Messick, J. M.: Crisis intervention: theory and methodology, ed. 3, St. Louis, 1978, The C. V. Mosby Co.

Alcoholism, addiction, depression: a nurse's story, Nurs. Outlook 13:48-49, 1965.

Andrews, L., McKenzie, L., and Chotlos, J.: The "game" and the alcoholic patients, Am. J. Nurs. 67:1672-1674, 1967.

Bales, R. F.: Cultural differences in rates of alcoholism, Q. J. Stud. Alcohol 6:480, 1946.

Block, M. A.: Alcoholism is many illnesses, Nurs. Outlook 13:35-37, 1965.

Byrne, M.: Resocialization of the chronic alcoholic, Am. J. Nurs. 68:99-100, 1968.

Canning, M. G.: Care of alcoholic patients, Am. J. Nurs. 65:113-114, 1965.

English, H., and English, A.: Psychiatric dictionary, New York, 1958, David McKay Co.

Field, W. E., and Reutke, W.: Hallucinations and how to deal with them, Am. J. Nurs. 73:638-640, 1973.

Fitzig, C.: Nursing in an alcohol program, Am. J. Nurs. 66:2218-2221, 1966.

Fowler, G. R.: Understanding the patient who uses alcohol to solve his problems, Nurs. Forum 4(4):6-15, 1965.

Freed, E. X.: The crucial factor in alcoholism, Am. J. Nurs. 68:2614-2616, 1968.

Glover, E.: The etiology of drug addiction, Int. J. Psychoanal. 13:298-328, 1932.

Jellinek, E. M.: In World Health Organization Technical Report Series No. 48, 1952.

Knight, R. P.: The psychodynamics of chronic alcoholism, J. Nerv. Ment. Dis. 86:538-548, 1937.

Kogen, K. L., and Jackson, J. K.: Role perception in wives of alcoholics and nonalcoholics, Q. J. Stud. Alc. 24:627-639, 1963.

Kolb, L. C.: Modern clinical psychiatry, ed. 8, Philadelphia, 1973, W. B. Saunders Co., pp. 204-222.

McNatt, J., and Sahler, S.: Alcoholism: caring for the alcoholic on a medical unit, Am. J. Nurs. **65:**114-116, 1965.

Menninger, K. A.: Man against himself, New York, 1938, Harcourt, Brace & Co.

Morton, E. L.: Nursing care in an alcoholic unit, Nurs. Outlook **14:**45-47, 1966.

Mueller, J. F., and others: The role of the nurse in counseling the alcoholic, J. Psychiatric Nurse **12:**26-32, 1974.

Parry, A. A.: Alcoholism, Am. J. Nurs. **65:**111-114, 1965.

Price, G. M.: Alcoholism—a family, community, and nursing problem, Am. J. Nurs. **67:**1022-1025, 1967.

Rado, S.: The psychoanalysis of pharmacothmia, Psychoanal. Q. **2:**1-23, 1933.

Tahka, V.: The alcoholic personality, a clinical study, Helsinki, 1966, The Finnish Foundation for Alcoholic Studies, pp. 15-16.

Tamerin. J. S., and Mendelson, J. H.: The psychodynamics of chronic inebriation: observations of alcoholics during the process of drinking in an experimental group setting, Am. J. Psychiatry **125:**886-899, 1969.

Thompson, G. N.: Acute and chronic alcoholic conditions. In Arieti, S., editor: American handbook of psychiatry, vol. 2, New York, 1959, Basic Books, Inc., pp. 1203-1221.

Trice, H. M.: Alcoholism in America, New York, 1966, McGraw-Hill Book Co.

World Health Organization, Expert Committee on Mental Health, Technical Report Series, No. 48, 1952.

ADDITIONAL READINGS

Alcoholism, alcohol: a hidden factor in physical illness, RN **37:**31-34, 1974.

Beck, R. A.: The diabetic alcoholic, RN **37:**35, 1974.

Beigel, A.: Drug abuse patients in a general hospital, Hospitals **48**(20):65-68, 70, 1974.

Bier, W. C.: Problems in addiction; alcohol and drugs, New York, 1962, Fordham University Press.

Blane, H.: The personality of the alcoholic; guises of dependency, New York, 1968, Harper and Row, Publishers.

Dickinson, C.: The alcoholic: an unperson? Nurs. Forum **14**(2):194-203, 1975.

Dickson, M.: Involvement of the spouse in treatment of the alcoholic, Nurse Mirror **139:**77-79, 1974.

Diethelm, O.: Etiology of the chronic alcoholic, Springfield, Ill., 1955, Charles C Thomas, Publisher.

Estes, N. J.: Counseling the wife of an alcoholic spouse, Am. J. Nurs. **74:**1251-1255, 1974.

Funston, F. D.: Detoxification: an alternate in transition, Can. Nurse **69:**27-29, 1973.

Heinemann, M. E.: Caring for patients with alcohol problems, J. Psychiatr. Nurs. **12**(6):34-38, 1974.

Irgens-Jensen, O.: Problem drinking and personality, No. 9, 1971, The National Institute for Alcoholic Research, pp. 9-15.

Jackson, K. M.: Chronic alcoholism, a case study, Nurs. Times **70:**1104-1107, 1974.

Laman, K. J.: Selected behavior characteristics of alcoholics and their spouses, Can. J. Pub. Health **65:**221-223, 1974.

Mueller, J. F.: Treatment for the alcoholic: cursing or nursing, Am. J. Nurs. **74:**245-247, 1974.

Orr, J.: Nursing care study. Frank—an environmental alcoholic, Nurs. Times **71**(19):726-727, 1975.

Rosen, E., and Gregory, I.: Abnormal psychology, Philadelphia, 1965, W. B. Saunders Co., pp. 397-421.

Schonbeck, J. M.: Christmas is, Am. J. Nurs. **74**(12):2192-2193, 1974.

Seixas, F. A.: Uncovering and counseling the alcoholic, RN **37:**36-37, 1974.

Slater, A. M.: Nursing care study: David—an alcoholic, Nurs. Times **71**(6):214-216, 1975.

CHAPTER 16

Patients who abuse other substances

Overdoses of drugs cause many health and mental health emergencies. The substances that act on the mind and influence behavior include not only narcotics and other illegal drugs but also prescribed medications such as tranquilizers and sedatives and even over-the-counter drugs such as Sominex. The overdoses may occur as a suicide attempt, by accident during periods of confusion or alcoholic intoxication, or from unsupervised self-medication. A related tragedy is the accidental poisoning of young children by drugs prescribed for adults in the family.

The first line of defense against substance abuse is prevention. The prescribing physician has the primary responsibility of preventing patients from acquiring large amounts of dangerous drugs. Any prescribing of large drug quantities to disturbed patients on an outpatient basis is unwise and unjustifiable. Unfortunately, the potentially lethal dose of some drugs is much lower than most physicians realize. Patients with depression are known to be high risks for suicide. In prescribing antidepressant therapy, the physician should be aware that an overdose consisting of a normal 10- to 14-day supply of the drug can be fatal. Therefore, the physician must decide whether it is feasible to treat seriously depressed individuals as outpatients. If a responsible relative cannot supervise the administration of the drug, admission to a hospital may be preferable. Another problem is that patients receiving long-term drug treatment frequently fail to take their medication regularly. This failure not only deprives them of the drug's therapeutic effect but also allows them to accumulate potential supplies for an overdose attempt.

The first rule of prevention is to use caution and common sense in prescribing psychotropic drugs. They are not harmless compounds, especially the newer tranquilizers and antidepressants.

Even when a physican makes every effort to prescribe drugs conscientiously, suicide attempts are still possible. Patients can mislead their physicians, and no physician should be so naive as to assume that this cannot happen. Also, patients with chronic anxiety or depression may seek care from two or more physicians at one time, receiving prescriptions from each.

Impulsive suicide attempts might be discouraged by packaging drugs individually. A hundred tablets are easily poured from a bottle and swallowed; it takes more time to take the same number from individual foil wrappers and it may be frustrating and time-consuming. The use of child-proof bottles for drugs offers a hopeful note in reducing accidental drug deaths of children.

A suicide associated with psychotropic drugs may take several forms. The patient may be discovered in a comatose or heavily sedated state by a friend, relative, or policeman. Another patient may be highly excited, agitated, or delirious. Or the patient may exhibit psychotic behavior and be out of contact with reality. In many cases, serious physical signs, such as hypotension, shock, pulmonary edema, or respiratory failure, may dominate the clinical picture and obscure the underlying cause of the problem.

Often one can pinpoint drug overdose as the cause of the emergency simply from the history given by the patient. He may admit to substance abuse or say that he has taken medications in a suicide attempt. Information can also come from relatives or friends, especially if the patient is unable to communicate coherently. Sometimes a suicide note or an open bottle of medication is found at the scene. In these circumstances, if the patient is heavily sedated or comatose, one should assume, at least tentatively, that a drug overdose is responsible for the condition. One should always remember that drug poisoning frequently occurs in conjunction with alcohol intoxication.

The treatment of drug overdose involves three basic methods: (1) the prevention of further absorption, if possible, (2) supportive therapy, and (3) specific antidotal measures.

Prevention of further absorption is useful only with poisoning from recently ingested drugs. In the case of a conscious patient, induced vomiting is more effective than gastric lavage and should be attempted when possible. This method should not be used with unconscious patients who may aspirate the vomitus. Another method involves the use of activated charcoal, a substance that binds with many drugs and can be effective in reducing further absorption. It should be instilled in the stomach with a lavage tube following drug-induced vomiting or gastric aspiration. The use of cathartics to promote excretion of any drug residual is of unproved value. These three conservative measures, combined with careful observations, are usually sufficient in mild drug poisoning.

In more severe cases, the most important aspect of care is supportive treatment. The management of complications associated with large overdoses, such as coma, shock, or respiratory failure, requires skilled medical care. It is important to monitor cardiac function, blood pressure, central venous pressure, respiration, temperature, renal output, level of consciousness, and other parameters of body function.

DRUG LETHALITY

To gain some understanding of the lethality of drugs, it is essential to have some idea of the principles of drug action. By definition, drugs are chemicals taken into the body to alter bodily physiology and to gain certain effects. The *main action* of the drug is its action on the primary target organ; however, drugs have more than one action and therefore act on multiple target organs; this is known as the *side effects*. Some more terms should be defined for clarity:

habituation the repetitive use of a drug for psychologic purposes.

addiction state characterized by severe physiologic changes that take place when use of a chemical agent is stopped. This results in the withdrawal or abstinence syndrome, such as sneezing, coughing, tremor, restlessness, insomnia, retching, sweating, tearing, etc.

tolerance state in which use of a chemical agent requires more of that agent, with time, to achieve the desired effect. (An addict may use enough of a drug at one time to kill someone who has not developed an increased tolerance.)

potentiation combined use of two or more agents that has a greater effect than simple summation ($1 + 1 = 4$).

lethality the amount of drug that constitutes a fatal dose.

Lethality varies from drug to drug and has been studied retrospectively in humans by examining hospital records. Statistics have been developed showing the LD_{50} (lethal dose$_{50}$), or the amount of the drug necessary to produce lethality in 50% of the population. This is on a bell-shaped curve. The lethal dose depends on the following factors:

1. Sex or weight (a smaller dose is lethal in women)
2. Age (less of the drug is necessary in children and the older age groups)
3. Relationship to meals (a full stomach inhibits abosrption, an empty one increases the rapidity of absorption)
4. Method of administration (the less common intravenous route is four to five times more potent and can cause infections, thrombi, and emboli)
5. Combination of drugs (potentiation)
6. Degree of addiction

The lethal dose can thus have a great range, but an average dose that will kill half the population as been calculated. A concept illustrating the relative

safety margin of drugs describes the lethal dose as a multiple of the usual dose
(× usual dose). Thus some drugs have greater or lesser margins of safety.
Tables 5 to 8 present the lethality of current drugs for adults. Included are the
generic name, trade name, street name (when known), usual dose and form,
lethal dose, and the number of capsules or tablets that constitute a lethal dose.
The data presented are general guidelines *only*, and no attempt has been made
to discuss antidotes. Since medications are usually given three to four times
daily, the lethal dose is a factor times each individual dose. Some medications
(such as sedatives) are given only once, at bedtime; these are indicated.

Table 5 presents the data on alcohol (the most commonly used and abused
drug) and the barbiturates, both short-acting and long-acting. Table 6 presents
the lethality of the nonbarbiturates, analgesics, and narcotics. Table 7 presents
the lethality of the minor and major tranquilizers, and Table 8 presents the
lethality of antidepressants.

It is wise to remember that combinations of drugs (such as alcohol and barbiturates) potentiate each other and can result in lower lethal dosages than

Table 5. Lethality of alcohol and barbiturates

DRUG NAME		USUAL DOSE	FORM	LETHAL DOSE
GENERIC	TRADE			
Alcohol				
Ethyl (% = 2 × proof)		4 to 6 oz	Liquid	30 oz
Isopropyl rubbing alcohol		None	Liquid	2 to 8 oz
Methyl (denatured spirits, wood alcohol)		None	Liquid	1 oz
Barbiturates				
Short-acting				
Amobarbital ("blues")	Amytal	0.2 gm daily	0.2 gm capsule	2 to 4 gm (20 to 30 capsules)
Amobarbital/secobarb- ital ("half & halfs")	Tuinal	0.1 gm daily	0.1 gm capsule	1.2 to 2 gm (12 to 20 capsules)
Pentobarbital ("yellows")	Nembutal	0.1 gm daily	0.1 gm capsule	1.2 to 2 gm (12 to 20 capsules)
Secobarbital ("reds")	Seconal	0.1 gm daily	0.1 gm capsule	1.2 to 2 gm (12 to 20 capsules)
Long-acting				
Butabarbital	Butisol	50 to 100 mg for sleep	0.1 gm tablet	10 gm (100 tablets)
Phenobarbital	Luminal	0.1 gm for sleep; 32 mg t.i.d. for sedation	0.1 gm capsule	10 gm (100 capsules)

Table 6. Lethality of nonbarbiturates, analgesics, and narcotics

DRUG NAME		USUAL DOSE	FORM	LETHAL DOSE
GENERIC	TRADE			
Nonbarbiturates				
Bromide	Bromo-Seltzer	2 to 4 oz	Powder	Nonlethal; overdose causes delirium
Chloral hydrate ("knockout drops")		1 gm for sleep	0.5- or 1-gm capsules	12 to 24 gm
Ethchlorvynol	Placidyl	500 mg for sleep	0.5-gm capsules	10 gm (20 capsules)
Flurazepam	Dalmane	30 mg for sleep	15- to 30 mg capsules	90 mg
Glutethimide	Doriden	0.5 gm for sleep	0.5-gm tablet	10 gm (20 tablets)
Methaqualone ("sopors")	Quaalude, Parest	150 to 300 mg	150- to 300-mg tablets	4.5 gm (15 tablets)
Methyprylon	Noludar	0.3 gm	0.3-gm capsules	10 gm (30 capsules)
Analgesics				
Aspirin and aspirin combinations	Empirin, Bufferin, Anacin	0.6 gm every 4 hr	0.3-gm tablets	30 to 60 gm (100 to 200 tablets)
Dextropropoxyphene	Darvon	65 mg every 4 hr	65-mg capsules	6.5 gm (100 capsules)
Narcotics				
Codeine (heroin)		0.05 to 1 gr	0.05- to 1-gr tablets	Lethal dose of narcotics depends on concentration, etc.
Dihydrohydroxy-codeinone	Percodan	5 to 20 mg for pain	1-ml ampules	
Dihydromorphinone	Dilaudid	2 to 4 mg t.i.d. for pain	1- to 4-mg tablets	
Meperidine	Demerol	50 to 150 mg for pain	50- to 150-mg tablets	
Methadone	Dolophine	2.5 to 10 mg t.i.d. for pain	5- to 10-mg tablets	
Morphine		¼ to 1 gr	¼- to 1-gr tablets	
Pantopium	Pantopon	5 to 20 mg for pain	1-ml ampules	

those shown in the tables. In general, a dose half the lethal dose described here will generally be nonlethal. Variations on the bell-shaped curve must be taken into account. If the drug taker is elderly, a child, a small woman, or has taken other drugs, this must be reconsidered, since the figures in the tables are standardized to apply to a male adult weighing 150 pounds.

Table 7. Lethality of minor and major tranquilizers

DRUG NAME		USUAL DOSE	FORM	LETHAL DOSE
GENERIC	TRADE			
Minor				
Chlordiazepoxide	Librium	10 mg t.i.d.	10-mg capsules	0.5 to 1.5 gm (50 to 150 capsules)
Diazepam	Valium	10 mg. t.i.d.	10-mg capsules	0.5 to 1 gm (50 to 100 capsules)
Meprobamate	Miltown, Equanil	0.5 gm q.i.d.	0.5-gm tablet	14 to 25 gm (28 to 50 tablets)
Oxazepam	Serax	30 mg t.i.d.	30-mg tablets	3 to 6 gm (100 to 200 tablets)
Major				
Chlorpromazine	Thorazine	10 mg t.i.d.	10-, 25-, 20-mg tablets	Essentially nonlethal; lethal dose 1,000 times usual dose
Chlorprothixene	Taractan	25 mg t.i.d.	25- to 100-mg tablets	
Haloperidol	Haldol	1.5 mg b.i.d.	½- to 2-mg tablets	
Hydroxyzine	Atarax	25 mg t.i.d.	10- to 100-mg tablets	
Mesoridazine	Serentil	50 mg t.i.d.	10- to 100-mg tablets	
Perphenazine	Trilafon	8 mg t.i.d.	4- to 16-mg tablets	
Prochlorperazine	Compazine	10 mg t.i.d.	5- to 10-mg tablets	
Promazine	Sparine	50 mg t.i.d.	10- to 200-mg tablets	
Thioridazine	Mellaril	100 mg t.i.d.	10- to 200-mg tablets	
Thiothixene	Navane	2 mg t.i.d.	1- to 10-mg capsules	
Trifluoperazine	Stelazine	2 mg b.i.d.	1- to 2-mg tablets	

Exact lethal doses have not been exactly established in all categores (especially new drugs) and are obtained by extrapolation. In general, no guarantees can be made about the correctness of the data, though they are based on current literature. In case of doubt, one should *always* consult with a physician experienced in matters of overdose.

NARCOTICS

Substance abusers refer to narcotics as "hard stuff" and indicate these to be the exalted heights that the neophyte may attain in substance abuse. Opi-

Table 8. Lethality of antidepressants

DRUG NAME		USUAL DOSE	FORM	LETHAL DOSE
GENERIC	**TRADE**			
Stimulants				
Dextroamphetamine sulfate	Dexedrine	5 to 10 mg	5-mg tablets or capsules	200 to 500 mg (40 to 100 tablets)
Methamphetamine ("speed")	Desoxyn	10 to 15 mg	5- to 15-mg tablets	200 to 500 mg (40 to 100 tablets)
Methylphenidate	Ritalin	10 mg b.i.d.	10-mg tablets	0.4 to 2 gm (40 to 200 tablets)
Racemic amphetamine	Benzedrine	5 to 10 mg	5-mg tablets or capsules	200 to 500 mg (40 to 100 tablets)
Monamine oxidase inhibitors				
Isocarboxazid	Marplan	These drugs rarely used at present; dangerous		
Nialamide	Niamid			
Tranylcypromine	Parnate			
Tricyclics				
Amitriptyline	Elavil	25 mg 3 to 6 times daily	25-mg tablet	2 to 4 gm (75 to 150 tablets)
Desipramine	Norpramin, Pertofrane	25 mg 3 to 6 times daily	25-mg tablet	2 to 4 gm (75 to 150 tablets)
Doxepin	Sinequan	25 mg 3 to 6 times daily	25-mg tablet	2 to 4 gm (75 to 150 tablets)
Imipramine	Tofranil	25 mg 3 to 6 times daily	25-mg tablet	2 to 4 gm (75 to 150 tablets)
Nortriptyline	Aventyl	25 mg 3 to 6 times daily	25-mg tablet	2 to 4 gm (75 to 150 tablets)

um and its derivatives have long been used by humans to produce a euphoric sense of well-being and tranquility. The most commonly used opiate is heroin. The pharmacologic substitutes for opiates, dihydromorphinone (Dilaudid), metopon, and meperidine (Demerol), are also used, depending on their availability. Having been exposed to the comforting effects of the drug, individuals resort to it repeatedly when under stress and pressure, until the habit is firmly established. Although the habitual use of these drugs results in physical and psychologic dependence, not all addicts show signs of major or minor mental illnesses. However, the continued use and dependence on narcotics often results in numerous physical discomforts, particularly when the drug dose is not readily available. Their ability to function and assume responsibility for self and family becomes an area of serious conflict. The abuser withdraws into his own world and seeks out his own kind for understanding and as a means of assuring knowledge of where the drug may be secured. His need for increased amounts of the drug demands more money. His inability to hold a job makes him beg or steal money from his family and friends. When this is not possible, he is driven to crimes of prostitution, assault, burglary, and even murder.

Narcotic addiction is related to the opportunity to acquire the drug and to the need for it. In some instances the first experience of the drug's effects is related to a prescribed dosage by a physician for an illness. The habit is more likely to be developed through association with other substance abusers, with whom a source of supply for the drug is established. For physicians, nurses, and other health workers, the availability of drugs presents a serious temptation, particularly in times of stress.

The prolonged use of morphine tends to result in social isolation and deterioration of personal habits. The patient's physical dependence on the drug and his inability to tolerate the anxiety and physical symptoms that go with a lack of morphine drive him to almost any lengths to secure it. Because of this and because the Harrison Act makes the possession and use of the opium derivatives without a license a criminal offense, the morphine abuser often comes into conflict with the law. The patient becomes increasingly less efficient and devotes less energy to ordinary goals and ambitions. His life becomes increasingly oriented to securing an adequate supply of his drug, and the amount needed tends to increase gradually as the body builds a tolerance. Many addicts take enough morphine in a single dose to kill a person not accustomed to the drug. The physical picture of the patient is rather typical: emaciation, grayish complexion, tremors, constricted pupils, poor speech coordination, coated tongue, halitosis, and marked constipation.

The abrupt withdrawal of morphine or other opium alkaloids produces a definite withdrawal or abstinence syndrome. The severity of the symptoms will depend on the length of time the patient has been an abuser and the dosage to which he is accustomed. Initial symptoms are yawning, lacrimation, sneezing, perspiration, and restlessness, followed by anorexia, muscular pains, and tremors. More severe manifestations are fever, increased restlessness and irritability, insomnia, and elevated blood pressure. Vomiting, diarrhea, weight loss, and prostration mark the most severe reactions. Because of the dangers of the withdrawal reaction, the sudden and complete removal of narcotics has been possible only since the use of methadone and other drugs has given evidence of the ability to control the symptoms of withdrawal.

Narcotic antagonists are new and experimental. They are being used in conjunction with methadone as a means of eliminating the pleasurable effects of the opiates. Experimenters have found that with the use of cyclazocine and naloxone patients are able to reduce their need for opiates and return to their work and home activities. Narcotic antagonists have also been used with methadone to alleviate the painful withdrawal symptoms. They have helped the patient to use psychotherapy and rehabilitation services more effectively for restoration to his family and community. Continued experimentation and validation need to be done. However, dependency on methadone has been noted.

The intensity of the withdrawal symptoms is directly related to the degree of physical dependence and the amount of the drug customarily used. Usually, the symptoms increase 8 to 12 hours after the last dose. This is followed by a peak reached between 36 and 72 hours and a gradual diminution over the following 5 or 10 days. It is not unusual for weakness, insomnia, nervousness, and muscle aches and pains to continue for several weeks. In severe cases, death has been known to occur. Some reports reveal that chlorpromazine has effectively alleviated the withdrawal syndrome in narcotic addiction and has made it possible for patients to participate more easily in psychotherapy.

Among users of narcotics, a whole new culture exists with its own jargon to exclude and confuse the uninformed outsider. Among other names, heroin is junk, H, horse, and smack; morphine is Miss Emma, M, and white stuff. It is not unusual to find groups forming with their own particular jargon and rituals. The nurse and therapist in attempting to reach the substance abuser must understand his terminology and the meaning of his experiences as opposed to values and practices of the "straight" life.

SEDATIVES AND DEPRESSANTS

Man's proclivity to use of and dependence on barbiturates has a long history. The use of barbiturates has become a major social problem because of the extensive prescription of the drugs by the medical profession, the calming effect of the drugs, and the ease with which the drugs can be obtained. Various preparations are widely used for their quieting effect and to produce sleep. Patients with neurotic tendencies find them a comfortable prop to allay anxiety and apprehension. Barbiturate preparations such as pentobarbital (Nembutal), amobarbital (Amytal), secobarbital (Seconal), and phenobarbital (Luminal) are prescribed over long periods of time.

Overdoses of barbiturates within a short period can cause a typical acute toxic reaction with delirium or death. Prolonged use may cause dullness and lethargy, and if continued for years, it may also result in gradual personality deterioration accompanied by organic symptoms such as memory defect, confusion, disorientation, poor judgment, and reduced intellectual capacity. This, however, is not the inevitable outcome; some persons use barbiturates for years without personality or intellectual deterioration. When the drug is stopped, the anxiety and tension return. Reliance on barbiturates is rather extensive among people who are familiar with their effects. The nurse who takes amphetamine (Benzedrine) to stay awake on night duty and barbiturates for sleeping during the day is not so rare as one might wish.

Another group of depressants, the nonbarbiturates, is also popular. Some commonly used nonbarbiturates are glutethimide, ethchlorvynol, ethinamate, and methyprylon, to name a few. This group and the barbiturates—commonly referred to as goof balls, barbs, birds, rainbows, and others—are widely used by substance abusers.

With individuals accustomed to a steady dosage of these drugs by prescription or by abuse, their abrupt withdrawal may precipitate severe convulsions. It is imperative that the person come under the supervision of a physician during the withdrawal process because lifesaving methods may be necessary.

During the initial 8 to 12 hours after the last dose, there is an indication of improvement. This is followed by the withdrawal pattern, including increasing nervousness, headache, anxiety, muscle twitching, tremor, weakness, insomnia, nausea, and a sudden drop in blood pressure when the person stands abruptly. These symptoms become severe at about 24 hours. Convulsions that may be severe enough to cause death and encephalographic changes develop within 36 to 72 hours. A period of mental confusion, delirium, and hallucination, similar to alcoholic delirium tremens, may also develop. This delirium, which may be accompanied by agitation and eventual exhaustion, may continue over a period of several days. When the particular drug cannot be identified in time to counteract its effect, the patient may die.

The individual who seeks help to reverse his dependence on drugs should be given sincere encouragement. The dread of the withdrawal experience is a great factor in deterring addicts from seeking help. The methadone maintenance program has helped in lessening the withdrawal symptoms and in maintaining the person on a functional level, so he is able to participate in social and work rehabilitation. Although there are many who advocate the principles underlying methadone maintenance, there are also those who claim it is trading one addiction for a more convenient one.

Methadone as a synthetic narcotic is relatively inexpensive, long lasting in effect (24 to 36 hours), and usually administered orally. Small doses are used to alleviate the expected withdrawal symptoms, and then the dose is gradually increased from 80 to 120 mg. This maintenance dose is said to relieve the craving for the "hard stuff." The proponents of methadone therapy prefer to provide treatment on an outpatient basis. The opportunity to work with the patient in his natural setting, the community, and to help him as he encounters the pressures of survival within his own social configuration is a more realistic approach. Treatment in the hospital does remove the abuser from a source of easy supply, and at times, this may be necessary. However, without continued support after he returns to his home base, the abuser may not be able to deal with or survive the pressure of his peer group. In a methadone clinic, the multidisciplinary team usually consists of a wide spectrum of professionals and semiprofessionals; physicians, nurses, psychologists, social workers, and clergy are included on this team. It is not unusual to find a number of former substance abusers who, as members of the working team, give validation to the patient who says: "*You* don't know what it's like."

With the alarming increase in the use of drugs, it has been evident that abusers may resort to hallucinogens for mind expansion, speed pills (amphetamines) for mood elevation, and depressants to come down. Under such circumstances, it is quite possible that the user will take an indiscriminate dose and be a victim of an overdose (OD). It is vitally important to ascertain the drugs that were used in the overdose to effectively treat the victim. The symptoms of overdose with barbiturates, heroin, and tranquilizers may be similar. A critical sign to look for is the pupil size—dilated with barbiturates and constricted with heroin. The telltale needle marks on the arms or legs may also be indicators of heroin addiction.

TRANQUILIZERS

Tranquilizers are relatively new drugs. They have had widespread use in American society because of their comforting and efficient effects. Although they reduce tension and anxiety, unlike the barbiturates they do not produce sleep or greatly impair mental and physical function. Generally, tranquilizers may be classified as major (those with antipsychotic activity) or minor (those that do not affect psychotic conditions).

The major tranquilizers include phenothiazines and the reserpine type drugs. These drugs do not appear to cause physical dependence and are not known as drugs of abuse.

The minor type of tranquilizers are chemically different drugs that have extensive use in the reduction of anxiety and tension. Some are used as muscle relaxants. Meprobamate and chlordiazepoxide are minor tranquilizers that have been occasionally misused. The symptoms evident in use and in withdrawal are similar to those seen with barbiturates.

STIMULANTS

The varieties of stimulants have increased since the 1930s. Cocaine was the usual addicting agent; however, synthetic drugs having greater potency have been produced in large amounts. These latter drugs have become readily available in the treatment of obesity, colds, and hay fever. Substance abusers sometimes refer to cocaine as "snow" and to the amphetamines and amphetamine-like drugs as "pep pills." These drugs are favored for their mood-lifting qualities and for the overall energetic feeling of well-being they impart.

Cocaine may be taken by hypodermic injection, by sniffing the powder form through the nostrils, or by swallowing it in pill form. Patients under the influence of cocaine experience euphoria accompanied by motor restlessness. Prolonged use results in habit deterioration, a dulling of the ethical and moral judgment, confusion, and somatic delusions. The expression "cocaine bug" is derived from a rather common somatic delusion of worms or bugs crawling under the skin. Physical symptoms include dilated pupils, weakness, and emaciation. The withdrawal of cocaine is not accompanied by a definite syndrome, since the drug does not include physical dependence. There is, however, a strong psychologic dependence that causes the user to become an abuser. It is not unusual for abusers to combine a depressant like heroin with a drug like cocaine or to alternate the two. Cocaine is commonly known as coke, snow, and star dust.

Amphetamines and other stimulant drugs (phenmetrazine) have had widespread therapeutic effects, but the feeling of well-being and other exhilarating experiences they create cause psychologic dependence in abusers. Physical dependence and an abstinence syndrome have been seen when the drugs are withdrawn. Generally, the stimulants are favored for the "high" feelings experienced by susceptible individuals who ordinarily feel depressed, fatigued, and apathetic. These drugs are known as cartwheels, bombitos, and by other special terms.

Amphetamine sulfate (Benzedrine) and dextroamphetamine (Dexedrine) are also widely used for their stimulating effect. Nurses, physicians, and students are frequent users. These drugs are commonly known among abusers as bennies, footballs, coast-to-coasts, copilots, eye openers, and pep pills.

Apparent "speeding" behavior includes overactivity, both motor and verbal, with flight of ideas, irritability, and rapid mood swings. In some cases, great fear and anxiety are present, followed by hallucinations and other manifestations of a psychosis. Physically, the findings are rapid pulse, blood pressure elevation, pupil dilation, muscular twitching, high fever, and convulsions. Thorazine is helpful in reducing the overactivity and quieting the patient. When these symptoms result from ingestion of very large doses of drugs, attempts to save the individual's life are futile.

HALLUCINOGENS

Hallucinogens have been used mainly in research studies and rarely in clinical medical use. Some hallucinogens, such as dimethyltryptamine (DMT) and lysergic acid diethylamide (LSD), are relatively new, while mescaline and psilocybin have been known and used in religious ceremonies for many centuries. Marijuana is also considered to be a hallucinogen but it is not a narcotic, although it is controlled under most laws with similar impositions.

Marijuana is widely known throughout the world by many names: pot, grass, bhang, ganja, dagga, masconha, djamba, and hashish. It has had only minor use for medicinal purposes in the United States because other, more effective drugs have been found to replace it. However, in a few countries (like India and Pakistan) it may still be used as a remedy. The most effective and quickest method of using marijuana is by smoking cigarettes made of it. These are made from the leaves of the female plant and are called reefers, joints, or sticks. Hashish, which is stronger and imported from the Middle East, is usually used in powder form. It is made from the resin of the flowering tops of the plants.

The marijuana abuser is attracted and subjugated to the euphoria, exaltation, and dreaming experiences it offers. These feelings are accompanied by a free flow of ideas. The abuser experiences a sense of unreality, a slowing of the sense of time, distortion in hearing, and disturbances in vision and distance. At times, apprehension and fear to the point of panic may also be experienced. Hallucinations occur with large doses, while restlessness, laughter, and over-talkativeness are the more desirable sensations experienced. Drowsiness usually follows the exhilarating periods. Physiologic signs that may be evident include dizziness, dry mouth, dilated pupils, burning eyes, urinary frequency, diarrhea, nausea, and vomiting.

Although there is not physical dependence on marijuana, there is a strong psychic dependence for abusers. The deteriorating effect on the personality of the individual and the psychotic-like episodes manifested in the behavior of the habitual user have caused passage of laws for its control. The psychologic dependence on marijuana has caused many persons to commit crimes and to indulge in other amoral and asocial acts in order to acquire it.

LSD and other popular hallucinogens are potent drugs that, when ingested in small amounts, are capable of producing gross hallucinatory experiences. LSD is frequently taken in the form of impregnated sugar cubes, cookies, or crackers. It is less often administered by injection. The user of LSD is said not to be dependent on it, nor does he experience a serious craving.

Changes in perception, thought, mood, and activity are frequently evident in LSD users. The senses seem sharpened but distorted; colors and sounds intensify and change in dimension and quality. Voices and words are heard but not understood; auditory hallucinations of music and voices may occur. The sense of taste changes and the texture of food may be described as gritty. Cold and sweating sensations, light-headedness, emptiness, shaking, vibrations, and fogginess may also be experienced. There is a unawareness of the body accompanied by a "floating feeling." An LSD trip usually lasts 4 to 12 hours, but it may continue longer. Time seems erratic; it slows, races, stops, or even moves backward. Bizarre ideas are free-flowing and minor events seem greatly important. Some users have described religious, inspirational, and insightful experiences while under the influence of LSD.

The mind expansion effect and the varied mood changes are unpredictable for each person and, possibly, for each trip. The bizarre behavior and the psychotic episodes related to LSD use have resulted in many casualties. Delayed reactions have resulted in injury and suicide. Reasearch has shown that chromosomal abnormalities have been found at least twice as often in LSD users as in other individuals. Congenital and birth defects have been reported on infants born of mothers using LSD.

SOLVENTS

The greatest danger in the use of solvents is that their abuse has become a practice of some children between the ages of 10 and 15. They inhale the fumes from glue, gasoline, paint thinner, and lighter fluid to produce a sense of intoxication. The youngster usually inhales the solvent via a bag over his nose and mouth or directly from the bottle or tank. The effects are similar to alcohol intoxication—blurring of vision, ringing of ears, slurred speech, and staggering. After about 30 or 45 minutes these symptoms are followed by drowsiness, stupor, and sometimes unconsciousness. The youngster does not usually recall the episode after he recovers. If the child tends to repeat this experience alone or in groups for "kicks," then serious consideration should be given to his need for such dependence.

NURSING INTERVENTION

The treatment of substance abuse has taken on considerably greater significance of late because citizens have become aware of the widespread use of drugs in their families, the schools, and the communities. The tragedies of substance abuse have hit home all too often. Federal and state legislation has been passed to facilitate the treatment and rehabilitation of drug victims.

Past practices in the treatment of abusers left a great deal to be desired. Today, treatment includes a number of considerations—controlled detoxification, psychiatric evaluation and therapy in hospitals and in community centers, continued medical supervision, counseling after return to the community, and job rehabilitation.

Treatment and rehabilitation answer only one phase of the problem after the fact. Prevention and education can have a significant influence in reducing the number of individuals who may come under the spell of drugs. Educational institutions on all levels—from the elementary schools to the universities—should do everyting in their power to reduce the number of persons who may become involved with drugs. This is not an easy task, but it is a vitally needed one. Public educational programs similar to the one illustrating the dangers of smoking could be helpful in reaching people in all walks of life.

Controlled withdrawal from drugs requires careful medical and nursing supervision. The physician and the team determine the method for each patient, depending on the substance and the individual's experience with it. For the patient, the withdrawal symptoms are rarely easy to cope with, and the nurse's role in this phase of treatment is important and demanding. Physical and psychologic needs are intertwined and are shared by the nurse with other members of the therapeutic team.

When detoxification has been concluded, the patient is reviewed with regard to the mental and emotional factors contributing to his dependence on drugs. Psychiatric consultation could result in the diagnosis and long-term treatment of the psychologic problem. This treatment usually begins in the hospital following detoxification and may be continued in the community mental health center or hospital clinic within the patient's community. The nurse's role in the treatment and continued care of the patient involves knowledge of substance abuse, individual and community factors that contribute to abuse of drugs, the various signs and symptoms giving clues to substance abuse, and the nurse's role in the prevention and teaching.

A personal caution for the student and nurse seems in order at this point. Both students and nurses have contributed to the growing numbers of substance abusers. Many students in colleges and universities are known to favor the use of drugs to relieve tension and anxiety, as well as for "kicks" and to be with the "in crowd."

Students in nursing need to ask themselves these questions: "Am I able to use my knowledge about drugs to control and restrain my own use of these drugs?" "Do I have enough personal strength and self-understanding to set my own goals rather than be dependent on the crowd's standards?" "Am I capable of helping others to recognize the dangers of drugs and to dissuade them from using and depending on them?" Drugs are a serious responsibility for nurses since they are easily accessible. If one is unable to maintain the legal and professional practices essential in their use, then the privilege and the responsibility of the therapeutic nursing role are violated morally, ethically, and legally.

Since nurses find themselves with people in various and multiple settings, they have the opportunity to observe and to interact with them in the home, the neighborhood, the hospital, the physician's office, the clinic, or other settings. Nurses are in a good position to recognize the signs and symptoms of substance abuse, to advise the abuser and his family, and to assist them in obtaining proper treatment.

A second aspect of prevention is teaching. This provides the opportunity to discuss the various medications and their tendency toward drug dependence and is part of helping the patient in self-care. Cautions on self-medication and misuse of drugs for relief of tension and anxiety should be stressed, particularly when the medication obviously does not take care of the cause. Young people who flaunt their drug experiences for "kicks" cannot be ignored. Nurses need to use their knowledge to discuss the dangers of drugs on the young people's level with facts and descriptions that will "get to them." The time and effort spent on prevention may seem futile in light of the enormity of the problem; however, every small effort can help.

In the hospital or clinic settings, the nurse's role in the care and treatment of patients with drug dependence requires sincere acceptance and understanding. The "hard core" abuser is not an easy person to deal with. He may be charming, intelligent, and likable in his attempt to gain favors with drugs and treatment. The very strong desire for the drug prompts him to use any and all ways to get it, and the nurse stands between the patient and the drug. A high degree of alertness, tact, and skill in the ability to differentiate true symptoms from pseudosymptoms are essential in the nursing of the substance abuser. To outwit the patient's efforts to circumvent the removal of dependence on drugs, while at the same time meeting his emotional needs, requires a diplomat of the first order.

In the hospital setting, the major focus is on control of the drug during withdrawal treatment. The surroundings, including all nurses and other personnel, should prevent the accessibility of the drug. The facility should be such that the treatment during detoxification provides the support the patient needs to overcome the withdrawal symptoms. The atmosphere should be realistic; after the physical symptoms have subsided, the patient should be given the opportunity to assist with self-care to his capacity. The environment should not be too stimulating but should include activities that provide meaningful diversion. Trained personnel with an understanding of the patient's illness are an absolute essential. In the community center, sincerity, realistic trust, and friendliness can go a long way in supporting the patient in his day-to-day progress.

The substance abuser is often described as an immature, insecure, dependent person who has an inherent inability to develop meaningful interpersonal relationships. Adolescent abusers have been found to have extreme difficulty in coping with the changes occurring in adolescence. Some youngsters are products of deprivation, while others have had overprotection. Most abusers have little or no confidence in themselves and a low tolerance for frustration. The patient needs relationships that contribute to his self-reliance and self-respect and that satisfy his emotional needs sufficiently to promote a feeling of comfort and to make socialization worth while. Particular problems center around evasion, negativism, hostility, dependence, and malingering. A relatively permissive atmosphere with firmness is indicated.

Evasion and escape from responsibility are rather typical, as would be expected. It is important to identify this and to accept it matter-of-factly while holding the patient to certain minimum standards, such as group participation, care of personal hygiene, and adequate diet intake. When negativism and hostility are manifest, the nurse should recognize them for what they mean but avoid any open issue on an authority basis. To accept behavior without sanctioning it and without punitive retaliation is the principle to be followed. If the patient's condition allows, an orientation early in his hospitalization to the purposes, rules, and procedures of the unit may serve as a basis for planning a routine with the patient and may serve to allay future misunderstandings as to what is expected of him.

The patient's need for confidence and security may be satisfied by nurses in carrying out their role. Their knowledge about the patient's illness and needs, their efficiency within the unit, and their confidence in themselves as persons contribute in reassuring the patient that the personnel are capable of helping him to help himself in resolving his problem. Hesitancy and uncertainty may be exploited by the patient, especially in evasion and malingering for the purpose of obtaining more medication or drugs. Dependence of the patient on the nurse is a frequent tendency fostered in the nurse-patient relationship and should be avoided. The nurse needs to be alert to this tendency and deliberately plan to build the patient's self-reliance and security. The patient needs acceptance, friendliness, and security.

The physical needs of the patient are related to the stage and degree of illness. Following an overdose of barbiturates, a stuporous patient needs the same care that any unconscious patient requires. Special attention should be given to respiratory difficulties associated with increased secretion of mucus and depression of the respiratory center that are the effects of barbiturate poisoning. With delirium or the withdrawal syndrome or morphine abuse, personal hygiene and good skin care are important. Fluids should be forced, and as soon as nausea subsides, an adequate diet of small frequent feedings should be instituted. The goal is to direct the patient to a regular, well-balanced diet.

Keen observation and tact are required in evaluating the patient's physical symptoms. The abuser is prone to exaggerate and pretend in order to secure medications over and beyond his real need; he is utterly amoral in this respect. Study of the patient and assessment of his actual physical condition require good judgment, which is developed through experience and practice. When the patient's behavior is judged to be intentionally deceiving, nurses need to understand the reason for this and to maintain a neutral attitude. If nurses do not understand, if they do not control their responses to the situation, and if they react with hostility and punitive action, the patient will be impelled to defensive and explosive behavior. Such an outcome will destroy the nurses' effectiveness and the patient's confidence in the nurses as therapeutic agents.

If the patient is receiving experimental drugs, very careful observation and recording of all aspects of behavior and physical condition are important. The patient's needs with respect to treatment will be determined on the basis of all the observations made.

Attention to personal hygiene, including every aspect of personal cleanliness and the establishment of a health routine, is usually necessary, since most patients have been careless in this respect for many years. It is not unusual for them to be unclean and disheveled because of poor living habits. The process of establishing habits of proper hygiene, good nutrition, and a balance of activities takes time and patience to be learned.

A protective atmosphere of acceptance and alertness is imperative in the care of a patient who is pathologically dependent on drugs. Protective needs fall into three categories—prevention of access to the drug of choice or any substitute, protection against injury during an acute episode, and protection against self-injury.

On admission, the patient and his personal effects should be thoroughly searched and his belongings, including money, should be removed until all possible sources of drugs are eliminated. Visitors and parcels should be subject to some form of control to prevent smuggling. Many trusting relatives and, unfortunately, some overly sympathetic personnel may be so misguided as to believe that they are doing the patient a favor by supplying him with drugs. Another source of danger is the person close to the patient who has a marked hostility toward him. Not understanding his own motivations, such a person may well contribute to the patient's difficulty by furnishing him with contraband. Pocketbooks and wallets of personnel should be locked away lest the patient steal money to purchase drugs through his friends.

Drugs in the hospital should be kept under strict control, and medications given should be taken under supervision at the time of administration to prevent hoarding. The patient's actual symptoms should be carefully evaluated to prevent unnecessary medication.

The patient may injure himself at any stage of his illness in an attempt to gain sympathy or to force the use of medication for the relief of pain. The danger is that the patient may injure himself more seriously than he intends. Emotional support, a program of activities to keep the patient busy, and close observation are protective measures. If depression or despondency is evident, precautions against suicide should be taken. To prevent injury during an acute episode, the nurse should remain close to the patient, observe him carefully, and utilize protective measures, such as side rails, whenever necessary.

One of the major problems of substance abusers is socialization or the "know-how" of establishing meaningful relationships with people. Group psychotherapy serves a twofold purpose: it helps the abuser learn self-examination and experience the socialization process. Treatment in hospitals, clinics, and the community has as its focus the return of the patient as a functioning member of society. Therefore the structure, plan, and routine activities of the patient and patient groups need to be centered around daily living, with the opportunity for the patient to learn self-reliance and to gain self-confidence.

The routine of the unit and the individual plan for the patient should focus on using every asset and resource the patient has toward the development of interpersonal relationships with other patients, personnel, and family. Being among patients with similar problems reduces the sense of isolation, and sharing feelings and experiences helps each patient realize that he is not alone in his problems. Insight into personal feelings and the courage to try to change can result from patient-to-patient support and professional assistance. Shared fears and difficulties are easier to face than fears kept to one's self. Ventilation and emotional catharsis in group discussions may be helpful, but careful attention should be paid to evidence of marked anxiety. Knowledge and skill in group process are necessary. It should be remembered that patients are more tolerant of each other than personnel are likely to realize. Sensitivity to how the patient feels, rather than how personnel feel about a situation, is the important criterion. In any instance, group interaction should be planned and encouraged and the patient should be discouraged from isolating himself.

The plan for rehabilitation is not the last consideration but the first. The whole purpose of treatment is to return the person to this family and community as a more effective participant and possibly as a contributor. The total plan for the treatment and care of the patient from the beginning is focused on the goal of removing his dependence on drugs and to replace this with independence and self-reliance in his ability to care for himself and those dear to him. All that he experiences during his hospitalization will influence how effective he will be and how soon he will be able to achieve independent functioning.

Following his discharge from the unit, continued support can be given by the community facilities, such as halfway houses, mental hygiene clinics, and mental health centers. Referrals and follow-up plans in these facilities are often needed as intermediate steps for the substance abuser. These facilities often provide educational and work programs for the development of meaningful skills leading to jobs for self-support. Halfway houses and night centers provide an extension of needed support by professional personnel while the patient tests his ability to reenter the competitive activities of society. The continued support of the patient is a must in his planned treatment.

REFERENCES

Aguilera, D. C.: Review of psychiatric nursing, St. Louis, 1977, The C. V. Mosby Co.

Caskey, K. K., Blalock, E. V., and Wauson, B. N.: The school nurse and drug abusers, Nurs. Outlook 18:27-30, 1970.

Condon, A., and Roland, A.: Drug abuse jargon, Am. J. Nurs. 71:1738-1739, 1971.

Fink, M., Freedman, A. M., Zaks, A. M., and Resnick, R. B.: Narcotic antagonists: another approach to addiction therapy, Am. J. Nurs. 71:1359-1363, 1971.

Fleming, J. W.: Recognizing the newborn addict, Am. J. Nurs. 65:83, 1965.

Foreman, N. J., and Zerwekh, J. V.: Drug crisis intervention, Am. J. Nurs. 71:1736-1737, 1971.

Fort, J.: Comparison chart of major substances used for mind alteration, Am. J. Nurs. 71:1740-1741, 1971.

Garb, S.: Narcotic addiction in nurses and doctors, Nurs. Outlook 13:30-34, 1965.

Golub, S.: Recognizing the drug abuser, RN 32:44-47, 1969.

Isler, C.: Narcotics addicts *need* nurses! RN 32:36-44, 1969.

Kolb, L. C.: Modern clinical psychiatry, ed. 8, Philadelphia, 1973, W. B. Saunders Co., pp. 509-529.

Kron, Y. J., and Brown, E. M.: Main line to nowhere; the making of a heroin addict, New York, 1967, World Publishing Co.

Lipp, M. R., Benson, S. G., and Allen, P. S.: Marijuana use by nurses and nursing students, Am. J. Nurs. 71:2339-2341, 1971.

Masters, R. E. L., and Houston, J.: Varieties of psychedelic experiences, New York, 1966, Holt, Rinehart & Winston.

McDermott, Sr. Raphael: Maintaining the methadone patient, Nurs. Outlook 18:22-26, 1970.

Morgan, A. J., and Moreno, J. W.: The practice of mental health nursing, Philadelphia, 1973, J. B. Lippincott Co., pp. 149-165.

Morgan, A. J., and Moreno, J. W.: Attitudes toward addiction, Am. J. Nurs. 73:497-501, 1973.

Muhlinkamp. A. F.: Personality characteristics of drug addicts, Perspect. Psychiatr. Care 6:213-219, 1968.

Nelson, K.: The nurse in a methadone maintenance program, Am. J. Nurs. 73:870-874, 1973.

Nowlis, H. B.: Why students use drugs, Am. J. Nurs. 68:1680-1685, 1968.

Rodman, M. J.: Drugs for pain problems, RN 34:59-69, 1971.

Sankot, M., and Smith, D. E.: Drug problems in the Haight-Ashbury, Am. J. Nurs. 68:1686-1689, 1968.

Solomon, D., editor: The marihuana papers, Indianapolis, 1966, The Bobbs-Merrill Co., Inc.

Sparratto, G. R.: Toward a rational view of drug abuse, J. Sch. Health 40:192-196, 1970.

ADDITIONAL READINGS

Armstrong, E.: Use or abuse? Can. Nurs. 71(3):107-108, 1975.

Cotroneo, M., and others: Addiction, alienation and parenting, Nurs. Clin. North Am. 11(3):517-525, 1976.

Dy, A. J., and others: The nurse in the methadone maintenance program: expansions and transitions in role, J. Psychiatr. Nurs. 13(3):17-20, 1975.

Fairclough, F.: Drug abuse, Nurs. Mirror **143**(5):67-68, 1976.

Henderson, E. H.: Problems of children with drug abusing parents, Nurs. Times **70**(49):1890-1892, 1974.

Morris, M. L., and others: The drug dependent patient and the nurse, Nurs. Care **7**(12):29-31, 1974.

Odom, C.: The enigma of drug abuse, J. Pract. Nurs. **24**(9):19-21, 1974.

Siegel, M. A.: Los Angeles teen challenge: a resocialization program for drug abusers, J. Psychiatr. Nurs. **12**(6):21-24, 1974.

Valentine, N. M.: An approach to staff development for the delivery of care to drug-addicted patients, Nurs. Clin. North Am. **11**(3):227-240, 1976.

CHILDREN: THEIR BEHAVIORS AND PROBLEMS

CHAPTER 17

Developmental problems of children

The extent to which there are increasing numbers and kinds of psychiatric–mental health services for children is witness to one aspect of progress our society has made toward mental health. People have become more attuned to behavior that may be indicative of emotional trouble. Nurses play a significant role in the identification of children and families who need psychiatric assistance. Community health, school, office, and hospital-centered nurses, in their encounters with children and families, have numerous opportunities to observe behavior and to detect signs of impending problems.

Primary and secondary levels of prevention are within the scope of nurses. They interact with children and parents in the community and in such facilities as prenatal clinics, well-child facilities, nursery schools, daycare centers, and elementary and secondary schools. Crisis situations and stressful happenings may come to the attention of nurses, who are in a good position to assist the parents and children toward psychiatric services. The care and treatment of children who are severely emotionally disturbed are complex and should be left to child psychiatrists and psychiatric nurses who have studied child psychiatry.

HISTORICAL REVIEW

Although evidence is available that peoples of ancient times and numerous cultures had concern for children and their welfare, no period in history has contributed so much to the understanding of children as has the twentieth century. Therefore it is not strange that many refer to it as the century of the child.

In the past, the role of the child was to obey, to serve, to honor, and to conform to his parents. His individuality and personal feelings were suppressed

375

lest he be considered a bad child. The will of the parents or guardians dominated the child's life. Rigid religious codes often determined the morality of right and wrong. Children were loved but were needed more. From a very early age, children were given specific chores essential to the vitality of family life; thus they developed strong feelings of being needed.

During the eighteenth and nineteenth centuries several writers drew attention to the natural development of children, their problems, and their pedagogy. Some began to look at children as individuals. Pestalozzi (1774) observed and recorded the behavior of his young son and emphasized the individuality of children as human beings. Similarly, Tiedemann in 1787 published the observations of the total growth and development of his children. In 1877, Darwin described the forces of human survival as evident in child development. The work of Preyer on the mind of the child is said to have been the beginning of child psychology. There were many others who contributed to the interest and study of children during these centuries and who thus set the stage for further progress in the twentieth century.

In the first half of the twentieth century, tremendous progress was made in the study of the child and his problems. Several forces were at work concomitantly to create this impetus. First, the scientific method had become an established method of enlightenment and had permeated the realms of medicine and the social sciences. The social sciences were accepted as respectable areas of knowledge within institutions of higher learning and were acknowledged for their professional value. Pedagogy, education curriculums, and methods were examined and questioned. Past theories on child-rearing were shaken.

Alfred Binet made a breakthrough when he published his famous scale of measuring intelligence in relation to mental age in 1905. The Binet-Simon scale demonstrated an important individual difference among children and stimulated the serious examination of human intelligence and the learning processes. Terman adopted this scale for use with American children and initiated much activity in further scientific study. Arnold Gesell and his associates contributed greatly to the objective observation and study of children through the use of modern and scientific techniques.

The nature-nurture controversy is no longer a subject for debate, since all schools of thought recognize the importance of both factors in human development. No one seriously contends that development is on an either/or basis, or that one variable excludes the other. Emphasis on the predeterministic view is still viable and has contributed important concepts to current developmental theory. The tabula rasa (blank slate) approach, on the other hand, with its emphasis on the role of the environment and experience in determining developmental outcomes, is becoming increasingly prominent in social learning theory.

Psychiatry and pediatrics witnessed many important changes in their knowledge and practice. In pediatrics, medical care became a planned routine for young children and preventive care became a concern. Dynamic psychiatry recognized the need to understand the whole person—his early experiences and his life's experiences, as well as his symptoms. A biographic history is now an essential component of the patient's personal data.

All of these factors and others led to a clearer understanding of youngsters as individuals, of their behavior, and of the underlying motives for their problems.

Today child psychiatry is accepted as a special and important field of psychiatry to be included in medical, nursing, and teacher education. Child psychiatrists are partners with pediatricians in the care of children in hospitals and clinics. Schools, juvenile courts, nurses, teachers, lawyers, and other institutions and individuals involved with children are more cognizant of the resources available to help youngsters with disturbing behavior. And most importantly, the public and the parents or guardians of children are being educated with respect to children's behavior problems and the various means available to **help** them to help their youngsters.

CHILDHOOD AND PARENTHOOD

The first year of life is one of almost total helplessness and dependence. The infant must learn to trust parental figures and become able to allow them out of his sight without fear or rage. He must also be able to develop confidence in the sameness and continuity of his environment and to internalize it through his developing tactile, auditory, olfactory, and visual senses. Deprivation in any one or a combination of these senses could lead to maladaptive response patterns affecting his biopsychosocial development.

During this stage, the symbiotic relationship that develops between the infant and the parental figure forms a foundation for the behavioral patterns of later personality development. This relationship goes beyond the symbiosis of mutual dependence for biologic survival; in the psychosocial development of the infant it implies that the parent is willing and ready to assume responsibility for the infant, who in turn accepts this care passively without reciprocating.

During infancy the mouth is the primary organ of gratification and exploration; feeding becomes an important aspect of meeting needs. This is controlled by someone else, usually the mother, and her consistency in meeting her infant's needs for oral gratification is the beginning of his development of trust in his environment.

As a result of the varied experiences that he and his parents share, the infant develops confidence that his needs will be met. Through their own dependability, the parents structure these situations so that there is a basis for a mutual sense of confidence. For example, if the infant is fed regularly at times when he has come to expect a feeding, his sense of trust is encouraged. But should the feedings become sporadic, he will become uncertain and anxious about his environment, and a sense of mistrust will begin to appear. His resulting fretful, anxious behavior may inspire further inadequate parenting. Another essential component of the healthy symbiotic relationship is the comfort brought by the parent; if discomfort is inflicted, any continued trust can be destroyed.

Environmental consistency and stimulation are important for cognitive and effective growth. The infant usually becomes aware of his parents as persons by 9 months; by the age of 4 weeks absence of parenting can provoke symptoms of insecurity such as crying and rocking, followed by withdrawal, depression, and even death.

Piaget (1963) describes the infant's development of intelligent behavior in this stage as *sensorimotor*. During the first year the reflex patterns he was born with are repeated and strengthened with practice. As a newborn, he is capable of grasping, sucking, auditory and visual pursuit, and other stereotyped behavior patterns. These can be activated by nonspecific stimuli in the environment; after being activated a number of times the response becomes spontaneous without further external stimulation. For example, at birth the infant is able to suck at the breast; continued practice improves his coordination and facility until this ability becomes well adapted to the goal of taking nourishment.

These primary reflex actions become coordinated into new actions. For example, the hand accidentally coming in contact with the mouth and initiating sucking movements may lead to more coordinated actions and to thumb-sucking as an established form of behavior. Later actions become oriented toward objects in the environment that stimulate his seeing and hearing, and intentional behavior emerges as he seeks to repeat these actions. He learns to begin meaningful actions in sequence and to explore new objects within his reach, thus developing goal-oriented activity. In this way physical activity patterns develop into mental activity patterns of response.

By the end of the first year the stage of purposeful behavior is reached, and exploration of further boundaries of the environment is begun. Motor actions have gradually become internalized as thought patterns. During this period the trend is toward a higher level of sensory experiences and related mental activities. By the end of the second year there is a functional understanding of play, imitation, causality, objects, space, and time. By the age of 2 years a child can truly imitate such behavior as eating, sleeping, washing himself, walking, and so on.

If the child does not develop the beginnings of trust, in later life there may be a sense of chronic mistrust, dependence, depressive trends, withdrawal, and shallow interpersonal relationships.

During the second year the child begins a struggle for autonomy. He shifts from dependence on others toward independent actions of his own. As his musculature matures, it is necessary for him to develop the ability of coordination such as holding on and letting go. Since these are highly opposing patterns, conflict may occur; one example is the conflict arising over bowel and bladder control. A power struggle may develop betwen the child and his parents, since elimination is completely under his control, and approval or disapproval become strong influences because of his parents' attitudes toward eliminative habits. The child is expected to abandon his needs for self-gratification and substitute ones that meet the demands of his parents, representing the later demands of society.

Cognitive development in this stage includes the first symbolic substitutions, words and gross speech. The child begins to manipulate objects and will look for hidden items. He recognizes differences between I, me, and mine and you and yours. He also begins to manipulate others by words such as no, and the origins of concrete literal thinking are developed; this is the period of *preoperational thought* that continues to the age of 7 years (Piaget, 1963). One of its characteristics is egocentrism, in which the child is unable to take the viewpoint of another person; at the end of this period, egocentrism is replaced by social interaction. The child has now formed concepts in primitive images, thing to thing. He cannot cope intellectually with problems concerning time, causality, space, or other abstract concepts, although he understands what each is by itself in concrete situations. His perceptions dominate his judgments, and he operates on what can be seen directly.

The psychosocial task during this stage is to develop self-esteem through limited self-control. The achievement of bowel and bladder control within the prescribed cultural expectations allows also for self-control without loss of self-esteem.

This is an important time for establishing a ratio between love and hate, cooperation and willfulness, and freedom of self-expression and its suppression. Failure during this stage is manifested in childhood by feelings of shame and doubt, fear of exposure, and ritualized activity; in later adulthood the failure to achieve autonomy is seen in the individual who is a compulsive character, with an irrational need for conformity and for approval.

PRESCHOOL

Erikson (1950, 1959, 1963) believes that in the preschool stage the child has the task of developing *initiative*. He will discover what kind of person he is going to be, he learns to move around freely and has an unlimited radius of goals, his language skills broaden, and he will ask many questions. His skill in using words is not matched by his skill in understanding them, and he is thus faced with the dangers of misinterpretation and misunderstanding. Language and locomotion allow him to expand his imagination over such a broad spectrum that he can easily frighten himself with dreams and thoughts.

The prerequisites for masculine and feminine initiative are developed. Infantile sexual curiosity and preoccupation with sexual matters arise. Oedipal wishes can occur as a result of increased imagination, and terrifying fantasies may develop, along with a sense of guilt about them.

Initiative becomes governed by a firmly established conscience. The child feels shame not only when he is found out but also when he fears being found out; guilt is felt for thoughts as well as deeds. In this stage anxiety is controlled by play, by fantasy, and by pride in the attainment of new skills.

He is ready to learn quickly and to share and to work with others toward a given goal; he begins to identify with people other than his parents and will develop a feeling of equality of worth with others despite differences in functions and age.

At 4½ to 5 years of age the shift from infantile to juvenile body build is rapid, and the beginning of hand-eye coordination and an intellectual growth spurt occur. The social base of gender role is firmly laid down by the end of the fifth year. If this stage is successfully accomplished, the child develops the fantasy of "I who can become"; but if the child is excessively guilt-ridden, his fantasy is "I who shouldn't dream of it." The desired self-concept at the end of this stage is "I have the worth to try even if I am small."

Failure or trauma at this time leads to confusion of psychosexual role, rigidity and guilt in interpersonal relations, and loss of initiative in the exploration of new skills.

PREPUBERTY

Prepuberty years are characterized as the learning stage; that is, "I am what I learn." The child wants to be shown how to do things both alone and with others; he develops a sense of industry in which he becomes dissatisfied if he does not have the feeling of being useful or a sense of his ability to make things and make them well, even perfectly. He now learns to win recognition by producing things. He feels pleasure when his attention and diligence produce a completed work.

There is a slow but steady growth as maturation of the central nervous system continues. In terms of psychosexual development there is reduced pressure in the exploration of sensuality and the gender role while other skills are developed and exploited.

The cognitive phase of development includes the mastery of skills in manipulating objects and the concepts of his culture. Thinking enters the period of *concrete operations* (Piaget, 1963), and the ability to solve concrete problems with this ability increases, so that toward the end of this period the child is able to abstract problems. The solution of real problems is accomplished with mental operations that the child was previously unable to perform. By puberty the child exhibits simple deductive reasoning ability and has learned the rules and the basic technology of his culture, thus reinforcing his sense of belonging in his environment.

Self-esteem is derived from the sense of adequacy and the beginning of "best" friendships and sharing with peers. This also marks the beginning of the individual's friendships and loves outside of his family, as he begins to learn the complexities, pleasures, and difficulties of adjusting himself and his drives, aggressive and erotic, to those of his peers. By learning and adjusting he begins to take his place as a member of their group and social life. In making this adjustment he seeks the company of his own sex and forms groups and secret societies. The gangs and groups, especially the boys, fight each other in games, baseball, and cops and robbers, working off much hostility and aggression in a socially approved manner.

Feelings of inadequacy and inferiority may begin if the child does not develop a sense of adequacy. Family life may not have prepared him for school, or the school itself may fail to help him in developing the necessary skills for competency. As a result, he may feel that he will never be good at anything he attempts.

NURSES AND ATTITUDES

Nurses have numerous opportunities to observe the behavior of children and parents. In their work and as members of the community, they develop relationships with children. However, a great deal is missed or lost unless nurses are perceptive and are equipped with a fine antenna to pick up and identify subtly expressed or camouflaged behavior. Observed behavioral cues, verbal and nonverbal, have to be seen for their true meaning.

In addition to observing behavioral cues, nurses in the clinical situation must report these accurately. An anecdotal record should be written, and where necessary, the nurse's reaction or interpretation may be included, if it is identified as an interpretation or personal reaction. Nurses need to develop the ability to know, to define, and to accept their own personal reactions. When there is confusion or great emotional involvement, the nurse should seek resources for assistance, such as psychiatric nurses, clinical specialists, supervisors, psychiatrists, and psychologists. Self-understanding is essential to helping others.

Nurses whose positions bring them into close contact with children would benefit by asking themselves several questions. "How do I feel about children?" "Why do I feel this way?" "Do I like or dislike children?" "What is my usual behavior as a nurse with children?" "What major purpose do I serve as a nurse with children?" "How do I feel about the various types of parents I encounter?" "Do I tend to blame parents or accept them in their roles?"

As nurses are human, so are parents. Some parents' behavior toward their children may be very disturbing and arouse much anger and hostility in nurses. When seeing the child's behavior toward the parents, nurses may very easily judge and blame the parents for the child's problems. This judgment is inescapably reflected in their treatment of the parents and child and renders them ineffectual in helping either party. Usually both parents and child need help. It is important to accept this fact and to recognize that the parents' behavior is often an expression of their problems, which require understanding and therapy. Often the recognition of the child's behavior problem serves as the clue of underlying deep, complex family problems. Family therapy attempts to provide the means for removing the child as the focal point of the parent's marital maladjustment or other familial disturbances. It attempts to consider the needs of all the family members relative to the whole problem.

NURSES AND PREVENTION

Preventive medicine is an integral part of the pediatrician's practice today, and it includes consideration of both physical and psychologic aspects. However, prevention of serious emotional problems and mental illness deals with many subtle and diverse factors. It includes conditions that enhance emotional well-being and those that contribute to the child's malfunctioning, such as slum housing, broken homes, sensory and cultural deprivation, school conditions, poverty, racial discrimination, and many other social conditions found in our affluent society.

Nurses as members of their communities and in their functions within a health agency are in a strategic position to participate in prevention. The potential of school nurses to fulfill their role in the prevention and early detection of emotional disturbances in school children has been vastly neglected. School boards and school officials contribute to school nurses' ineffectiveness by defining their duties and the use of their time, knowledge, and skills. School nurses should be aware of their role in primary prevention in the school environment as well as secondary prevention with the early recognition and treatment of emergency disturbances. School nurses have no excuse for not meeting these prime responsibilities.

In addition, the community mental health movement, which has expanded at a surprisingly rapid pace, holds promise of increased comprehensive mental health programs and services for children. Planning for these programs means coordination in such areas as urban renewal and public housing, juvenile delinquency, the proverty program, and mental retardation programs so that all programs and services within the community work together to meet the multiple and varied needs of the child and the family with mental health problems. Such a program should set its goals to provide diagnostic and treatment services and to prevent and reduce mental illness within the community.

In planning for community mental health programs, certain key factors may be helpful.

1. The needs of the emotionally disturbed child may be met more effectively when there is a wide range of educational, preventive, diagnostic, and treatment facilities within the community.

2. Therapeutic services provided for children in the early ages or at early stages of emotional illness are usually more effective, shorter in duration, and have more promising results than they do if these services are delayed and the problems become gross disturbances.

3. Continuity of treatment for the child and his family is a major factor. This means collaboration among the various agencies and the persons cooperating in the child's treatment.

Neither nurse nor individual can afford to abdicate responsibility to do his or her part in community mental health, particularly with respect to the needs of children.

REFERENCES

Chapman, A. H.: Management of emotional problems of children and adolescents, Philadelphia, 1965, J. B. Lippincott Co.

Christina, Sr. Mary: The role of the nurse in child caring institutions, J. Psychiatr. Nurs. **2:**281-285, 1964.

Erikson, E. H.: Growth and crises of the healthy personality. In Senn, M. J. E., editor: Symposium on the healthy personality, New York, 1950, Josiah Macy, Jr., Foundation.

Erikson, E. H.: Identity and the life cycle, Psychological Issues, vol. 1, no. 1, New York, 1959, International Press.

Erikson, E. H.: Childhood and society, New York, 1963, W. W. Norton & Co.

Fagin, C., editor: Nursing in child psychiatry, St. Louis, 1972, The C. V. Mosby Co., p. 183.

Field, W. E., Jr.: Watch your message, Am. J. Nurs. **72:**1278-1289, 1972.

Hyde, N. D.: Playtherapy—the troubled child's self-encounter, Am. J. Nurs. **71:**1366-1370, 1971.

Howells, J. G.: Modern perspectives in child psychiatry, Springfield, Ill., 1965, Charles C Thomas, Publisher, pp. 251-284, 336-349.

Kanner, L.: Child psychiatry, ed. 4, Springfield, Ill., 1972, Charles C Thomas, Publisher, pp. 1-133.

Lesser, A. J.: Accent on prevention—through improved service, Children **11**:13-18, 1964.

McBride, A. B.: The anger-depression-guilt go-round, Am. J. Nurs. **73**:1045-1049, 1973.

Morgan, A. J., and Moreno, J. W.: The practice of mental health nursing: a community approach, Philadelphia, 1973, J. B. Lippincott Co., pp. 114-128.

Piaget, J.: The child's conception of the world, Potowa, N.J., 1963, Littlefield, Adams, & Co.

Salerno, E. M.: A family in crisis, Am. J. Nurs. **73**:100-103, 1973.

Shufer, S.: The pediatric mental health nurse clinician, Nurs. Outlook **19**:543, 1971.

ADDITIONAL READINGS

Baker, P.: Social development during the first two years of life, Nurs. Mirror **142**(24):70-71, 1976.

Brenton, A. G., and others: Helping a child develop, Nurs. Times **71**(27):1052-1055, 1975.

Eddington, C., and others: Sensory-motor stimulation for slow-to-develop children: a home-centered program for parents, Am. J. Nurs. **75**(1):59-62, 1975.

Edgcumbe, R.: Development of aggressiveness in children, Nurs. Times **72**(13)(Suppl. VII):15, 1976.

Geller, J. J.: Developmental symbiosis, Perspect. Psychiatr. Care **13**(1):10-12, 1975.

Heinz, L.: The nurse in role in a parenting process program, J. Psychiatr. Nurs. **13**(2):27-30, 1975.

McDonagh, M. J.: Creative process and its relation to sense of self, separateness, and reality, Perspect. Psychiatr. Care **14**(2):68-74, 1976.

Miller, K.: A fable, Perspect. Psychiatr. Care **14**(2):66-67, 1976.

Pinkerton, P.: Emotional development and the clinical implications, Nurs. Mirror **141**(25):48-50, 1975.

Solomon, R.: The gifted child—a problem of recognition, Nurs. Times **71**(24):940-941, 1975.

CHAPTER 18

Children with functionally based behavior problems

Although the underlying dynamics of mental disorders in children are closely allied to those of adults, a child's behavior must be analyzed and evaluated in light of his development. This task is difficult and depends on the child's communication skills, imagination, and cooperation. A child's problems are manifested in behavior that disrupts the routine of his daily living, his relationships with his parents and family, and sometimes the affairs of the community. The disturbance created by the child is his way of saying he has deep, personal discord and that he needs help. The behavior is a sign, a symptom, and not an inherited tendency or a weakness. During childhood, numerous, rapid changes take place that are often accompanied by normal problems. These normal problems are associated with the activities of daily living.

FEEDING-EATING PROBLEMS

The feeding problem is the mother's; the eating problem is the child's. It is often difficult to distinguish which caused the situation. The mother's problem may be related to her desire to give the best care to her infant or child and to the anxiety resulting from her attempts. Time schedules and specified foods and the maximum amounts of each, rigidly adhered to, are causes to stir even a young infant to rebellion. As the infant or child expresses his objection to the feeding routine, the mother becomes more convinced that the child has a problem and tries harder, increasing anxiety and tension. Several research experiments with infants and children have been carried out that demonstrate the child's ability to select satisfactorily his nourishment in the kind and amounts to meet his optimal needs.

Anorexia is usually caused by psychologic disturbances when there is no evidence of physical illness. Some frequent clues may be the child's preference for specific foods only, his refusal of food at mealtime but not between feedings, and his refusal of food from his mother or father and acceptance of food from other sources. On the other hand, the child may refuse all food. The cause for loss of appetite should be examined from the point of view of the child and the end he hopes to achieve by his behavior, from the point of view of the mother or other adult who feeds the child (her relationship to the child and her attitude toward his feeding), and, last, from the point of view of the feeding technique.

The child's refusal of food may be his method of gaining the fondling, cuddling, and attention of an otherwise unaffectionate mother who feeds and cares for him automatically. He may have learned that his refusal to eat gives him control over the household and permits him to have his way. Or he may use this negative behavior to express his unhappiness or depression. The parent-child relationship is basic to all considerations. The mother's method of feeding the child could be controlled by her underlying feelings, such as rejection, overprotection, anxiety, lack of knowledge, adherence to a set routine, confusion, and fear.

The treatment of children with feeding-eating disorders must obviously involve the child, his symptoms, and his parents. Very often, anxiety over the child's malnourished condition results in symptomatic treatment, while the underlying causes are overlooked. Therefore the symptoms may recur frequently. Mothers need guidance in dealing with the problem and are often advised to ignore the symptoms. Their anxiety and oversolicitude may prevent this approach from being successful. Between-meal feedings are discouraged, and the child's favorite foods are offered at mealtime as a means of interesting the child in eating. Small portions are recommended until he requests more. When the eating habit is reestablished, other foods may be introduced gradually. Concomitant with the direct attention to the problem is study of the child's underlying motivation. The mother is helped to understand her feelings and the contribution that she makes to the problem.

Anorexia nervosa is a general term used to designate severe loss of appetite and self-denial of food. This condition occurs more often in adolescents than in younger children and suggests a serious emotional disorder. The self-imposed starvation may jeopardize the child's life. Hospitalization and psychotherapy in a controlled setting are recommended.

Another eating disorder is *excessive eating*. The reasons for overeating are related to some of the causes discussed previously. The oversolicitude of a well-intentioned mother may establish the habit of excessive eating. It may well be the best way a child has of gaining approval and expressions of affection from his parents. He may use large amounts of food to compensate for unsatisfied desires and frustrations. Treatment involves the child and his parents, his symptoms, and his purpose for eating as he does. For the adolescent, obesity may be a problem of great magnitude because our society places considerable emphasis and significance on being trim and slim—the "diet-cola" generation. The parents view the situation as a serious handicap since it affects the child's social relationships and activities among his peers and in the community.

Pica designates a disorder characterized by the ingestion of substances having no apparent nutritional value. The reasons for this condition are not fully understood. An infant often places toys and other objects (including the bedrails) in his mouth. Often the ingestion of paint causes serious lead poisoning. Bugs, worms, dirt, pebbles, strings, hair, buttons, and paper are some other objects that children may ingest habitually, which result in a variety of disorders. Preventive measures are indicated when this condition is first observed.

The nursing care of children with undereating and overeating disorders involves the observation of the child's behavior and recording the behavior as a means of identifying the underlying causes. The nurse's warmth, interest, and affection for the child will go far in gaining his trust and perhaps cooperation in his psychotherapy. The child's projection of his maternal attitudes to the nurse should be recognized and handled matter-of-factly, without retaliation and hostility. Keeping the child occupied, particularly an older child, will help to distract his attention and conversation from his symptoms. Patience and understanding are essential in the management of these patients.

SLEEP DISTURBANCES

Sleep patterns of normal children show some variations, but when a child is disturbed, sleep behavior becomes a problem that is manifest in a wide range of symptoms from mild restlessness to wakefulness, insomnia, excessive drowsiness, and variations of these. When no physical disorder is present, emotional factors must be carefully examined. A brief period of psychotherapy may be indicated since sleep disturbances very often accompany other conditions such as anxiety, jealousy, insecurity, fear, and psychoneurosis.

The complex function of speech requires the use and synchronization of certain areas of the brain, the organs of vocalization and hearing, the intelligence and comprehension, and the emotional components involved in understanding and responsiveness. An impairment or disturbance in speech may denote trouble in any of these areas. When the speech disorder has no organic basis, the cause is usually associated with the child's parental and family situation and his emotional maladjustment. Delayed speech, prolonged baby talk, lisping, and stuttering are conditions that have strong emotional implications. Present-day studies tend to support the theory of their psychologic origin.

Stuttering is the involuntary hesitation, the repetition of words, or the prolongation of sounds in speech. The frustration of the stutterer frequently causes him to go through certain body movements. Tossing of the head, facial grimaces, swallowing, gasping, clenching of the fists, jerking arm motions, and stamping of the feet are frequent when the child attempts to control or relieve his stuttering. Although it is recognized that stuttering indicates some underlying emotional disturbance, the manifestations of this behavior contribute additional difficulty to the development of his personality. A child who stutters becomes sensitive and self-conscious and shies away from social activities. Ridicule from children and insensitive adults causes him to withdraw and become seclusive—all of which, of course, contribute more to the child's tension and stuttering. Treatment should begin as soon as the stuttering becomes acute. If the child can be helped to resolve his emotional disorder early, his stuttering habit can then be relieved and further emotional trauma can be avoided.

Mutism is the inability to speak and is associated with other complex disorders such as childhood schizophrenia, early infantile autism, and hysteria. Nonverbal communication is a challenge to the nurse and requires alert attention, imaginativeness, understanding of the child, and sympathetic patience. Care of the child should not be an automatic routine in which things are done to him but should provide an opportunity for the child to participate to the degree that he is able. Direct questions should not dominate the conversation; rather, inflections in sentences should convey the invitation for the child to respond.

PROBLEMS IN JUVENILE DELINQUENCY

Children who violate the law frequently come to the attention of the courts. These children are classified as juvenile delinquents. At the present time, the rate of juvenile delinquency is shamefully high. Although many persons have studied this problem, little understanding has been gained as to how delinquent children may be helped and rehabilitated. The reasons for the troublesome behavior are closely allied to the feelings and needs of the child.

The range of delinquent behavior is very demeanors, stealing, sexual acts, destruction of property, and cruelty and more serious crimes, such as injury to persons, substance abuse, and murder. The motives causing such crimes are inherent in the child's personality and background. The responsibility and contribution of the parents, family, and community to the child's problem are inescapable and are demonstrable in most cases.

Classification of delinquents is difficult because of the great diversity of problems and the involvement of sociologic, psychologic, anthropologic, psychiatric, and legal components. Each discipline approaches the problems from a particular viewpoint, categorizing them within its own terminology. Generally, classifications of delinquency are of three types: those directly related to the offender's behavior, those related to his personal qualities and motivation, and those related to his interaction with others.

Although the courts attempt to help children in trouble, the available aid is far from satisfactory. Judges and other individuals involved with cases of juvenile delinquency are often unprepared to understand the etiologic and psychologic factors. The preparation of judges, probationary officers, and correction school personnel should contain knowledge and experience with children and their problems as well as study of those conditions in the family, the community, and society that contribute to juvenile delinquency.

CHILDREN WHO CONTROL ANXIETY WITH PHYSICAL SYMPTOMS

In the process of growth and development, children are setting up and reinforcing the building blocks of their personalities. In the course of this process, the dynamic ingredients, such as security, that contribute to the foundation and strength of this structure may be threatened. The consequence is anxiety manifested in behavior symptoms similar to those in adults, as well as in other symptoms peculiar to children. The infant's holding his breath, the child's temper tantrums, and night terrors are evidences of underlying anxiety. Somatic symptoms are also used by children to express anxiety.

A specific event may precipitate an episode of anxiety in a child, but this event is rarely the entire cause of the symptom. Fear of death, anxiety related to a previous illness, or anxiety over a parent's health or welfare may create an underlying anxiety of long duration that can be touched off by a precipitating event. The anxiety attack has many physical components that are frequently evident in cardiac, respiratory, and digestive complaints. Although these attacks are usually temporary, they may return at the occurrence of another precipitating event.

Another manifestation of anxiety is commonly known as *hysteria*. This condition includes a wide variety of physical symptoms that do not have an organic cause and toward which the individual shows relative emotional indifference. The child's attempt to suppress or repress some painful experience may result in some type of somatic behavior pattern. The range of hysterical behavior is wide and difficult to categorize. The symptom may involve the sensory, motor, visceral, and vasomotor functions. Rarely are the somatic manifestations true to the pathologic conditions they resemble, evident when the patient is sleeping, or harmful to the handicapped individual.

The child who develops somatic symptoms, episodic states, or fugues on a hysterical basis is believed to show certain personality characteristics. He often dramatizes his thoughts and feelings. His moods may change rapidly from depression to elation. He is superficial and tends to overimitate and play-act. It is not unusual to trace his behavior to a previous experience or the observation of another sick person whose symptoms he has adopted.

A better organized and more lasting pattern of somatic symptoms may also occur in children. The underlying anxiety is usually constant and the cause exists within the child's environment. A child, infected by the parent's control of anxiety by physical symptoms, often adopts this pattern as his own. Pleasure and affection gained during illness may make somatic symptoms a blessing in disguise. Unbearable conditions in school or at home may encourage him to seek the solace of illness and invalidism. In essence, physical symptoms are used by the child to ease the pressures of his anxiety and thus meet needs not otherwise satisfied.

School phobia and *learning inhibitions* are associated with anxiety present in children under considerable stress in the school situation. With school phobia, the major cause may be attributable to the separation of the child from his mother and home. The learning inhibitions diagnosis is usually associated with the child's loss of self-confidence, which lowers his motivation, interest, and capacity to learn. Anxiety and other emotional components may be present as the result of traumatic experiences that can reduce or impede the child's learning capacity. The need to identify the underlying cause and to help the child regain security and self-confidence is the task of the psychiatrist, the nurses, and the teachers, who need to include parents and family in the process.

Children react to their physical symptoms in various ways. Some worry about them and discuss them constantly. Others delight in them as they give a blow-by-blow account of their aches and pains. Some may not discuss the matter but obviously display the limitations imposed by the symptom. The physical complaints take on a variety of patterns and may simulate, to a degree, a real physical illness. Headaches, dizziness, weakness, fainting, nausea, indigestion, diarrhea, and constipation are frequent generalized complaints.

The treatment and nursing care of children with this disorder are very sensitive. These children are developing patterns of adjustment, and it is important to discourage this behavior. Somatic complaints as patterns of behavior can be fixated or obviated, depending on the wisdom of the treatment plan instituted.

A word on prevention seems apropos. Nurses who care for children in pediatric wards or in other parts of a general hospital should be aware of the dynamics that encourage the development of this pattern of adjustment. Treatment of the whole child rather than of his appendectomy or his tonsillectomy is crucial. Time must be spent with the child if nurses are to know him and if they are to understand how he feels. The way they allay his fears, the way they prepare him for an operation or treatment, and the understanding and warmth they display will influence the child's reaction to his illness. The parents' role and their part in helping the child at this time are most important. Nurses are in a position to help parents by talking with them, by referring them to the physician, and by alerting the physician to the parents' needs.

The child who has developed this behavior pattern is greatly helped by psychotherapy. Given the opportunity, the child will discuss his troubles and soon discover the related causes for his basic anxiety. The somatic complaints quickly disappear since he no longer has any need for them. The part that parents play in the development of this pattern must also receive attention from the therapist. The goal is to make being well more fun and more satisfying than being sick.

If the child is hospitalized for his somatic complaints, the nurse should minimize attention to the symptoms, be guided by the psychiatrist's advice, and plan activities appropriate for the child's age. Reassurance often encourages the child to take a step forward, but nurses should be alert as to whether they have achieved this encouragement. Sometimes a child cannot accept reassurance any more than an adult can. When the child shows signs of fear or anxiety, nurses need to be understanding and to provide an adequate explanation to alleviate the fear. Socialization and activities with other youngsters should be a part of the planned care. A matter-of-fact attitude toward the physical symptoms is probably better than ignoring them.

CHILDREN WHO CONTROL ANXIETY THROUGH RITUALISTIC PATTERNS

The psychodynamics of obsessive and compulsive behavior for children are similar to those for adults. These factors are discussed in Chapter 11.

Ritualistic activities and play are very much a part of the normal behavior of children. Counting white cars, walking on the line of the pavement, and spitting on the bat for luck in baseball are common acts of children at play. However, when the pattern is systematized and dominates the child's daily activities, such as eating and dressing, the behavior becomes a disorder. If the obsessive thoughts and compulsive behavior consume most of the child's waking hours, his school work, his play, and his general health may suffer. Whereas an adult can indulge his obsessiveness and compulsiveness alone, a child often requires and involves other persons. Usually it is the mother who is closest to him and on whom he is dependent for assistance in his daily needs. He imposes on her his repetitious thoughts and demands that she participate in his compulsive acts. This is distressing to the mother, who is usually a rigid, perfectionistic person herself. Her criticism and annoyance add to the child's guilt feelings and to his dilemma. The perfectionism and obsessiveness of the mother or of the father could be etiologic factors of the child's behavior.

Psychotherapy has great value for these children. Primary in therapy are the atmosphere and relationship that provide the child with the freedom to talk about his thoughts, feelings, and acts without judgment and ridicule. His parents are too involved and critical of his behavior to provide this need. Understanding and acceptance, regardless of his behavior, are the basis for all relationships with this child. This fact is helpful for nurses to remember since they, like the mother, may be drawn into the child's pattern of behavior. Patience with respect to the time needed and the peculiar compulsive activity is essential. A plan of daily living as pleasant and close to normal as possible should be followed in order to avoid any secondary gains from reinforcement of the ritualistic pattern.

Since obsessive and compulsive tendencies are rooted in parental behavior, psychotherapeutic help for the parents is certainly indicated. Being able to help the mother or father understand and overcome these tendencies is sometimes a difficult project; however, it is important if the child is to be freed of the pattern.

PSYCHOTIC BEHAVIOR IN CHILDREN

In recent years, more investigations and studies have been made of children whose symptoms defy understanding and diagnosis. It is extremely difficult to recognize and detect psychotic behavior in very young children; however, some investigators have reported such findings in infants less than 1 year of age. Since the life activities of infants and children involve interaction with their environment and principally the people in the environment, it is in this area that signs occur.

In 1944, Kanner reported on early infantile autism in which withdrawal behavior was observed very early in infancy. In the 150 children studied, some common characteristics were detected. The children tended to be self-sufficient and content to be left alone and ignored the presence of individuals around them. Mothers reported their disappointment when a child did not respond to being picked up. Speech was learned by rote; the child recited poems and words with unusual accuracy, but he lacked the ability to use words to convey appropriate meaning. Autistic children sought to keep things the same and related to objects rather than to people. Their activities were centered around their toys or other objects, and they rarely responded to the persons in the room. Their intelligence appeared to be good, if not superior. It was recognized that all of the 150 autistic children studied had highly intelligent parents who were interested and preoccupied with their professions or with art rather than with people and their families.

Symbiotic infantile psychosis was described by Mahler in 1952. This condition becomes obvious at a later age than autism. The major symptoms revolve around the intense, close relationship of a child to his mother. The child never learns to relate to other people, and his own identity is lost. The child never separates himself from his mother in identity and proximity.

Since there is so little known about psychotic conditions in children, treatment is equally puzzling. However, each day more knowledge is gained from the investigations and experiences of those persons working with children. Drugs and shock therapy have not been effective. The current treatment of these psychotic conditions includes residential care with an intensive one-to-one relationship with selected staff members, in order to establish a positive and consistent milieu for the child; family therapy; multiple-impact therapy, with the total family participating in concentrated, brief periods of psychotherapy; and behavior modification using either positive reinforcement such as candy or food to reward acceptable behavior or negative reinforcement to extinguish undesirable behavior.

REFERENCES

Chapman, A. H.: Management of emotional problems of children and adolescents, Philadelphia, 1965, J. B. Lippincott Co.

Chess, S., and Thomas, A., editors: Annual progress in child psychiatry and child development, New York, 1968, Bruner and Mazel, Publishers, pp. 281-321, 540-565.

Christina, Sr. Mary: The role of the nurse in child caring institutions, J. Psychiatr. Nurs. 2:281-285, 1964.

Engel, G.: Psychological development in health and disease, Philadelphia, 1963, W. B. Saunders Co., pp. 29-220.

Fagin, C., editor: Nursing in child psychiatry, St. Louis, 1972, The C. V. Mosby Co., p. 183.

Field, W. E., Jr.: Watch your message, Am. J. Nurs. 72:1278-1280, 1972.

Fisher, W., Mehr, J., and Truckenbrod, P.: Human services: the third revolution in mental health, New York, 1974, Alfred Publishing Co.

Freud, A.: Adolescence. In Eissler, R., and others, editors: The psychoanalytic study of the child, vol. 13, New York, 1958, International Universities Press, Inc., p. 255.

Howells, J. G.: Modern perspectives in child psychiatry, Springfield, Ill., 1965, Charles C Thomas, Publisher, pp. 251-284, 306-333, 336-349.

Hyde, N. D.: Play therapy—the troubled child's self-encounter, Am. J. Nurs. 71:1366-1370, 1971.

Kalman, M., and Davis, A., editors: New dimensions in mental health: psychiatric nursing, ed. 4, New York, 1974, McGraw-Hill Book Co.

Kanner, L.: Child psychiatry, ed. 4, Springfield, Ill., 1972, Charles C Thomas, Publisher, pp. 1-133, 165-254.

Kolb, L. C.: Modern clinical psychiatry, ed. 8, Philadelphia, 1973, W. B. Saunders Co., pp. 530-550.

Lesser, A. J.: Accent on prevention—through improved service, Children **11**:13-18, 1964.

Lippman, H. S.: Treatment of the child in emotional conflict, ed. 2, New York, 1962, McGraw-Hill Book Co.

Mahler, M. S.: On child psychosis and schizophrenia. In Eissler, R., and others, editors: The psychoanalytic study of the child, vol. 7, New York, 1952, International Universities Press, Inc., pp. 286-304.

McBride, A. B.: The anger-depression-guilt go-round, Am. J. Nurs. **73**:1045-1049, 1973.

Morgan, A. J., and Moreno, J. W.: The practice of mental health nursing: a community approach, 1973, Philadelphia, J. B. Lippincott Co., pp. 114-128.

Ohman, E. N., and Walano, D.: An approach to the nursing diagnosis of behavior in a pediatric specialty clinic, Nurs. Sci. **2**:152-159, 1964.

Petrie, A., McCulloch, R., and Kasdin, P.: The perceptual characteristics of juvenile delinquents, J. Psychiatr. Nurs. **1**:142-151, 1963.

Salerno, E. M.: A family in crisis, Am. J. Nurs. **73**:100-103, 1973.

Shufer, S.: The pediatric mental health nurse clinician, Nurs. Outlook **19**:543, 1971.

Simpson, E. S.: A better tomorrow for disturbed children, Am. J. Nurs. **69**:1031-1033, 1969.

Turner, R.: A method of working with disturbed children, Am. J. Nurs. **70**:2146-2151, 1970.

ADDITIONAL READINGS

Comley, R.: Self-injuries behavior in a retarded child, Nurs. Mirror **142**(12):66-68, 1976.

Davis, C.: Nursing care study: personality disorder, Nurs. Times **72**(18):695-697, 1976.

Haus, B. F., and others: The effect of nursing intervention on a program of behavior modification by parents in the home, J. Psychiatr. Nurs. **14**(8):9-16, 1976.

Jones, L.: The role of the hospital nurse in the therapeutic team, Nurs. Mirror **143**(2):66-67, 1976.

Lesser, S. R.: Psychiatric management of the deaf child, Can. Nurse **71**(10):23-25, 1975.

CHAPTER 19

Children with organic behavior disorders

It has been noted that physical illnesses could be the sources for behavior problems in children, particularly if they result from unsatisfactory parent-child relationships. There are other behavioral changes primarily caused by organic pathology and secondarily influenced by the parent-child relationship. These organic behavior problems require considerable knowledge and skill in physical and psychiatric nursing care. The causes for these conditions are numerous and sometimes nebulous. They may include congenital anomalies, birth injuries, brain tumors, metabolic and endocrine dysfunction, and infections. Invariably children with these conditions require medical care, psychiatric and psychologic guidance, and ingenious nursing care.

The physical assessment of the newborn in the nursery is a routine but highly significant process. This examination and the nurse's expertise in knowing the range of normal could result in early detection of abnormalities. Early diagnosis of pathologic conditions could be the first step toward the prevention of future complications and maladjustment.

The infant's stay in the newborn nursery should be more than just an automatic feeding, cleaning, and sleeping routine. The cry of the infant, his sleep pattern, how he takes his feedings and the amount, and his response to individuals are manifestations of his early behavior and need to be attentively observed rather than taken for granted. Professional nurses, and maternity nurse specialist's in particular, need to provide the guidance and teaching of other personnel in the nurseries to be alert for infant behavior that may be signs of possible pathology.

CONGENITAL ANOMALIES

Congenital anomalies become apparent early in the infant's life, and his development is often marred by some physical deformity and intellectual impairment. Blindness, contractures, paralysis, deafness, and ataxia are commonly observed. The life span of this child is conditioned by the area of the brain involved and the nature of the deformity. The causative factors for malformation of the fetus include genetic factors, intrauterine complications during pregnancy (Rh factors, drug addiction, toxemias, maternal syphilis, and x-ray of pregnant uterus), and premature birth. Drugs, such as the much-publicized thalidomide, administered to women during pregnancy also can cause the deformity or death of an infant.

Malformation of the brain renders the child, if he survives, intellectually deficient and, to a greater or lesser degree, dependent on others for his physical needs and daily care. Porencephaly is the absence of part of the brain tissue, sometimes forming a cavity. Death occurs early in infancy. Microcephaly indicates an abnormally small brain and head formation. Hydrocephalus is characterized by ⌐n unusually large head caused by an increased accumulation of cerebrospinal fluid in the ventricles or subarachnoid space. Infants with these conditions are seen and treated in pediatric nurseries. Their nursing care requires diligent attention to physical needs for the maintenance of health and the prevention of infections since their physical stamina is usually decreased. Although these infants may have a distorted appearance, it is important for the nurse to be aware of and respond to their emotional and psychologic needs, which are the same as for other infants. Microcephalic and hydrocephalic children who survive infancy are mentally retarded and require continued detailed care at home or, more often, in an institution.

Mongolism (Down's syndrome) is a congenital condition that is more evident because these children grow to adolescence and adulthood. The mongoloid has a characteristic physiognomy and accompanying mental deficiency. Studies have shown that these conditions involve chromosomal abnormalities.

The characteristic appearance of a mongoloid child is marked by a small head flattened posteriorly, eyes with oblique palpebral fissures and vertical folds of skin at the inner canthus, and a flat bridge on a short nose. Other body features are also observable: the limbs are short, the hands are fat and stubby with small fingers, the palms show unusual line markings, the toes and thumbs are abducted from the other digits, and the tongue has deep fissures and often protrudes. Other anomalies may also be present. Mental and physical development is often impaired. The behavior of this child presents few problems since he is usually cheerful, affectionate, and obedient. When institutionalized, he adjusts readily and seems content in his environment. He is susceptible to numerous infections, particularly upper respiratory. Although death has frequently occurred at adolescence, improved medical and institutional care have prolonged life. Depending on his intellectual level, the ability to learn is limited. However, he tends to imitate the behavior of others and takes great pleasure in doing this.

Many of these children, because of their affectionate nature, are dearly loved by their parents and siblings. Consequently they are retained in the home. The increased demand for the mother's time and attention may create problems for the other children. Public health nurses can be of great assistance to the mother and family by their availability and teaching. Day schools and special classes for the mentally retarded in the community are beneficial for many mongoloid children.

METABOLIC AND ENDOCRINE DISORDERS

Some metabolic disorders, brain tumors, toxic infections, and head injuries result in rapid physical and mental degeneration and death in a relatively short period of time. Tay-Sachs disease is a hereditary degenerative disease that becomes apparent after the sixth month of life. Its onset is rapid; the changes, both physical and mental, are progressively debilitating; death occurs at about the third year. A cherry red spot on the retina is diagnostic. Muscular weakness and atrophy, blindness, convulsions, and emaciation, if the child has had inadequate food intake, require imaginative and intensive nursing care.

Phenylketonuria (PKU) is a disturbance in protein metabolism that is not as devastating as Tay-Sachs disease. It can now be detected and prevented in early infancy. Blood tests for large amounts of phenylalanine and a simple urine test with ferric chloride for urinary phenylpyruvic acid are tests that could signal early treatment and thus prevent brain damage. A low protein diet, which reduces the phenylalanine in the blood, has proved most therapeutic. Convulsive occurrences and feeblemindedness are major symptoms as the sick child grows and develops. It is common to find several children in the same family afflicted with this disorder, which tends to be transmitted from parents to children. Early detection in the nursery and by the public health nurse in the home is of primary importance. When the nurse discovers a child with phenylketonuria, an inquiry should be made about many, if not all, of the family relatives to help prevent the progressive course of this disorder.

TOXIC DISORDERS

During the developmental years, normal children may fall victims to a number of factors that could result in brain damage. The causative factors include infections, poisons, tumors, mechanical trauma, and others.

Meningitis, encephalitis, brain abscesses, and skull fractures are serious illnesses for the growing child. In general the toxic factor invades the brain tissues, often causing edema, and produces physical, mental, or emotional changes depending on the site involved. The symptoms vary. Drowsiness and lethargy may be present in some patients, whereas hyperactivity and restlessness may be seen in other patients. Vital signs that may be observed early include changes in respiration and pulse. Projectile vomiting and slow pulse and respirations are diagnostic of intracranial pressure as seen in brain abscesses. As these conditions progress, delirium, convulsions, and coma are serious symptoms. Hallucinations, when they are present, arouse great fear. Constant supervision of these patients is essential to prevent injury, to keep the patients as comfortable as possible, and to observe any changes in their condition. In patients with encephalitis, ocular changes are common, and postencephalitic symptoms, including changes in the sleep pattern, speech impairment, palsies, tics, ptosis, and convulsions, often persist because of the original brain damage.

During the acute phase of these conditions, the children are very sick and often unresponsive. Their physical care requires extensive medical and nursing procedures to reduce toxicity and to relieve physical discomfort. Nutrition and fluid intake are of primary importance to maintain the child's physiologic needs. When he is immobile for long periods, change in body position alleviates pressure areas. In overactivity, padding the crib or bed helps to avoid injury.

After the acute stage, the child's behavior changes slowly because of the physical exhaustion caused by the disease. An assessment of the physical and mental residual impairments should be a prerequisite for planning his convalescence and rehabilitation. Physical impairments require medical and specialized therapy. Mental impairment and behavioral changes will require psychologic evaluation and psychiatric follow-up.

Personality changes that may result vary considerably with the severity of the illness and the damage incurred. Children who were once well behaved become restless, unruly, aggressive, and explosive. They are difficult to manage at home and at school. Antisocial acts, such as stealing, lying, destructiveness, profanity, and rages, may be seen. Although they say they feel remorseful, they also state that they cannot help themselves. Their moods change rapidly, conveying tenderness at one moment and hostility and destructiveness at the next.

Mental growth and intellectual retardation vary with each patient. Some children may suffer no intellectual loss, whereas others may retain the level of achieved development but progress no further. Still other children may lose a great deal of their previous achievement and regress further with time.

Infants and toddlers have been notorious for their tendencies to lick and ingest paint known for its lead content. Lead is neurotropic in action. In lead poisoning, when the child is resuscitated following cardiac arrest, severe brain damage often results. Preventive steps have been taken by requiring manufacturers to provide nonlead paint for toys, furniture, and home use.

Brain tumors are less frequent in children than in adults. Head injuries are found more frequently and are caused by birth injuries, falls, accidents, or intentional abuse from parents or siblings. The symptoms of these conditions include headache, dizziness, nausea, projectile vomiting, slow pulse, stupor, and seizures. Specific symptoms are related to the area involved and to the size of the tumor or injury to the tissues. Personality changes as prodromal symptoms may be evident to the alert observer. These may include restlessness, irritability, apathy, depression, or confusion. However, these signs may escape the mother, who sees and accepts variability in the child's daily behavior. It is only when more pronounced symptoms occur that she becomes alarmed. The nurse who may see the child in the doctor's office or clinic may engage the mother in conversation about the child and by so doing identify the onset of gradual behavioral problems or changes. Mental retardation is relative to the pathologic disorder and the success of therapy.

BEHAVIOR DISORDERS WITH CONVULSIONS

Fainting, jerking and twitching movements, and convulsions or seizures are not uncommon in children. They may be associated with a physical illness or they may occur spontaneously and without repetition. However, when convulsions are recurrent in children, parents become greatly distressed. They are sure the child is doomed to insanity, mental retardation, or at least moral depravity. It is difficult to erase these ignorant beliefs handed down from the past.

The cause for the convulsions requires serious and thorough investigation. A diagnosis should be made only after careful tests have been taken. The electroencephalogram is considered to be the best current diagnostic tool for epilepsy. Once the certainty of idiopathic epilepsy has been established, medication and treatment can be instituted. Most adults with epilepsy experienced its onset in childhood or adolescence.

Regardless of the cause for the convulsions, there are two attack phenomena observed in children—grand mal and petit mal. The psychic equivalents are rare. The grand mal attacks manifest themselves to a greater or lesser degree in the following manner. An aura or sign may or may not be felt by the child prior to loss of consciousness. Some children give out a shrill cry. The child falls into a tonic spasm, making his body stiff and rigid. In a few seconds, clonic movements occur over the entire body; these include twitching, jerking, and kicking movements. Mouth and tongue movements and gasping and gargling sounds are exhibited. Tongue biting may occur. The eyes are rolled back and the pupils change from occlusion to dilation. The corneal reflex is absent and the Babinski sign is positive. Involuntary urination and defecation may result. Increased salivation is apparent and sometimes forms a froth on the lips. This stage is followed by relaxation and deep sleep. When the child awakens, he may be confused, weak, and drowsy. The child does not remember the attack but becomes aware that something has happened to him from the manner and facial expression of his parents and others around him. The pattern and regularity of the attacks are not the same, and all attacks do not follow the typical picture just described. Variations among patients and in each individual patient may be observed. The jacksonian type has specific, characteristic movements, indicating a focal cortical lesion.

Petit mal is used to describe a brief loss of consciousness without seizures. These episodic staring, vacant spells last only a few seconds, and the child is not aware of them at all. A parent, teacher, or playmate may notice the behavior, particularly if he or she is conversing with the child at the time.

As soon as diagnosis is established, an anticonvulsant medication is usually prescribed. The type and the dosage depend on the individual and on the ability to control the convulsions. The child's reaction to the medication should be watched carefully, particularly when the drug or dosage is changed or varied. When the drug is to be discontinued, the dose is gradually diminished over a period of time. Some of the more common drugs used are phenobarbital (Luminal), phenytoin (Dilantin), phenantoin (Mesantoin), trimethadione (Tridione), phenacemide (Phenurone), and paramethadione (Paradione).

A ketogenic diet, containing a low carbohydrate and high fat composition, is more beneficial for children than for adults with epilepsy. The child may find this diet unpalatable unless some imagination and care are used in its preparation. The mother and the nurse may need the expert assistance of a dietitian. Fluids may need to be restricted since some children have shown a decrease in convulsions when dehydration is present.

The child with epilepsy has problems that grow out of the nature of his illness. Parents, siblings, relatives, playmates, teachers, and others convey mixed attitudes toward the child, particularly when they witness his seizure. Fear, pity, and revulsion may be portrayed in their faces as their words attempt to mislead the child. It is not unexpected, then, that the child reacts and thus manifests problematic behavior. This is often interpreted as the epileptic personality. The parental reaction to the child and his condition is vitally important in his adjustment. These children have similar needs for love, security, acceptance, and happiness as other children. Emotional disturbances have been known to trigger convulsions in some children.

Mental deterioration is not a natural concomitant of epilepsy, as was once believed. Mental retardation, when evident, is attributed to many varied causes, which usually fall into five areas: (1) constitutional makeup of the child, (2) injury to the brain before the onset of epilepsy, (3) increased frequency of grand mal seizures, (4) toxicity caused by overdosage of bromides or phenobarbital, and (5) psychologic and social mistreatment resulting in self-centeredness and severe discouragement. Dostoevski, Flaubert, and other persons are witness to the fact that superior intelligence and epilepsy can be compatible. The legendary epileptic personality is a myth rather than a reality.

MENTAL RETARDATION

Mental retardation does not define a single disease but a syndrome that can be produced by many causative factors, alone or in combinations. There is a considerable variety of conditions falling under the category of mental retardation. Very often, mental deficiency and mental retardation are used interchangeably.

Impairment of intelligence is a cardinal symptom of this syndrome. Standardized tests are used to measure the level of the person's intelligence quotient. Mentally retarded individuals are usually found to have an I.Q. below 70. Impairment is usually observable in maturation, learning ability, and social adjustment. Retardation varies in degree and in the capacity for mental performance. Severe retardation could force the child to a vegetative existence of complete dependence. Individuals who are less retarded, capable of training for self-care and social interaction, are incorporated into the family and the protected environment of a home. Still others may be able to attend special classes in public schools and go on to job training. The particular capabilities of each retarded child should be evaluated as one basis for establishing a suitable plan for his development and social adjustment.

Mental retardation has been with mankind for many ages. In the past much pity was shown for these children because of the hopelessness in knowing what to do. Attitudes have changed with the use of proven techniques to help the retarded person reach his maximum potential. Research has increased and resources and facilities have been provided that have improved the care and training of mentally retarded children, adolescents, and adults. The late President Kennedy's support gave great impetus to the movement. Public and parental education has helped to change some of the negative attitudes and the hopelessness surrounding the mentally retarded. Many of these patients, of all ages, who were confined and forgotten in back wards of large public psychiatric institutions have been moved to special facilities for their care and thus helped to develop to their full potential.

The Accreditation Council for Facilities for Mentally Retarded (1971) has attempted to help the mentally retarded toward a more normal life pattern. This new attitude—that the retarded are deserving of a normal environment— reflects hope rather than despair, that the retarded are human beings with the same rights and privileges as others. This normalization principle is also the goal of behavioral therapy.

Behavioral therapy has been found to be effective for all levels of retardation including the profoundly and severely retarded. Fox and Azrin (1972) indicate that two major phases are part of the program: (1) treatment training and setting criterion performance and (2) maintenance which provides the environment and opportunities to ensure that the newly acquired skills will be used in the activities of daily living. The concepts and techniques of behavioral therapy can be valuable tools for the psychiatric nurse. Caplan (1961) points out, "Knowledge is limited on the organic factors that have an etiologic role in the production of mental disorders in children. Research has produced valuable information that could result in improved primary prevention were it more generally used. . . . Current scientific interest promises a brighter future for the children yet to be born."

THE CARE OF CHILDREN

The nursing care of children generally is not a simple task. Children and their behavior problems are as varied as the individuals. Physical and mental symptoms add to the needs that must be considered in their nursing care, whether at home or in an institution.

Nurses' attitudes and knowledge of children, in illness and in health, should result in acceptance of children as they are and in intelligent, creative nursing care. This can happen only if they like children and have studied the children's needs. Management of behavior problems requires special attention to child psychiatry and learning experiences with children manifesting behavior problems. Nurses soon realize that to help the mentally handicapped child they need the assistance of many other professional and nonprofessional personnel as much as the others need theirs. It is important that they care for the child and his total needs; therefore, they must work, cooperate, and plan with his parents and others who are essential for his complete care. If they do not, the child will suffer.

Physical needs. The dependence of children on adults for their physical needs is related to their age and their physical and mental capacities. When they are sick, their dependence is greater. This is particularly true with organic behavior disorders.

The physiologic and medical needs of the child with organic behavior disorders are dictated by the physician. How these are implemented for each child depends on the nurse and the child. It is unfortunate that in some instances the nursing care directed toward meeting physical and medical needs is a brisk routine imposed in exactly the same manner on every young patient. The care of children requires time and personal involvement.

Comfort aspects for patients with physical abnormalities and behavior disorders require intelligent, imaginative management. The child with cranial and brain trauma may be completely or partially paralyzed, necessitating constant attention. Oral hygiene, skin care, exercise of muscles, and other body movements periodically during the day and night maintain the child's well-being. Management of a child with an enlarged head (hydrocephalus), a paralyzed limb, or total body paralysis (children with Tay-Sachs disease) should be thought through and planned before action is taken. Injury must be avoided. Nurses should instruct and supervise other personnel who assist in the care of these children.

Nutritional needs entail the composition of the diet, the method of preparation, and the manner of feeding. Special diets, such as the ketogenic diet, must contain the necessary nutrients and must be adequate in amount to provide its therapeutic effect. Special and regular diets must be of the consistency for easy ingestion and must be palatable to the child. Appetite is usually poor with illness; nothing should add to this difficulty. Feeding of the child is the direct responsibility of the nurse. The nurse, like the mother, should find the one particular way suitable for feeding each child. Supporting a wobbly head by holding the child in a special position comes with experimentation. The child's swallowing reflex may be impaired, and very small spoonfuls and an adequate length of time at feedings may be required. Tube feeding, when necessary, should include care of the membranes of the nose and the child's general comfort when the tube is inserted or retained in place. The amount of food taken should satisfy the child's hunger as well as maintain his weight and health. Feeding time should be made into a pleasurable experience for the child.

Protection from injury is necessary at all times. The nurse must evaluate the environment to see what may be hazardous before any accident or injury happens. The child with convulsions should be in a low bed with a padded headboard if necessary. The spastic child may need constant assistance when walking.

The nurse's responsibility does not end with the child's discharge; the mother and sometimes the entire family must be instructed in how they can best meet the sick child's needs. Referrals to public health nurses for continued care and supervision of this child in the home can contribute much to his well-being and to parents' reassurance.

Psychotherapeutic needs. The child's mental defect is devastating to most parents. Their feelings may be a mixture of guilt, self-pity, revulsion, rejection, and shame. Parental feelings and attitudes need to be considered early in order to facilitate acceptance of the child as he is. Only then can the parents and family make a logical plan for his care, growth, and development. Acceptance and understanding are not always achieved and remain a stumbling block in the child's progress. Overprotective parents can also cause harm by fostering overdependence of a trainable child and perhaps by neglecting the other children.

As mentioned previously, the psychologic needs of these children are the same as for normal children. The parent-child relationship is equally important. Several authors have written that behavior problems in children with organic brain disorders are stimulated by emotional conflicts growing out of parent or sibling relationships rather than directly from the pathologic disorder. Acceptance and love can go a long way with these children. For the child who is institutionalized, the female nurse often becomes the mother figure. Her feelings, attitudes, and behavior toward the child are equally as important as those of parents. The male nurse similarly can play the role of father figure and help in parental relationships with children. Like other children, children with organic behavior disorders benefit by firm but tender care supported by love and affection.

Since most behavior problems arise within the social and parental relationships of the child, careful study and analysis can detect the true motive underlying the troublesome behavior. Unfortunately, all too often the surface behavior is considered, and the real cause is not unearthed. In young children psychotherapeutic conversations and play sessions help to reveal the underlying problem rather quickly. In older children, it may require more time, closer observations, psychologic testing, and numerous psychotherapeutic sessions. When child-parent relationships are acutely difficult, the removal of the child from home may be best. Hospitalization should then provide the permissiveness for self-expression and acceptance that were lacking in the home. Older children will test the nurse and therapist time and again for their objectivity and true acceptance. The nurse's knowledge of the child's background could be helpful in avoiding pitfalls.

REFERENCES

Adams, M. L.: Care of the retarded child in the home, Nurs. Forum 6:403-418, 1967.
Barnard, K., and Powell, M. L.: Teaching the mentally retarded child, St. Louis, 1972, The C. V. Mosby Co.
Caplan, G., editor: Prevention of mental disorders in children, New York, 1961, Basic Books, Inc., pp. 1-51.
Fagin, C. M.: Nursing in child psychiatry, St. Louis, 1972, The C. V. Mosby Co.

Fox, R., and Azrin, N.: Restitution: a method of eliminating aggressive disruptive behavior of retarded and brain damaged patients, Behav. Res. Ther. **10**:15-27, 1972.

Joint Commission on Accreditation of Hospitals: Standards for residential facilities for the mentally retarded, Accreditation Council for Facilities for Mentally Retarded, 1971.

Kanner, L.: Child psychiatry, Springfield, Ill., 1972, Charles C Thomas, Publisher, pp. 255-440.

ADDITIONAL REFERENCES

Azrin, N., and Armstrong, P.: The mini-meal—a method for teaching eating skills to the profoundly retarded, Ment. Retard. **11**:9, 1973.

Salerno, E. M.: A family in crisis, Am. J. Nurs. **73**:100-103, 1973.

Schaefer, H. H., and Martin, P. L.: Behavioral therapy, New York, 1975, McGraw-Hill Book Co.

Shufer, S.: The pediatric mental health nurse clinician, Nurs. Outlook **19**:543, 1971.

APPENDIXES

APPENDIX A

Condensed classification of mental illnesses with diagnostic criteria*

DISORDERS CAUSED BY OR ASSOCIATED WITH IMPAIRMENT OF BRAIN TISSUE FUNCTION

    I. Mental retardation

Subnormal intellectual functioning that originates during the developmental period and impairs learning and social adjustment.

        Borderline—I.Q. 68 to 83†

        Mild—I.Q. 52 to 67

        Moderate—I.Q. 36 to 51

        Severe—I.Q. 20 to 35

        Profound—I.Q. under 20

        Unspecified—has not or cannot be evaluated

      A. Following infection or intoxication

Results from residual cerebral damage from intracranial infections, serums, drugs, or toxic agents.

      B. Following trauma or physical agents

Includes mechanical injury at birth, asphyxia at birth, and postnatal injury.

---

*Summarized from Diagnostic and statistical manual of mental disorders, II, seventh printing, Washington, D.C., 1974, The American Psychiatric Association.

†Some of the problems of quantification are revealed by the fact that differentiation depends on judgments that may be hard to defend. An I.Q. of 68 means borderline and one of 67 means retardation. An I.Q. of 36 means moderate and an I.Q. of 35 means severe retardation.

409

C. With disorders of metabolism, growth, or nutrition

Includes Tay-Sachs disease, Niemann-Pick disease, phenylketonuria, and hypoglycemosis.

D. Associated with gross brain disease (postnatal)

Includes all diseases associated with neopasms that are not secondary to trauma or infection, also including postnatal conditions in which structural reaction is evident but etiology uncertain.

E. Associated with diseases and conditions due to unknown prenatal influence

Includes conditions known to have existed at the time of or prior to birth for which definite etiology cannot be established. Primary cranial anomalies and congenital defects of undetermined origin are included.

F. With chromosomal abnormality

Includes those with an abnormal number of chromosomes and chromosomal abnormalities of morphology.

G. Associated with prematurity

Includes those with a birth weight of less that 2500 grams (5.5 pounds) or a period of gestation less than 38 weeks and an etiology that cannot be classified under another category.

H. Following major psychiatric disorder

Includes those who show mental retardation following psychosis or major psychiatric disorder in early childhood when cerebral pathology cannot be demonstrated.

I. With psychosocial deprivation

Includes those who show a definite history of deprivation but no evidence of organic disease or pathology.

J. With other and unspecified conditions

II. Organic brain disorders

Organic brain disorders are characterized by the evidence of brain damage and the following symptoms: (1) defects in orientation, (2) impairment of memory, (3) impairment of intellectual functions such as comprehension, knowledge, and learning, (4) impairment of judgment, and (5) the lability and shallowness of affect. Acute brain disorders result from temporary, reversible impairment of brain functioning and thus have a good ultimate prognosis. Chronic brain disorders are caused by relatively permanent impairment of the brain and thus the ultimate prognosis as to the return of previous levels of adjustment limited.

A. Senile and presenile dementia

Includes senile brain changes ranging from the mild, with self-centeredness, difficulty in assimilating new experiences, and labile emotionality, up to the severe, including the state of vegetative existence.

B. Alcoholic psychosis

Includes a wide variety of responses ranging from the acute and immediate to the chronic and irreversible. In this category are delerium tremens, Korsakoff's psychosis, hallucinosis, paranoid state, acute intoxication, deterioration, and pathologic intoxication.

C. Psychosis associated with intracranial infection

Includes psychoses with general paresis (syphilis), with other syphilis of the central nervous system, with epidemic encephalitis, with other and unspecified encephalitis, and with other unspecified intracranial infection.

D. Psychosis associated with other cerebral condition

Includes psychoses with cerebral arteriosclerosis, with other cerebrovascular disturbance, with epilepsy, with intracranial neoplasm, with degenerative disease of the central nervous system, with brain trauma, and with other unspecified cerebral conditions.

E. Psychosis associated with other physical condition

Includes psychoses with endocrine disorders, with metabolic or nutritional disorder, with systemic infection, with drug or poison intoxication other than alcohol, with childbirth, or with other undiagnosed or unspecified physical condition.

F. Nonpsychotic organic brain syndromes

Includes all of the preceding in which there is demonstrable brain damage but in which psychotic behavior is not a major consideration.

DISORDERS OF PSYCHOGENIC ORIGIN OR WITHOUT CLEARLY DEFINED PHYSICAL CAUSE OR STRUCTURAL CHANGE IN THE BRAIN

Psychotic disorders: characterized by personality disintegration, inability to use reality testing in situations, and inability to relate effectively to other people and to handle own work.

I. Schizophrenia

Reactions characterized by disturbances in reality relationships, concept formations, affective responses, intellectual function, and behavior patterns. Frequent occurrences are strong tendency to retreat from reality, emotional disharmony, stream of thought disturbances, regressive behavior, and sometimes deterioration.

A. Schizophrenia, simple type

Characterized by reduction in external attachments and by impoverishment of human relationships. Apathy and indifference occur. Severity of symptoms increases over a long period of time with mental deterioration. Hallucinations and delusions are infrequent.

B. Schizophrenia, hebephrenic type

Typified by inappropriate and shallow affect, silly behavior and mannerisms, giggling, delusions, hallucinations, and regressive behavior.

C. Schizophrenia, catatonic type

Significant motor behavior; generalized inhibition shown in stupor, mutism, negativism, and waxy flexibility. Excessive motor activity and excitement also occur.

D. Schizophrenia, paranoid type

Characterized by autistic, unrealistic thinking, delusions of persecution or of grandeur, ideas of reference, and hallucinations. Behavior is unpredictable, but an underlying hostility and aggression are often constant.

E. Acute schizophrenic episode

Acute onset of symptoms characterized by confusion, perplexity, ideas of reference, emotional turmoil, dream-like dissociation, excitement, depression, or fear. Recovery may occur or the patient may progress to the other types of classic schizophrenia.

F. Schizophrenia, latent type

Clear symptoms of schizophrenia but no history of a psychotic schizophrenic episode. Included are incipient, prepsychotic, pseudoneurotic, pseudopsychopathic, or borderline schizophrenic behavior.

G. Schizophrenia, residual type

Signs of schizophrenia shown following a psychotic episode, but the patient is no longer psychotic.

H. Schizophrenia, schizoaffective type

A mixture of schizophrenic symptoms with pronounced elation or depression.

I. Schizophrenia, childhood type

Occurs before puberty and may be manifested by autistic, atypical, and withdrawn behavior; failure to develop self-identity; and gross immaturity and inadequacy in development.

J. Schizophrenia, chronic undifferentiated type

Mixed schizophrenic symptoms with schizophrenic thought, affect, and behavior not classifiable under other types.

K. Schizophrenia, other and unspecified types

Any type of schizophrenia not previously described.

II. Major affective disorders

Characterized by disorder of mood, extreme elation or depression, that dominates the life of the patient. Onset is not ordinarily related to a definite precipitating life experience.

A. Involutional melancholia

Occurs in the involutional period and is characterized by worry, agitation, and severe insomnia. Feelings of guilt and somatic preoccupations may grow to delusional proportions.

B. Manic-depressive illnesses

Marked by severe mood swings and a tendency to remission and recurrence.

1. Manic-depressive illness, manic type

Consists of manic episode marked by excessive elations, irratibility, talkativeness, flight of ideas, and accelerated speech and motor activity.

2. Manic-depressive illness, depressed type

Consists of depressive episodes characterized by severely depressed mood and by mental and motor retardation. Uneasiness, apprehension, perplexity, and agitation may be present.

3. Manic-depressive illness, circular type

Characterized by at least one depressive and one manic episode.

4. Other major affective disorder

Includes those not classified above, as well as affective disorders in which manic and depressive episodes appear simultaneously.

5. Unspecified major affective disorder

III. Paranoid states

Essential abnormality: a delusion generally persecutory or grandiose in nature. Disturbances in mood, behavior, and thinking are derived from the delusion.

A. Paranoia (rare)

Characterized by gradual development of intricate, complex, and elaborate paranoid system, usually based on the misinterpretation of an actual event.

B. Involutional paranoid state

Characterized by delusional formation with onset in the involutional period.

C. Other paranoid state

IV. Other psychoses

A. Psychotic depressive reaction

Depressive mood attributable to some experience.

B. Reactive excitation or confusion

C. Acute paranoid reaction

D. Reactive psychosis, unspecified

E. Unspecified psychosis

V. Neuroses

Chief characteristic: anxiety expressed directly or controlled by psychologic mechanisms. Mechanisms produce symptoms of subjective distress from which the patient wants relief. There is no gross distortion or misinterpretation of reality or gross personality disorganization. Contact with reality is maintained.

A. Anxiety neurosis

Characterized by anxious overconcern extending to panic and often associated with somatic symptoms. It may occur under any circumstances and is not restricted to specific situations or objects.

B. Hysterical neurosis

Characterized by involuntary psychogenic loss or disorder of function; begins and ends in emotionally charged situations and is often symbolic of the underlying conflicts.

C. Phobic neurosis

Characterized by intense fear of an object or situation that the patient consciously recognizes as no real danger. This is generally recognized as fears displaced to the phobic object or situation from some other object of which the patient is unaware.

D. Obsessive compulsive neurosis

Characterized by the persistent intrusion of unwanted thoughts, urges, or actions that the patient is unable to stop.

E. Depressive neurosis

Characterized by an excessive reaction of depression to an internal conflict or to an identifiable event such as the loss of a love object or a cherished possession.

F. Neurasthenic neurosis

Characterized by complaints of chronic weakness, easy fatigability, and sometimes exhaustion.

G. Depersonalization neurosis

Characterized by a feeling of unreality and of estrangement from the self, body, or surroundings.

H. Hypochondriacal neurosis

Characterized by preoccupation with the body and with fear of presumed diseases of various organs that persist despite reassurance.

I. Other neurosis

J. Unspecified neurosis

VI. Personality disorders and certain other nonpsychotic mental disorders

A. Personality disorders

Characterized by deeply ingrained maladaptive patterns of behavior.

1. Paranoid personality
   Characterized by hypersensitivity, rigidity, unwarranted suspicion, jealousy, envy, excessive self-importance, and a tendency to blame others and to ascribe evil motives to them.
2. Cyclothymic personality
   Characterized by recurring and alternating periods of depression and elation.
3. Schizoid personality
   Characterized by shyness, oversensitivity, seclusiveness, avoidance of close or competitive relationships, and often somewhat eccentric behavior. The inability to express hostile and aggressive feelings is common.
4. Explosive personality
   Characterized by gross outbursts of rage or of verbal or physical aggressiveness that are strikingly different from usual behavior.
5. Obsessive compulsive personality
   Characterized by excessive concern with conformity and adherence to standards of conscience that lead to rigidity, inhibition, overconscientiousness, and inability to relax easily.
6. Hysterical personality
   Characterized by excitability, emotional instability, overreactivity, and self-dramatization.
7. Asthenic personality
   Characterized by easy fatigability, low energy level, lack of enthusiasm, marked incapacity for enjoyment, and oversensitivity to physical and emotional stress.
8. Antisocial personality
   Characterized by unsocialized behavior patterns that tend to bring them into conflict with society. Such patients are incapable of loyalty, grossly selfish, callous, irresponsible, impulsive, and unable to learn from experience or punishment.
9. Passive-aggressive personality
   Characterized by both passivity and aggressiveness. Aggressiveness may be expressed passively.
10. Inadequate personality
    Characterized by ineffectual response to intellectual, emotional, social, and physical demands.

B. Sexual orientation disturbances
   Characterized by persons whose sexual interests are directed toward objects other than people of the opposite sex, and toward sexual acts

not considered normal or not performed under normal circumstances.

    1. Homosexuality
       Sexual interest in the same sex.
    2. Fetishism
       Loving an inanimate object.
    3. Pedophilia
       Sexual interest in young children.
    4. Transvestitism
       Masquerading in the clothes of the opposite sex.
    5. Exhibitionism
       Indecent exposure.
    6. Voyeurism
       Morbid desire to look at the sexual organs.
    7. Sadism
       Pleasure found in inflicting pain.
    8. Masochism
       Sexual pleasure heightened with mistreatment and beating.
    9. Other sexual deviation

VII. Alcoholism
Characterized by enough alcoholic intake to damage physical health or personal or social functioning or to become a prerequisite to normal functioning.

    A. Episodic excessive drinking
       Alcoholism plus intoxication as frequently as four times a year.
    B. Habitual excessive drinking
       Alcoholism plus intoxication more than twelve times a year or under the influence of alcohol more than once a week.
    C. Alcoholic addiction
       Characterized by direct or strong presumptive evidence that the patient is dependent on alcohol.

VIII. Drug dependence
Addicted to or dependent on drugs; habitual use of or a clear sense of need for the drug.

    A. Drug dependence, opium, opium alkaloids, and their derivatives
    B. Drug dependence, synthetic analgesics with morphine-like effects
    C. Drug dependence, barbiturates
    D. Drug dependence, other hypnotics, sedatives, or tranquilizers
    E. Drug dependence, cocaine
    F. Drug dependence, *Cannabis sativa* (hashish, marijuana)

    G. Drug dependence, other psychostimulants (amphetamines and so on)

    H. Drug dependence, hallucinogens

    I. Other drug dependence

IX. Psychophysiologic disorders

Characterized by physical symptoms caused by emotional factors and involving a single organ system, usually under autonomic nervous system innervation. Physiologic changes are those that normally accompany emotional states but are more intense and sustained. The patient may not be consciously aware of his emotional state.

    A. Psychophysiologic skin disorders

        Includes neurodermatosis, pruritus, and atopic dermatitis.

    B. Psychophysiologic musculoskeletal disorders

        Includes backaches, muscle cramps, myalgias, and tension headaches.

    C. Psychophysiologic respiratory disorders

        Includes bronchial asthma, sighing, hyperventilation syndromes, and hiccups.

    D. Psychophysiologic cardiovascular disorders

        Includes paroxysmal tachycardia, hypertension, and migraine.

    E. Psychophysiologic hemic and lymphatic disorders

        Includes any such disorders in which emotional factors play a causative role.

    F. Psychophysiologic gastrointestinal disorders

        Includes peptic ulcers, chronic gastritis, ulcerative or mucous colitis, hyperacidity, or pylorospasm.

    G. Psychophysiologic genitourinary disorders

        Includes disturbances in menstruation and micturition, dyspareunia, and impotence.

    H. Psychophysiologic endocrine disorders

        Includes any disturbance in which emotional factors play a causative factor.

    I. Psychophysiologic disorders of organ of special sense

    J. Other types of psychologic disorders

X. Special symptoms

    A. Speech disturbance

    B. Specific learning disturbance

    C. Tic

    D. Other psychomotor disorder

    E. Disorder of sleep

    F. Feeding disturbance

    G. Enuresis

    H. Encopresis

    I. Cephalalgia

    J. Other special symptom

XI. Transient situational disturbances

More or less transient disorders of any severity that occur in individuals without any apparent underlying mental disorders and that represent an acute reaction to overwhelming environmental stress.

    A. Adjustment reaction of infancy

        Example: grief reaction associated with separation from the mother.

    B. Adjustment reaction of childhood

        Example: jealousy associated with the birth of a younger child.

    C. Adjustment reaction of adolescence

        Example: irritability and depression associated with school failure.

    D. Adjustment reaction of adult life

        Example: resentment with depressive tone associated with unwanted pregnancy.

    E. Adjustment reaction of later life

        Example: feelings of rejection associated with forced retirement and manifested by social withdrawal.

XII. Behavioral disorders of childhood and adolescence

Disorders that are more stable, internalized, and resistant to treatment than transient situational disturbances.

    A. Hyperkinetic reaction of childhood (or adolescence)

        Characterized by overactivity, restlessness, distractibility, and short attention span.

    B. Withdrawing reaction of childhood (or adolescence)

        Characterized by seclusiveness, detachment, shyness, timidity, and inability to form close relationships.

    C. Overanxious reaction of childhood (or adolescence)

        Characterized by chronic anxiety, excessive and unrealistic fears, sleeplessness, nightmares, and exaggerated autonomic responses.

    D. Runaway reaction of childhood (or adolescence)

        Characterized by the escape from threatening situations by running away from home for a day or more without permission.

    E. Unsocialized aggressive reaction of childhood (or adolescence)

        Characterized by overt or covert hostile disobedience, quarrelsomeness, physical and verbal aggressiveness, vengefulness, and destructiveness.

     F. Group delinquent reaction of childhood (or adolescence)

          Acquisition of the values, behavior, and skills of a delinquent peer group to which the patient is loyal.

     G. Other reaction of childhood (or adolescence)

XIII. Conditions without manifest psychiatric disorder and nonspecific conditions

    Includes individuals with social maladjustments who are psychiatrically normal but who have problems severe enough to call for a psychiatric examination.

     A. Marital maladjustment

          Characterized by significant conflicts or maladjustments.

     B. Social maladjustment

          Includes individuals thrown into an unfamiliar culture, cultural shock, or conflict caused by divided loyalties to two cultures.

     C. Occupational maladjustment

          Gross maladjustment in work situation.

     D. Dyssocial behavior

          Not classifiable as antisocial, but predatory with a tendency to follow more or less criminal pursuits; includes racketeers, dishonest gamblers, prostitutes, and dope peddlers.

     E. Other social maladjustment

     F. Nonspecific conditions

          Not classifiable elsewhere.

     G. No mental disorder

Standards of psychiatric–mental health nursing practice*

Standard I. Data are collected through pertinent clinical observations based on knowledge of the arts and sciences, with particular emphasis upon psycho-social and biophysical sciences.

Standard II. Clients are involved in the assessment, planning, implementation and evaluation of their nursing care program to the fullest extent of their capabilities.

Standard III. The problem-solving approach is utilized in developing nursing care plans.

Standard IV. Individuals, families and community groups are assisted to achieve satisfying and productive patterns of living through health teaching.

Standard V. The activities of daily living are utilized in a goal directed way in work with clients.

Standard VI. Knowledge of somatic therapies and related clinical skills are utilized in working with clients.

Standard VII. The environment is structured to establish and maintain a therapeutic milieu.

Standard VIII. Nursing participates with interdisciplinary teams in assessing, planning, implementing and evaluating programs and other mental health activities.

Standard IX. Psychotherapeutic interventions are used to assist clients to achieve their maximum development.

*From American Nurses' Association: Standards of psychiatric–mental health nursing practice, Kansas City, Missouri, The Association.

Standard X. The practice of individual, group or family psychotherapy requires appropriate preparation and recognition of accountability for the practice.

Standard XI. Nursing participates with other members of the community in planning and implementing mental health services that include the broad continuum of promotion of mental health, prevention of mental illness, treatment and rehabilitation.

Standard XII. Learning experiences are provided for other nursing care personnel through leadership, supervision and teaching.

Standard XIII. Responsibility is assumed for continuing educational and professional development and contributions are made to the professional growth of others.

Standard XIV. Contributions to nursing and the mental health field are made through innovations in theory and practice and participation in research.

Glossary

aberration deviation from what is natural or normal.

acculturation the process by which an individual adapts himself to the culture in which he is reared or adapts himself to another culture.

acting out expressing certain kinds of unconscious conflicts through behavior.

acute hallucinosis mental illness associated with the use of alcohol and characterized by predominantly fearful auditory hallucinatory experiences and accompanied by a clear sensorium.

addiction psychologic and physical dependence on a drug.

affect generalized feeling tone distinguished from emotion in being more persistent and pervasive.

affective psychosis a psychotic reaction in which the predominant feature is a disturbance in emotional feeling tone, usually depression or elation.

aggression a feeling or action that is hostile or self-assertive.

agitation the psychomotor expression of uncomfortable feelings (pacing, picking at the skin, restless movement of the hands or legs).

altruism behavior motivated predominantly by an interest in others.

Alzhiemer's disease a condition with marked brain atrophy of a senile type occurring at an early age and characterized by a high degree of dementia.

ambivalence opposing emotions, desires, or attitudes existing at the same time toward an object or person.

amnesia a loss of memory that may vary in length of time or degree of loss.

antidepressants drugs with the selective action of lifting the mood, calming disturbed behavior, and restoring vitality.

anxiety a state of apprehensive tension caused by real or imagined danger.

apathy a state of indifference in a situation that would ordinarily arouse some response.

association connecting one thought or feeling with another.

attitude a predisposition to react in a manner conditioned by personal endowment and past experience.

autism an introspective absorption in fantasy with a complete exclusion of reality.

autoerotism sensual self-gratification as through thumb-sucking, stroking, or masturbation.

behavior the actions of an individual or group.

behavior deviation behavior interpreted as falling outside the accepted limits of the culture.

blocking a sudden stoppage in the stream of thought.

blunting dullness of emotional response.

castration literally, the loss or damage of the genital organs. Symbolically, a state of powerlessness or psychologic impotence.

cathexis the emotional investment in a person, an object, or an idea.

cephalalgia headache of recurring, unilateral type following the distribution of the external carotid artery, usually occurring at night in persons at middle age and after.

character the personality traits or behavioral style of an individual.

childhood a collective term denoting the growth period from infancy to the end of puberty.

circumstantiality the quality of being circumstantial; minuteness of detail.

cognitive pertaining to the mental processes of judgment, memory, comprehension, and reasoning.

community a group having mutual interests or a population within geographic boundaries.

complex a group of associated ideas that have a strong emotional tone and generally are unconscious.

compulsion an uncontrollable urge to think or act against one's better judgment.

confabulation the filling-in of memory gaps with made-up episodes.

conflict a painful state resulting from the existence of opposing desires, emotions, or goals.

confusion a state of perplexity characterized by lack of clear thinking. In organic states this may include a clouded sensorium.

congenital inherent at birth.

congruence consistency in thinking, feeling, and actions.

consciousness a division of the mind or being aware of one's environment and one's self.

constitution the psychologic and physical endowment of an individual; his potential or physical inheritance from birth.

conversion the process by which an emotional conflict is expressed as a physical symptom.

counter-transference the feelings and reactions of the therapist toward the patient that are derived from early experiences.

crisis intervention short-term therapy designed to reduce the impact of the crisis and to help the patient develop more effective coping behavior.

culture the social organization characteristic of a particular group of people.

defense mechanisms processes by which the mind seeks relief from emotional conflict.

déjà vu a feeling of familiarity with a place or situation that one has never actually been to or been in.

delirium a state of mental disturbance characterized by confusion, disordered speech, and often hallucinations.

delirium tremens delirium induced by prolonged and excessive use of alcohol.

delusion a fixed false belief that cannot be corrected by reason or evidence.

dementia a deterioration of intellectual capacities.

dementia praecox a diagnostic term becoming obsolete and being replaced by the term "schizophrenia" (see **schizophrenia**).

denial a defense mechanism by which the mind refuses to acknowledge a thought, feeling, wish, need, or reality factor.

dependency needs essential needs for mothering, love, affection, shelter, protection, security, food, and warmth that begin at birth.

depersonalization the experiencing of feelings of unrealness about the self or the environment.

depression a feeling of sadness or dejection.

deprivation, emotional lack of adequate human or environmental experience.

deprivation, sensory lack of adequate perceptual stimuli, such as may occur to a confined prisoner.

descriptive psychiatry a system of psychiatry based on the study of observable phenomena; to be differentiated from dynamic personality.

deterioration an impairment in quality or character.

discrimination separation of one person or group from another by the use of preferential characteristics.

disfranchise to deprive of a right, privilege, or power.

displacement a mechanism whereby the emotions associated with one idea or object are unconsciously attached to another.

dissociation the detachment of certain aspects or activities of the personality from the control of the individual.

dream mental activity during sleep that is dissociated from the self and consciousness of the waking state.

drive motivation or basic urge in man; to be distinguished from the purely biologic concept of drive.

dynamic forceful, active, or in progress.

dynamic psychiatry the study and interpretation of emotional processes and the changing factors in human behavior and its motivation.

dynamics of behavior that which impels the patient to behave as he does, the significance and meaning of his behavior, and the purpose of his behavior.

eclectic selecting from various systems.

ego the conscious self; that part of the mind that develops to deal with reality.

ego ideal that part of the psychic structure that represents the ideal aims and goals of the individual.

egocentric self-centered.

electroconvulsive therapy electric treatments to produce a grand mal convulsion in an individual.

electroencephalogram a record or tracing measured by a specific instrument that indicates the rate of electric discharges in the brain.

electroshock a form of treatment in which a convulsion is produced in a patient through the application of electric current to the temporal region of the head.

elopement in psychiatric experience, an escape from the hospital by a patient.

emotion a distinctive feeling tone, such as love, hate, or fear.

empathy the capacity of feeling in communion with others.

empirical based on observation and experience rather than on scientific theory.

encopresis the involuntary passage of feces.

enterprise an undertaking that involves activity, energy, and courage.

epilepsy a disturbance in consciousness that may be accompanied by convulsive phenomena.

euphoria an exaggerated sense of well-being.

exhibitionism a personality trait characterized by the pleasure of being noticed by others.

extraversion the direction of interest and emotions toward the environment.

fabrication made-up events to fill in gaps of memory.

fainting temporary loss of consciousness.

fantasy indulgence in daydreaming or fancy; usually used in the sense of contrast with reality.

fear an emotional response to perceived danger; to be distinguished from anxiety, which does not necessarily identify the danger.

feminist movement movement advocating legal and social changes to establish political, economic, and financial equality of the sexes.

fixation psychoanalytic term to indicate an arrest at a particular stage of psychosexual development.

flight of ideas a rapid succession of ideas in which the goal idea is not reached.

free association a psychoanalytic technique whereby the patient must say whatever comes into his mind.

fugue state a dissociative state characterized by amnesia and actual physical flights from an intolerable situation.

functional mental illness a mental illness in which organic change cannot be demonstrated as a consistent accompaniment or cause.

furor a fury or frenzy.

general paresis a syphilitic infection involving predominantly the cerebral cortex.

ghetto a section of a city in which members of a social group are segregated.

globus hystericus a symptom in which there is a sensation of having a ball in the throat; hysterical spasm of the esophagus.

grand mal a specific convulsive manifestation in epilepsy in which loss of consciousness, tonic spasm, series of jerky movements, and stuporousness follow each other in sequence.

grandiose that which is characterized by affectation, eminence, magnificence, or splendor.

grief a normal emotional response to recognized loss. It is self-limiting and gradually subsiding within a reasonable time.

group dynamics the study of the processes of small groups.

hallucination an imaginary sense perception.

heterosexual sexual attraction for or toward persons of the opposite sex.

holistic nursing nursing involving conscious and intentional consideration of multiple factors—cultural values, family customs, language, religion, socioeconomic conditions, and others—that are significant in looking at the totality of the individual, his needs, and his care.

homosexual sexual attraction for or toward persons of the same sex.

homosexual panic acute and severe feelings of anxiety based on unconscious homosexual conflict.

human that which is characteristic of man.

hydrocephalus a birth defect characterized by an abnormally large head caused by an increased accumulation of cerebrospinal fluid in the ventricles or subarachnoid space.

hypnosis an induced dissociative state.

hypochondriasis a morbid preoccupation with the state of health.

hypoglycemosis hypoglycemia with low blood sugar, hunger, sweating, nervousness, and dizziness.

hysteria a form of psychoneurosis that includes a wide variety of physical symptoms without organic pathologic changes and toward which the patient shows relative emotional indifference.

id a psychoanalytic term used to denote the unconscious part of the personality that contains primitive urges and desires and is ruled by pleasure principle.

ideas of reference the incorrect interpretation of incidents as having direct reference to the self.

identification a mechanism by which one feels or thinks as another person.

illusion a misinterpreted sensory perception.

incorporation a psychologic mechanism whereby a person symbolically takes in a part of another person to be part of his self. For example, the infant presumably fantasizes that mother's breast is part of him.

insight a reasonably accurate self-judgment including the emotional acceptance of self.

instinct inborn drive. Human instincts include self-preservation, sexuality, personality instincts, and social instincts.

insulin shock as a form of treatment often produces coma in a patient by the injection of sufficient amounts of insulin.

intellectualization a defense mechanism that employs reasoning and logic to defend against uncomfortable feelings.

intelligence the ability of a person to solve problems, adapt to new situations, and understand and integrate previous experiences.

intrapsychic that which takes place within the mind.

introjection the incorporation and acceptance as one's own behavior of patterns, attitudes, and ideals of others.

introversion the direction of interests and emotions toward one's self.

involutional psychosis a psychiatric disorder occurring during that period of life referred to as menopausal, climacteric, or involutional.

juvenile delinquency a legal classification of children whose actions and behavior violate the law.

kleptomania compulsive stealing.

Korsakoff's psychosis a chronic mental illness usually associated with the use of alcohol, characterized by polyneuritis, reduced intellectual capacities, and the marked use of confabulation to compensate for memory loss.

labile unstable.

latency period a psychoanalytic term for the developmental phase between the oedipal and adolescent phases of life (ages 7 to 11 years).

libido a psychoanalytic term meaning the vital force or psychic energy that motivates living.

malinger to deliberately pretend to have an illness that does not exist.

manic-depressive psychosis a class of mental disorders in which the most dramatic symptoms occur in mood disturbances.

megalomania a psychiatric syndrome characterized by delusions of great self-importance, wealth, or power.

melancholia severe depression.

mental mechanism characteristic ways of thinking that serve to meet the needs of the personality.

mental retardation an impairment in intelligence that makes the individual's intelligence quotient lower than average for the individual's development.

microcephaly a birth defect involving the formation of an abnormally small head and brain.

milieu the people and factors within an environment with which a person interacts.

motivation that within the individual that prompts him to action.

mutism inability to speak.

myalgia muscular pain.

narcissism a psychoanalytic term denoting self-love.

narcolepsy a condition in which the individual is overcome by an uncontrollable desire to sleep.

negative feelings unfriendly, hostile feelings.

negativism a generalized resistance to any suggestion from outside the self.

neologism literally, new words; a meaningless word coined by a psychotic patient.

nervous breakdown a nonmedical, nonspecific term for emotional illness.

neurasthenia psychoneurosis in which the predominant pattern is motor and mental fatigability.

neurosis a functional disorder without organic pathology in which the patient's behavior does not seem bizarrely different from accepted cultural patterns; used interchangeably with psychoneurosis.

Niemann-Pick disease enlargement of the liver and spleen with lipoid metabolic disturbances; usually occurs in Jewish infants.

object a psychoanalytic term meaning person.

object relationship the emotional bonds that exist between one individual and another.

obsession the uncontrollable urge to think some thought against one's will.

Oedipus complex a psychoanalytic phase of psychosexual development whereby the child (roughly ages 4 to 7) has feelings of attachment for the parent of the opposite sex and also feelings of envy and aggression toward the parent of the same sex.

operant conditioning a specific method of treating behavior in which desired behavior is enforced by reward and undesired behavior is extinguished by punishment or by being ignored.

oral eroticism pleasurable sensations obtained from the mouth.

oral stage a psychosexual phase of development that refers to both the oral-erotic and oral-sadistic phases of the first year of life.

organic mental illness a mental illness accompanied by or caused by organic change.

orthopsychiatry psychiatry concerned with the study of children in which the emphasis is placed on preventive techniques to facilitate normal, healthy emotional development.

overcompensation a defense mechanism whereby a physical or psychologic deficit produces exaggerated correction.

panic a term used in psychiatry to indicate acute, intense, and overwhelming anxiety.

paranoia a rather rare mental illness characterized by logical and well-systematized delusions of persecution; the personality well preserved.

paranoid similar to paranoia, but the delusions of persecution are not so systematized or logical as those of paranoia.

personality the organization of the sum of the behavior patterns of the individual.

perversion a maladjustment in which the sexual object or method of satisfaction deviates from the accepted social patterns.

petit mal a momentary loss of consciousness occurring in epilepsy; muscular twitchings may or may not be present.

phallic stage a psychosexual phase of development (roughly ages 4 to 6) during which the child's interest centers around issues of potency and strength.

phobia a compulsive or a morbid fear of an object, situation, or act.

pica the habitual ingestion of substances that have no nutritional value, such as worms, soil, paper, and paint.

play therapy a technique used in child psychiatry to establish interaction between the child and a therapist.

pleasure principle the regulation of activity with the purpose of avoiding pain or procuring pleasure.

porencephaly the absence of part of the brain tissue, sometimes forming a cavity.

preconscious that part of the psychic structure in which thoughts are not in immediate awareness but can be recalled by conscious effort.

prevention, primary all efforts involved in the promotion of health when the individual is in the prepathogenesis period. Its focus is on protecting man against disease agents (such as immunizations and personal and mental hygiene) or establishing barriers against the agents in the environment (such as environmental sanitation, air pollution control, and water purification).

prevention, secondary efforts made toward early detection of pathogenesis and prompt treatment. This has three major purposes: (1) to prevent the spread of disease, (2) to cure or arrest the disease, thus preventing complications or sequelae, and (3) to prevent chronic disability. These make case-finding an essential activity.

prevention, tertiary efforts made in the presence and progression of pathogenesis to reverse or correct the disease condition by means of therapy, hopefully to avoid sequelae and to limit disability.

projection a mental mechanism in which perceptions, motivations, desires, thoughts, and activities stemming from within the self are attributed to the external environment.

psychasthenia a form of psychoneurosis in which compulsive patterns of behavior predominate.

psychiatrist a doctor of medicine who has postgraduate training and experience in diagnosis and treatment of mental illness.

psychiatry the branch of medicine dealing with disorders of behavior and personality.

psychoanalysis (1) System of psychology elaborated by Freud that attributes abnormal behavior to repressions in the unconscious. (2) Method of treatment designed to investigate the unconscious mental processes.

psychoanalyst a psychiatrist or a lay therapist who has had additional training in psychoanalysis and who practices the techniques of psychoanalytic therapy.

psychodynamics the systematized knowledge and theory of human behavior, its motivation, and psychoanalytic principles.

psychogenesis the causation of symptoms by mental or emotional factors, as opposed to organic reasons.

psychologist a health professional who specializes in psychology and has earned a graduate degree (M.A. or Ph.D.).

psychology an academic discipline, a profession, and a science dealing with the study of man and his behavior.

psychoneurosis a psychiatric term used interchangeably with neurosis.

psychosexual development a psychoanalytic term that distinguishes phases of development of the person from birth to adult life.

psychosis mental illness in which the behavior deviations are bizarrely different from the socially accepted standards.

psychotherapy the planned measures undertaken to restore a patient to mental health.

psychotomimetics experimental drugs which, when taken, produce a hallucinogenic reaction.

rationalization a mental mechanism whereby the patient substitutes a plausible reason for the real one motivating his behavior.

reaction formation a defense mechanism operating unconsciously, whereby an opposite attitude or behavior takes the place of the real attitudes, impulses, or behavior the individual harbors either consciously or unconsciously.

reality the character of being true to life.

reality principle the regulation of activity in accordance with the demands of reality.

regression a mental mechanism whereby an individual reverts to patterns of behavior characteristic of an earlier phase of development.

rejection the act or state of refusing to accept.

repression a mental mechanism that operates unconsciously to keep from awareness unpleasant experiences, emotions, and ideas.

resistance a psychiatric term used to imply an individual's reluctance to bring repressed thoughts or impulses into awareness.

retrospective falsification the distortion of remote memory to fit personality needs.

role a pattern of expected behavior facilitated by interpersonal relationships in a specific setting.

Rorschach test a psychologic test designed to disclose conscious and unconscious personality traits and emotional conflicts. The person being tested tells what is suggested to him when viewing a series of standard inkblot patterns.

sadism pleasure derived from inflicting physical or psychologic pain on others.

schizoid resembling or like schizophrenia; usually applied to personalities that are predominantly introverted.

schizophrenia a class of functional mental illnesses characterized by lack of correlation between thinking and feeling and lack of correlation between the patient's experience and reality and with a rich variety of symptoms in thinking, feeling, and motor activities.

    catatonic type outstanding peculiarities of conduct with phases of stupor or excitement, the latter characterized by a compulsive or stereotyped pattern of behavior.

    hebephrenic type silliness, inappropriateness, bizarre delusions, and hallucinations, appearing early and deteriorating comparatively early.

    paranoid type form dominated by delusions, especially of persecution and grandeur.

    simple type apathy, lack of interest, and blunting of emotion with child-like behavior.

sedative drug used to calm, to induce sleep, and for the relief of anxiety.

self-system the organization of the self with its interrelationships of the organic, the emotional, and the social components; the balance of these interrelationships forming the personality orientation that will function to select the elements of experience to which the individual will react.

senescence the natural developmental process of growing old.

senile psychoses a group of mental illnesses associated with changes in the nervous system occurring in old age.

sibling brother or sister.

sibling rivalry the competition between siblings.

sociopathic personality a conduct disorder in which the integration of experience is apparently absent, inhibitory control is reduced, but the intellect remains intact.

soma the physical aspect of man as distinguished from the psychic.

somatic physical.

stall a loss in the amount of forward progress necessary to maintain the therapeutic process.

stereotypy the use of monotonous repetition of verbal, intellectual, emotional, or motor activities.

stuttering involuntary hesitation, repetition of words, or prolongation of sounds in speech.

style the distinctive and characteristic mode of one's behavior.

subconscious that part of the mind not immediately focused in awareness but that may be brought to awareness when desired.

sublimation a mental mechanism whereby the energy associated with primitive drives is successfully utilized in constructive social activities.

substitution a defense mechanism by which one attitude or emotion is replaced by another.

superego psychoanalytic term used to describe the critical aspect of the personality; usually equated with the popular term "conscience."

supervision in psychiatric nursing a teaching or educative process by which therapy is managed.

suppression a mental mechanism whereby unpleasant feelings and experiences are deliberately kept from awareness.

symbolization the investment of one idea, object, or experience in another.

Tay-Sachs disease familial idiocy accompanied by loss of vision.

therapeutic serving to cure or heal.

tic an uncontrollable repetitious gesture or muscular movement.

tranquilizers drugs that, when administered in proper dosage, calm the patient by reducing anxiety and disturbed behavior, thus facilitating his ability to perform his activities of daily living.

transference the unconscious identification with another person in a role with which an individual has had past experience.

unconscious that part of mental activity that is not accessible to conscious awareness.

undoing a defense mechanism by which something is verbalized or acted on in reverse in the hopes of "undoing" something the ego finds intolerable.

ventilation free verbal expression of feelings, worries, tensions, and problems.

waxy flexibility (cerea flexibilitas) a condition found in catatonic schizophrenia in which the extremities have a wax-like rigidity and will remain for long periods in any placed position, no matter how uncomfortable.

withdrawal a form of behavior that implies a retreat from reality.

Index